Think Yourself Thin

214 Mental Tricks, Habits, Inspirations, and Substitutions

Katherine Tallmadge, MA, RD

LifeLine
Press

A Regnery Publishing Company, Washington, D.C.

ISBN 0-8487-2771-1
Published in the United States by
LifeLine Press
A Regnery Publishing Company
One Massachusetts Avenue, N.W.
Washington, DC 20001

Portions of this book were previously published by Lifeline Press as _Diet Simple_.

Visit us at www.lifelinepress.com

Printed on acid-free paper
Printed in the United States of America

10 9 8 7 6 5 4 3 2 1

Books are available in quantity for promotional or premium use. Write to Director of Special Sales, Regnery Publishing, Inc., One Massachusetts Avenue, N.W., Washington, DC 20001, for information on discounts and terms or call (202) 216-0600.

The information contained in this book is not a substitute for medical counseling and care. All matters pertaining to your physical health should be supervised by a health care professional.

To my family and Jack

Contents

Part III

Fast and Delicious Batch Recipes from the Best Chefs

Appendices

Indices

Acknowledgments

Several years ago, I wrote a proposal for *Think Yourself Thin*, a culmination of what I had learned through many years of helping thousands lose weight and gain back their health and vitality painlessly. The publishers and agents who looked through the proposal said they loved the book and were impressed with my knowledge and credentials. But (there's always a "but") they said they couldn't publish it unless I found a major celebrity to endorse it or unless I came up with a "gimmick."

So my proposal collected dust for a couple of years. I kept sending it around, but always got the same response. Then one night I had dinner with Karen Anderson, the acquisitions editor at LifeLine Press, a new health publisher based in Washington D.C. Initially, Karen said the same thing as the other publishers ("It would be so great if you had a celebrity!"). But out of the blue, she called me a month later and asked if I would meet with the publishers and staff at LifeLine. There I met Mike Ward, who immediately loved the idea, and shared my vision that this book would help a lot of people. Over the next five months, we worked like mad to finish it.

I say five months, but I really mean twenty-five years! That's truly how long it's taken me to pull together the information in this book—getting my nutrition degree, my behavioral sciences degree, my journalism degree, keeping up with the scientific literature, going to conferences, and working with extremely qualified experts. These physicians, psychiatrists, counselors, even physical therapists and exercise experts, have all contributed to the knowledge, experience, and material you'll find in these pages. The USDA's Center for Nutrition Policy and Promotion gets a special mention. They held a series of fabulous conferences that gave me a great foundation of knowledge in children's research.

But I have to say my greatest influence is my clients: their successes and failures, ups and downs, reactions, suggestions, and support. I feel privileged every time someone calls me or walks into my office that they would put their health into my hands and give me their trust. I've had the opportunity to peer into the minds of some of the most interesting, insightful, fun, and loving people. Guiding them week after week, month after month, year after year, taught me what worked and what didn't. It gave me an appreciation for peoples' complexity, their strengths, weaknesses, and vulnerabilities. I am indebted to all of them for that.

I would like to thank my colleagues and friends at LifeLine Press with whom I've had the privilege to work over the past couple of years: Karen Anderson, Mike Ward, Marji Ross, Molly Mullen, Lauren Lawson, John Lalor, and LifeLine's president, Alfred Regnery, who has also been a great supporter. Thanks also to my patient and talented editors, Matthew Hoffman and Ernie Tremblay, and to publicist Cathy Lewis.

I thank the folks at Oxmoor House for their support and their belief in me and my program. I'm grateful that they're giving the American public credit for their intelligence and their realization that gimmicky, unhealthy, fad diets are not the way to go.

In June 2002, I was selected as a National Spokesperson for the American Dietetic Association. It's been one of the greatest privileges of my life. I have learned so much through the ADA and I thank the colleagues and friends that I've met there. My admiration grows every day for their professionalism and their absolute dedication to informing the public about important nutrition issues of the day. Lori Ferme, with whom I speak almost daily, has been a great help and support, as have Doris

Acosta, Bridget McManamon, Irene Perconti, and Ron Moen, the new CEO, whom I admire a great deal. I also want to thank the staff at the ADA's Washington office, who work tirelessly to promote the cause of good nutrition at government levels. I've relished the opportunity to become acquainted with my colleagues in the ADA spokesperson program, all experts in their fields, who have a wealth of knowledge I have had the privilege of benefiting from.

Thanks to Les Dames d'Escoffier and all the fine chefs who contributed their time and talents to making *Think Yourself Thin* a source for delicious, healthy food, and to Christine Palumbo, who patiently helps me nutritionally analyze my recipes.

I would like to thank my professors at the University of Maryland, The Catholic University of America and American University, who helped instill in me a respect for science, objectivity, accuracy and honesty.

And, of course, thanks to my family for having so much faith in me through the years. They taught me the value of honesty, integrity, fairness, hard work, and the arts. And thanks to my love, John (Jack) Shaw.

Why I Wrote This Book

I first started thinking about weight problems when I was a child in Ohio. One evening, everyone but my mother was at the table eating dinner. When I rushed into the kitchen to find her, I must have startled her. She had been weighing peas on a kitchen scale, but now the peas were spilling all over the floor. I helped her pick them up.

"Mom, what are you doing?" I asked. Weighing peas, after all, seemed like a very strange thing to do.

"I'm fat," she replied. She sounded upset. "I'm fat, I'm on a diet, and I have to lose weight."

Now, you have to understand that my mother was—and is—a beautiful Swedish woman. She married an American serviceman, my father, in France, and they moved to the United States when I was 18 months old. She was definitely a star—"the Swedish beauty"—wherever we lived. Friends referred to her as another Ingrid Bergman. That certainly was the way her admiring daughter saw her.

Yet here she was, weighing peas! And that's the way it was going to be throughout her life: a constant struggle to lose 20 pounds, regain it, plus more. Every time she went on a diet and lost weight, she'd gain back even more each time. It was a constant, demoralizing, losing battle. Her problem with weight began after her third child was born (my comment "Another stinkin' brother!" became neighborhood legend). Mom had a winning personality that included a fun, goofy side. She enjoyed lots of friends, and was also artistic. Everyone, then and now, loved her. But all she could focus on was how FAT she was. The shame and disappointment that she felt stayed with me.

Years later, when faced with choosing a major in college, I picked dietetics. I wasn't even aware of the inner voices affecting me at that time, of the reasons why I made that choice. It's only now, after years of reflection, that I realize why I'm so passionate about my work. I chose this as my life's vocation so that I could help people like my mother.

Like Mother, Like Daughter

Studies have shown that when parents are obsessed with weight problems, their children are also more likely to have weight problems in life. And when parents are not consistent in their attitudes toward food—when they alternate constantly between "off" and "on"—the children are more likely to develop eating disorders.

In my case, overeating became a way of life when I left home for college. I stuffed myself with sweets, chips, and other snack foods—all of the things I couldn't get that easily at home, but which now were readily available.

Visiting my Swedish grandparents one summer didn't help. We would start the day with a big breakfast bowl of strawberries—nothing wrong with that so far, but wait—with heavy cream poured over them. We'd end the evening with cookies and hot chocolate—made with cream, naturally. And I wasn't exactly starving between breakfast and bedtime. I cringe when I see a photo of me, standing between my grandparents, that was taken between my sophomore and junior years. With those chipmunk cheeks, I was a regular Swedish meatball!

My weight problem in college followed the classic yo-yo pattern. I'd gain weight, diet, gain the weight back, diet again, and so on. Eventually

I had a full-blown eating disorder. I was shocked at my own behavior, and sought help immediately.

I realize now that my eating disorder was a grief reaction to the death of my American grandmother, which left a great void in my life. It was also a result of a childhood spent with a mother with a poor body image who was constantly dieting. It was a very difficult time in my life, both personally and professionally.

I knew that my scientific knowledge of nutrition wouldn't be enough to solve my problems. I decided to pursue a master's degree in behavioral science because I had come to realize that our behavioral patterns lead to our physical problems. I wanted to learn how to change people's lives, including my own.

The bottom line, dear reader, is that I'm no sacrosanct preacher looking down at a congregation of sinners. I've been there! I had a weight problem and an eating disorder. And I know what it takes to come back from those depths of despair—and to stay on top!

It Will Work for You

My professional career has evolved in response to my desire to make a real difference in people's lives. I quickly realized, as a college intern with the National Institutes of Health, that a hospital setting was not for me. You meet most patients only once, and hand them a nutritional printout. Minimal impact, there. I longed to spend more time with them, but there weren't enough hours in the day to counsel the patients in the hospital.

Only marginally more satisfying was the year I spent managing the dietary program of a large nursing home. I needed this experience in order to get my certification as a registered dietitian—it was, in effect, a professional internship. But while I hired, trained, and managed a crew of 20, and was in charge of 130 patients' nutritional health, I wanted more personal interaction with those patients. And I knew that their nutritional problems had begun long before they arrived at that nursing home.

I soon realized that private practice was the only path that would give me the opportunity to help people turn their lives around. That was a scary move—my first year, I earned all of $4,000!—but I survived, and referrals from the doctors I worked with helped me build my practice to a sustainable level.

Watching my clients change negative patterns of behavior into positive ones has been a joy, and I've felt honored to be a part of that process. In particular, I enjoy hearing clients tell me that they never knew that losing weight could be so easy, or so positive. Many clients actually sit in my office saying, "It can't be this easy. Tell me that there's something more difficult I have to do." That's music to my ears!

I've also learned from my clients. In fact, most of the strategies in this book come from them, at least indirectly. When I give them suggestions, they invariably make changes and adaptations that work best for them. When I saw how a series of small, positive steps could lead to significant accomplishments, it seemed only natural to let others in on those secrets—first with articles in popular and professional publications, then with television and radio appearances, and now with this book.

I've done it. My clients have done it. And now you can too!

PART I

It's All in the Thinking

CHAPTER I

It's Easier Than You Think

Every year, publishers churn out dozens, if not hundreds, of diet and weight-loss books. Pick up any newspaper or magazine, and you're likely to see a few articles devoted to healthy eating and dieting.

I don't think it's an exaggeration to say that Americans have an insatiable appetite (forgive the pun) for information about losing weight. This is a good thing, in a way. Overweight and obesity are among the leading risk factors for dozens of chronic, serious health threats.

Then there are the social costs. In a society that celebrates thin, those of us who struggle to control our weight often feel marginalized, at best. If the plethora of weight-loss information helps even a few people lose weight, the cost of paper and ink seems well justified.

Alas, most of the people who read these books and articles won't lose much weight—and they'll be even less likely to keep it off permanently. Americans, regrettably, are getting heavier by the year. In fact, more than two-thirds of American adults (65 percent, to be exact) are overweight, and nearly a quarter of these are obese.

I've known a few people who woke up one day, stood in front of the mirror, and said to themselves, "This is it, I'm going to lose weight"—and

3

actually succeeded the first time. But they're the exceptions. Most people who try to lose weight will have a lot of false starts. They might lose weight for a while, but the weight slowly comes back. They're always switching diet plans—sometimes a new one each month. They take weight-loss supplements. They eat no fat, no carbs, no whatever—and the darned weight still won't budge.

It doesn't have to be this way. Losing weight isn't rocket science (even though a lot of big-name authors, with their infinitely complex plans, would like you to believe it is). It doesn't require memorizing long lists of foods and calorie contents. You don't have to quit eating chocolate or pumpkin pie. You don't even have to "diet" in any formal way. In fact, the less you diet, the more successful you're going to be.

About 30 seconds after starting my practice as a weight loss and nutrition counselor, I began hearing stories from clients about promising diet programs that went bad. It was puzzling. Some of the approaches, at least the ones I was familiar with, sounded reasonable. Why weren't they working?

Before I could help my clients lose weight, I had to understand where they were coming from. So I set aside some time to read the best-selling diet books. I spent weeks in the aisles of a huge bookstore in the Georgetown neighborhood of Washington, where I browsed through hundreds of books in the Diet and Nutrition section.

Most of the diet books focus on particular parts of the problem—calories, fat, lack of exercise, and so on. Few look at the big picture, and even fewer address the real-life situations and challenges that people find themselves in every day.

Another thing I've noticed is that many diet plans tend to insist on unnecessarily rigorous goals, along with complicated styles of eating that no sane person is going to follow for very long. All I can say is that the Puritan spirit is alive and well in the diet industry. No matter how much you want to lose weight, following these joyless programs almost guarantees failure.

Which brings us to *Think Yourself Thin*. It's comprehensive, in the sense that I have tried to provide all of the information that you need to lose weight. But it's not complicated. Quite the opposite. My feeling is that you already know the basics: that fruits and vegetables are good, too much food is a problem, and a little extra physical activity is always nice. I'm not going to waste your time talking about things that you already know. Rather, I have provided hundreds of practical (almost mindless!) ways to incorporate smart eating and exercise into your already busy life. Diet and nutrition are the core of the program, but you'll also find a lot of tips for managing stress, getting more physical activity (without really exercising), and controlling all of those emotional ups and downs that really put on the pounds.

You can think of *Think Yourself Thin* as an enticing buffet of easy-to-digest tips, strategies, and mental tricks. The advice is simple, but not simplistic. And it's very goal oriented. Rather than merely asserting that particular strategies—giving up the creamy dressing on a Caesar salad, for example—can be helpful, I took the next step and calculated the actual weight loss that you're likely to achieve.

No one is going to follow each and every piece of advice in this book. That's fine. I want you to pick and choose among them. Find the strategies that fit your personality and lifestyle. Check the amount of weight you can lose with each one. You may find that you only need a few of these tips—or a few dozen—to get your weight where you'd like it to be.

The *Think Yourself Thin* program is easy. It's based on solid science. And because it offers such a huge menu of choices, it can be customized to match your lifestyle, habits, and appetites.

Does it work? Don't take my word for it. See for yourself!

CHAPTER 2

Tiny Changes, Lasting Results

E very tip in this book is based on sound science. I've spent many years studying the different ways in which diet, exercise, behavior, and even emotions affect weight control. Incorporating water into your meals, for example, will reduce your appetite. How do we know? As you'll see below, scientists have researched the subject. They have also shown that avoiding late-night calories can reduce fat storage, and that allowing yourself to eat an occasional hot fudge sundae or any other treat you really love actually improves motivation. Follow these and other tips in this book, and you'll be more successful at losing weight than you ever imagined you could be. My experience, and the experience of the country's top experts, bears this out.

Adding Volume

I've found that when my clients eat more fruits and vegetables over the course of a week, they're more likely to lose weight. If during the week, they make a big purchase of beautiful produce at the farmers' market or cook up a batch of veggie soup, or on Sunday cut and chop veggies to snack on all week, they're likely to experience a 1-pound weight loss. As you can see, small changes produce big results.

Research backs up my experience. Every study analyzing the eating habits of successful weight-loss maintainers has found that they consume more fruits and vegetables than people who gain their weight back. One study showed that eating vegetables was one of the largest differences contributing to the success of people who lost weight permanently versus people who didn't. Another study found that adding low-calorie foods, such as water (0 calories), vegetables, and fruits into your recipes naturally reduces calorie intake by at least 100 per meal. That means if you add a high volume of fruits, vegetables, or water (i.e., water incorporated into foods, such as soups) to each of three meals a day, you'll create a 300-calorie deficit, which could lead to a 30-pound weight loss in a year.

Adding water, fruits, and vegetables to foods and meals works because it adds volume and helps you feel full and satisfied with fewer calories.

Lightening the Calorie Load

The longest-running, most comprehensive study of successful weight-loss maintainers, the National Weight Control Registry (NWCR), studies people who have won the battle of the bulge permanently. The average person in the registry has lost 70 pounds and kept it off for an average of 6 years. They're home free. So it's always interesting and important to see what their experiences are.

The NWCR and several other studies confirm the importance of fruits and vegetables in the diet and show that a reduction in calorie-dense foods such as fats, fatty meats, and sweets also plays an important role in success. After 12 to 24 weeks of eating fewer of these foods, a weight-loss maintainer will reach a point where her taste for calorie-dense foods changes. They begin to taste too sweet or too fatty. She'll often find herself avoiding deep-fried foods, and overeating and craving food in general will begin to take a less important place in her life. What she won't do, however, is eliminate sweet, fatty foods altogether.

This is an important aspect of keeping weight off. When I work with my clients, I get to know them pretty well, and find out a lot about their weight-loss struggles. So many of them failed because they followed rigid diets that left no room for error or fun. They would lose weight, but ultimately, following the diet would prove so difficult that they would gain all their weight back, and then some.

They were pleased with the *Think Yourself Thin* approach because they were able to lose weight with small dietary changes, but were still able to enjoy a night out in their favorite restaurant and to continue eating their favorite foods. They just picked their moments of indulgence more carefully.

On the other hand, one study found that people who relapsed typically felt deprived and set apart from the people around them. Whether they took medications or supplements, fasted, or went on Spartan diets, they found that denying themselves the foods they loved made them extremely vulnerable to giving up and going back to old eating habits. They wanted to be able to eat the same foods as their families and friends, not special meals that made eating seem more like work than pleasure.

But aside from keeping count of calories, several other aspects to losing weight and keeping it off permanently are supported by important scientific research, and I use them in my own practice.

Eating Style

I have found that eating regular meals is important in achieving weight-loss success. My clients who feed themselves well and regularly during the day are more likely to lose weight. Studies consistently bear this out. One study showed that weight-loss maintainers usually ate smaller, more frequent meals (about five a day), while those who relapsed were more likely to skip meals and snack on candies and chocolates more often.

Who prepares the food and where you eat it also makes a difference. Successful weight-loss maintainers prepared and ate most of their food at home, as opposed to a restaurant or fast food joint.

And breakfast! Your first meal of the day is *so* important. For years, I've been advising my clients to eat a hearty breakfast every morning. And when they do, they're amazed at how much better they feel. They have increased energy and attention span, and they're more likely to lose weight.

Studies have confirmed the importance of breakfast for the nutritional quality of your day, but also for weight loss. One study found that relapsers were more likely to skip breakfast. The NWCR found that a strikingly high number of their maintainers never skipped breakfast. This suggests that eating breakfast may be an important long-term behavioral goal for weight-loss maintenance.

My clients tell me and the researchers surmise that eating breakfast may prevent the ravenous hunger that leads to overeating later in the day. Breakfast eaters probably eat lighter foods later in the day than do those who relapse, which helps explain their successful weight loss and maintenance.

Oddly, the NWCR found that breakfast eaters also exercised more. The only explanation the researchers could come up with was that breakfast gave people more energy to be physically active. Organizational skills, however, may be the real answer. Other studies report that having these skills plays a role in making the time for exercise, so they may be a factor in making time for breakfast as well.

Tragically, skipping breakfast seems to have a marked effect on the weight of teens. Based on analysis of USDA food surveys performed by *Shape Up America!*, nearly 80 percent of heavier girls studied were failing to eat breakfast regularly, though the majority of thinner girls (60 percent) did eat breakfast.

Physical Activity

One of the most striking discoveries I've made while working with clients for the past 20 years is the high correlation between physical activity and weight. It almost never failed that when a client was going through a time in his or her life when he or she was gaining weight, they were more sedentary. And the times during which they were happiest with their weights were when they were very physically active.

This isn't rocket science, but if you want further evidence, every study that has analyzed the habits of successful weight-loss maintainers found an uncannily close connection with physical activity. And physical activity is especially necessary for weight-loss *maintenance*. Without it, most people simply put their weight back on.

As with diet, physical activity can be accomplished in small, manageable increments. Just 10 to 15 minutes in the morning can burn 100 calories. If we do the math, that can produce a 10-pound weight difference in just 1 year.

Self-Monitoring

Keeping a food diary has been shown to cause weight loss independent of any other factor, according to every major study. Whenever I ask a new client to record what they eat for 1 week—objectively and at the time of eating—without changing anything else, inevitably they lose weight. And it's always such a pleasant surprise because each one swears they ate normally and didn't give up a thing!

Studies show that self-monitoring through a diary is especially effective during stressful periods, family gatherings, or holidays, if you would like to lose weight or prevent the usual gain. At the back of this book, on page 485, you'll find some sample journaling pages that have helped many of my clients. Feel free to photocopy these pages and use them for your own diary entries.

Another way to monitor yourself is through regular weigh-ins. The successful NWCR subjects weighed themselves regularly. Keeping track of their weight helped them make sure that any minor weight gains were nipped in the bud immediately. They also kept track of how they felt and looked in their clothes. They rarely went over 5 pounds. On the other hand, people who relapsed seemed more willing to accept larger weight gains or didn't notice their weight creeping up until they had gained a substantial amount.

Coping Skills

While most people have a fairly substantial amount of stress in their lives, some handle it more effectively than others; this is yet another factor separating weight-loss maintainers from those who relapse.

One study found that people who were successful at losing weight and keeping it off faced the problems in their lives head-on, then did something about them. When they needed help, they sought it from family and friends. And when they felt overly stressed, they didn't turn away from the challenges ahead of them. Instead, they coped by using relaxation techniques, exercise, and working more. Those who relapsed, on the other hand, were far more likely to try to avoid their problems. They ate more, slept more, and spent a lot more time sitting around wishing their problems would solve themselves. And few felt they had many people to turn to for help. In other words, they behaved like victims.

Ways of Thinking and Living

Interestingly, having a less than interesting life can frustrate your weight-loss success. One study found that women who lived unchallenging and unrewarding lives secluded in their homes were more likely to be overweight. It wasn't until they got out and became more involved in activities outside the home that they were successfully able to shed pounds and keep them off.

Again, it must be very easy to feel stuck and alone—like a victim—if you're at home all the time with few social contacts and little to keep you occupied. One study showed, however, that women who managed to reach a higher stage of maturity in their thinking and realized that their weight was their own responsibility, not something that victimized them, began to take charge of their body size. They developed new eating habits, exercised more, and became more self-confident. They no longer thought of themselves as victims.

Obviously, the way you think about yourself and your efforts will affect your results. Recent research has demonstrated that people who maintain their weight loss, just like people who are normally thin, are far more likely to think of themselves more forgivingly, as "average" or "a little out of shape," unlike relapsers, who have a negative self-image and tend to think of themselves as "heavy" or "ugly."

Simple Changes, Lasting Results

Will everyone who follows these guidelines succeed right away or achieve model-thinness? Of course not. Losing weight requires commitment, motivation, and perseverance. Some people work toward their weight-loss goals with awesome intensity. Others need more cajoling and encouragement, and perhaps a failure or two before they're ready to go all the way.

It doesn't matter which group you fall into. After beginning the process of taking care of yourself, even if you achieve only minor weight losses in the beginning, you'll start feeling on top of the world. This is what I hear every day from my clients, and it's what I live for. The NWCR studies show more than 90 percent of successful weight-loss maintainers report an improved quality of life, level of energy, mobility, general mood, and self-confidence, and more than 60 percent experience improvements in their physical health and in interactions with others— *particularly with the opposite sex.*

So get started! Maybe you'll fail at first. So what? Nearly everyone who struggles with weight will succeed at times and fail at others. Doctors call this "weight cycling." You may know it as "yo-yo dieting." For a long time, researchers believed that people whose weight cycled up and down were almost condemned to failure. It was thought that yo-yo dieting made it increasingly difficult to lose weight over time. Because nearly everyone goes through this cycle at least a few times, the news seemed discouraging.

More recently, however, the National Task Force for the Prevention and Treatment of Obesity reviewed some 28 medical studies on weight cycling. The conclusion: "There is no convincing evidence that weight cycling in humans has adverse effects on body composition, energy expenditure, risk factors for cardiovascular disease, or the effectiveness of future efforts at weight loss."

In other words, a history of yo-yo dieting has *no* effect on your body's ability to shed pounds. That's the good news.

The bad news is that the more often people go on diets, fall off of diets, and move on to new diets, the harder it becomes emotionally to succeed. This is especially true when people attempt (and fail) to lose weight with very rigorous, low-calorie diets.

I hate fanatical diet programs. They take the joy out of eating. Heck, they take the joy out of living! And the research is pretty clear by now that too-tough diets simply don't work for most people. Even if you lose weight initially, you're going to get bored or frustrated with all of the restrictions. Every time you go off the diet, then try it again or do something similarly restrictive in the future, your odds for success drop even lower, and science bears this out every time.

Losing Weight Is Easy

Let me present some of the findings from the bible of obesity treatment practitioners, *Clinical Guidelines on the Identification, Evaluation, and Treatment of Overweight and Obesity in Adults*, published by the National Institutes of Health.

Your initial goal, say the guidelines, should be to lose 10 percent of your weight in 6 months. That's a relatively modest, achievable goal that *you* can achieve by implementing just a handful of the suggestions in *Think Yourself Thin*. Most of the report details the health benefits of losing weight, but here are some of their suggestions for how to reach that desirable goal:

• **Be yourself.** Look through the suggestions and tips in this book and choose the ones that seem to fit your personality. Everyone has different needs and appetites. We can't all follow the same weight-loss plan and hope for success anymore than we can all wear the same size shoes.
• **Be reasonable.** Don't expect to lose half your weight in a month and keep it off. It's far healthier to achieve and maintain a moderate weight loss than it is to lose a huge amount of weight and then gain it all back.
• **Be moderate.** Although diets that are extremely low in calories produce more weight loss at first than do moderately low calorie diets, the weight you lose on a more moderate diet is far more likely to stay off over the long term.

This is exciting news from the experts. But I didn't need to hear it from them. My own experience working with my clients has taught me that you don't have to go on depressing or demoralizing diets to lose weight. And the more you try, the more you learn. Your chances of succeeding are still great—even if you've tried and failed in the past.

The NWCR that I mentioned earlier found that 91 percent of the weight-loss maintainers that they study had failed at previous weight-loss attempts. "They tried all the wrong ways to do it," the study's authors noted, "and then they figured out the right ways to do it."

So, for good reasons, I take a radically different approach from the diet faddists. I don't encourage people to count up every calorie they consume. I don't insist you give up ice cream or a favorite restaurant. And I certainly don't push people to sign up at their local gym, as long as they're willing to get regular exercise in some other way.

What I do encourage people to do (and what I do myself) is to approach weight loss by making many incremental changes, changes they can live with. Eating one less take-out meal a week. Starting the day with oatmeal. Having a snack before settling in at happy hour. These and other simple changes add up to a lot of lost calories—and weight—over the course of the year. Why go through the misery of a super-tough diet when you can make tiny changes that will have even better results?

William Dietz, director of Nutrition and Physical Activity at the federal Centers for Disease Control and Prevention, put it very succinctly, "Even the population which has had the most massive weight increase over the last 30 years, that is, middle-aged females, the weight change of 18 pounds over this period can be accounted for by about a 13 calorie per day imbalance. So, the small differences that have occurred in the population may well be what is driving this [obesity] epidemic."

The same approach that I recommend for diet and nutrition—making a series of small changes over time—also works for physical activity. It's true that hard-core exercise is an excellent way to control weight. The drawback is that it's a real turnoff for most people. Jogging 4 miles a day will certainly burn impressive amounts of calories. But who does it? Most people find themselves only thinking about jogging, not actually doing it, and then feel guilty about it.

What's the alternative? According to the Centers for Disease Control and Prevention and the American College of Sports Medicine, people are more likely to stick with low- to moderate-intensity physical activities than all-out workouts. In other words, taking a few extra walks around the mall might be better for losing weight than attempting—and giving up on—more rigorous types of exercise. Moderate physical activity is just as good for your overall health as sweating through competitive aerobics classes or other high-intensity workouts.

You'll get excellent health and weight-loss benefits just by being active for a total of 30 minutes a day. Taking stairs instead of elevators. Walking to the corner store. Dancing. As long as it all adds up to 30 minutes—and if you do everything at about the same intensity as a brisk walk—you'll be in great shape.

It's the same idea, really, as making small, but consistent, changes in your diet. And that's the premise of *Think Yourself Thin*. I've found that people who make a series of small changes—so small, in many cases, that they hardly notice them—lose more weight over time than those who embark on all-or-nothing diet plans. It's also a lot more fun because they continue to live life to the fullest!

You Can Do It!

As I mentioned above, weight-loss experts agree that your initial goal should be to lose 10 percent of your weight in 6 months. That's not very much at all. It's a good goal because nearly everyone can achieve it, and when you've been successful once, you'll be more motivated to keep it up.

Unfortunately, the weight-loss industry is dominated by those who insist that the only road to weight loss is to follow absurdly detailed eating plans, or to exercise at a level that would tax trained athletes, let alone the "normal" men and women I see every day.

Terrible advice! In my experience—and the experience of today's top experts—the tortoise beats the hare every time.

The battle of your bulge will be won at the margins. Sweeping, life-transforming changes are impractical and won't work. Shrewd, small, concrete changes that can be easily incorporated into your daily routine are certain to lead to success.

That's the foundation of *Think Yourself Thin*. Set reasonable goals. Make small changes. Look for approaches that complement, not dominate, your life, and are changes you can live with. You will lose weight. I guarantee it!

Goals You Can Live With

So many of my friends and clients have tried, with varying degrees of success, to lose weight. Why does it have to be such a difficult and frustrating process?

Part of the problem, I think, is that so many diet plans make completely unrealistic promises. Instant weight loss! Look great in 30 days! Unless you're an expert in the field, it's almost impossible to know for sure what's real and what's not—what works and what's nothing more than marketing hype.

My approach is very different. When I first meet with clients, I emphasize that losing weight and keeping it off is a *journey*, not a once-and-done technique. I do spend a lot of time talking about calories, styles of eating, and so forth, but I'm more concerned with attitude. Once you understand the basic issues, such as the need to eat less excess food and be more physically active, successful weight loss mainly depends on motivation.

Ah, motivation—that's the hard part! It's easy to make the decision to lose weight, and it's easy to succeed for a while. But over time, everyone's motivation tends to flag a bit, and that's when the risk of gaining—or regaining—weight becomes a real issue.

Setting Goals, Keeping Goals

I've found that the best way for most people to stay motivated on their weight-loss journey is to have very specific goals at every step of the way. Goals change all the time, of course. If you've just started thinking about your weight, your goal might be as simple as to lose a few pounds this month. Over time, your goals may shift to things like, "I want to be as physically active as I used to be," or "I want to wear the same jeans I wore five years ago."

Goals are good. Specific goals are even better because they give you something concrete to aim for. Goals are also an excellent way to measure your progress along the way.

I can't stress enough that goals should be fun and liberating, not just another ball and chain that weighs you down and reminds you of your failures. (We all have them, believe me!)

Everyone's goals are different, of course. I don't presume to have a one-size-fits-all set of goals that works for everyone. Over the years, however, I have developed some goal-setting strategies that I think can make a real difference. To be helpful tools in losing weight, your goals should be:

• **Realistic.** Perfectionist goals set you up for failure. Permit yourself to be imperfect, and even plan imperfections in your program

• **Small behavioral steps.** You can't set a goal of losing 2 pounds, but you can set a goal of doing the things that will cause you to lose 2 pounds, such as eating a good breakfast, adding vegetables to your meals, or eating a light dinner. Set goals based on what you will "do," as opposed to what you will "be." Once you do the things you've outlined for yourself, the weight loss will fall into place.

• **Positive.** Instead of stating what you won't do ("I won't eat chocolate when I get home from work") state what you will do ("I'll prepare a beautiful bowl of raspberries when I get home from work").

• **Flexible.** Setting a goal to "exercise every day" may not be possible because of unforeseen circumstances. But saying instead, "I will be physically active five out of seven days," is certainly doable. And if you end up exercising every day, you get bonus points!

• **Measurable.** "I'll eat more fruits and vegetables" is a noble goal, but how will you know when you reach it? Give yourself some specific criteria so you can reward yourself for a job well done. For instance, "I'll add a vegetable soup or salad to every lunch this week." This way, you know exactly what you need to do to achieve your goal and deserve a reward at the end of the week.

• **Important to you.** If you've set a goal to "eat a light dinner" and you continually don't achieve it, reevaluate whether it's really important to you to eat a light dinner. Or is there some internal need for you to have a heavy dinner that you're not aware of?

• **Set in a supportive environment.** Do you need to have healthful, tasty foods in your refrigerator ready to heat up at a moment's notice? Take a look at your environment to determine if it is supportive enough for you to achieve your goal.

Your Personal Goal Worksheet

You can think of goals as interim steps on the journey to weight loss. Some goals are long term, some aren't, but all goals will serve to guide you to a particular place you want to be.

I ask all of my clients to think about where they'd like to be in 1 year. This sort of big-picture goal is a great way to help you choose the dozens of little goals that will help get you where you want to be.

Do you have a pencil or pen? Good! Let's decide where you want to be in a year.

Weight

One year from now I want to weigh _____ pounds. This will be a loss of _____ pounds from my present weight of _____. This translates to _____ pounds per week.

Shape

What is it about my appearance that I'd most like to change by losing weight? (Examples: the size clothes I'd like to wear; losing the belly bulge; a slimmer waist or thighs; more muscles, etc.)

_____

_____

_____

_____

Medical

One year from now I want my cholesterol to be _____.

I want my blood pressure to be _____.

I want better mobility in my (list the joints or body parts that you'd like to improve)_____.

Other health benefits I want to achieve include:

_____

_____

_____

_____

Energy Levels

One year from now I want more and better energy. My goals include (list specifics, such as "walk with a lighter step," or "be able to spend more time with my friends"):

_____

_____

_____

_____

Happiness

One year from now I want to feel better about myself in the following ways (Examples: "having more confidence," or "developing more rewarding relationships"):

_____

_____

_____

_____

Is every line filled in? Congratulations! You've made the first step toward achieving your goals: less weight, more strength, better energy—whatever you want!

Don't forget this page once you've filled it in. As the year progresses, look at it frequently. Assess your progress for each of the different goals. Add new goals or revise old ones as necessary. Think of this "goal sheet" as your road map for the coming year. You can change direction at any point. You can slow down or speed up. But at least you know where you're going!

Let your journey begin!

CHAPTER 3

Fed Up With Fads

Spend some time in the bookstore or just plug the word "diet" into your search engine and you'll be overwhelmed by the thousands of diet books and theories out there. How in the world can you evaluate which diets offer substance and which ones provide a large dose of snake oil? There may be a best way to lose weight while not damaging your health, but how do you find it? And which approach will provide you with a game plan you can stay with over the long haul?

Most books on the subject offer a hook or gimmick, a sort of magic wand to wave over the bathroom scale to make the numbers grow smaller by the day, but do any of these gimmicks actually work? The answer is simple: If a diet plan advocates eating fewer calories than your body burns, you'll lose weight. However, weight loss shouldn't be your only consideration. You need to know if the plan will help you *keep* the weight off and, more importantly, if it's safe.

Risky Business

Some of the currently popular diets are downright risky where your health is concerned. The most dangerous are those that advocate eating large quantities of unhealthy foods, cut healthy foods from the diet, include stimulants or "weight-loss herbs" or "supplements," or are just too low in calories.

For instance, high-protein/low-carbohydrate diets advocate eating unlimited quantities of meats and animal fats, which decades of respected research have shown us are known contributors to heart disease and cancer. They also advocate eating a limited array of vegetables, and almost no fruits or whole grains. Yet over 200 scientific studies have shown a diet high in vegetables, fruits, and whole grains dramatically enhances health and prevents disease.

The most extreme diet of this type is the Atkins Diet. Even though the Atkins Diet has received some positive press lately, if you look deeper and beyond the public relations hype, you will find some troubling facts. While it's true that studies show this diet, like many other unhealthy fads, will temporarily help you lose weight and lower your cholesterol (losing weight with any method will), it has far-reaching short-term and long-term negative health consequences.

Atkins says the essence of the diet is to eat all the meat and fat you want, but keep your carbohydrate intake to a minimum—about 20 grams per day (virtually zero vegetables, and no fruits or whole grains)—in order to produce a condition in your body called "ketosis." Ketosis is an unnatural physiological state your body goes into when you are ill or starving. It disrupts acid/base balance, causing the blood to become too acidic, leaching calcium from the bones, and causing dehydration, bad breath (from the ketone bodies), and poor appetite, among other symptoms. Atkins' own 6-month study reported many unhealthy side effects: 1) Urinary calcium excretion and uric acid excretion significantly increased, showing the increased acidity of the blood and possible leaching of calcium from bones (think: osteoporosis). 2) The researchers estimated the loss as 44 percent muscle and water loss (only 66 percent fat lost). 3) Significant adverse effects were reported by the subjects: 68 percent experienced constipation, 63 percent bad breath, 51 percent reported headaches, 10 percent noted hair loss.

And those were just the short-term consequences. The long-term consequences are even more dangerous.

Armed with this information, even if you decide to try it, I recommend you only do it temporarily. Once you stop losing weight, continuing on this style of diet—with unlimited meats and animal fats and low quantities of fruits and whole grains—will increase your risk for high cholesterol, heart disease, and many cancers. New evidence suggests that a diet such as the Atkins Diet, which causes high levels of blood cholesterol and high blood pressure, may increase the risk for Alzheimer's and dementia. The studies show diet may be even more influential than carrying the "Alzheimer's gene." Decades of research has confirmed that a Mediterranean- or Asian-style plant-based diet containing lean meats, fish, and healthy plant-based oils and fish oils, is the one most highly correlated with health, slimness, vitality, and longevity.

The Zone, Carbohydrate-Addict's, Protein Power, and Sugar Busters diets also advocate limited vegetables, fruits, and whole grains, but they're not as radical in cutting back the carbs as Atkins and they advocate eating leaner meats. This makes them a small step above Atkins, but still nothing I would recommend. I don't agree that any fruits, vegetables, or whole grains should be eliminated categorically from the diet (nobody became overweight from eating too many carrots!).

Atkins and other no-carb gurus also have people believing that carbohydrates and high insulin levels cause diabetes. But the fact is that what causes diabetes and insulin resistance is being overweight or being sedentary. And weight gain is caused by an imbalance in the calories you take in versus the calories you burn. As soon as you start losing weight—using any method, particularly if you're exercising—your blood glucose and insulin will drop dramatically.

Research confirms that people who eat more fruits, vegetables, and whole grains are the successful weight-loss maintainers. These low- to no-carb diets are more of the same—diets you can't stick with because of their rigid, unhealthy rules and regulations.

For all of these reasons, I would categorize these diets, especially the Atkins Diet, as dangerous. They're also monotonous, which means they're hard to stick with. Any diet you can't stick with for life, and enjoy, won't keep your weight off.

At the other end of the scale are the (unnecessarily) extreme low-fat/high-carbohydrate category of diets, such the Dean Ornish Plan, the Pritikin Plan, the Gabe Mirkin Plan, and the Fat Gram Counter, all of which take your fat intake to under 20 percent of your total calories. While research shows successful weight-loss maintainers eat a low-fat diet because fats are so calorie-dense, it's all relative. People who are walking weight-loss success stories still eat 20 to 30 percent of their calories as fat, which will amount to 35 to 75 grams for most people.

Not all fats are created equal. Current research suggests that for maintaining good health, the most important fats to reduce in the diet are saturated fats and trans fatty acids. These are mainly found in animal products and processed foods and are correlated with an increased risk of coronary heart disease and cancers. Some fats, particularly monounsaturated fats and polyunsaturated fats such as omega-3 fatty acids, are actually good for you.

Finally, eating a low-fat, high-carbohydrate diet in itself won't make you shed pounds. You'll lose weight only if your total calorie intake is lower than your burn rate. Though studies show most weight-loss maintainers do eat a high-carbohydrate diet, they mean *relatively* high, and the carbohydrates they're referring to are fruits, vegetables, and whole grains, not giant bagels, frozen yogurt, and fat-free cookies. Obviously, a low-fat/high-carb diet is not a magic bullet, especially if it's loaded with sugar and white flour products.

Food-combining diets, blood-typing diets, grapefruit diets, fruit-only diets, cabbage soup diets, don't-mix-protein-with-starch diets, and detox diets are all based on pseudoscience, which is a nice way of saying *no* science. There is absolutely no evidence that grapefruit burns fat or that eating certain combinations of foods increases your metabolism rate. In one popular "detox plan," the Fat Flush, the author claims "evening primrose oil mobilizes the metabolically active fat known as brown adipose tissue," and this in turn "burns off extra calories and boosts energy." The author says evening primrose oil "revs up the metabolism." If losing weight were that easy, why isn't everyone doing it? Because it's a bunch of hooey. The meal plans in this approach are all extremely low in calories, and if anyone follows them they'll lose weight for that reason. Ultimately, however these are silly, unnecessarily complicated approaches to eating, so there is little chance anyone will follow them for long.

In the "most likely to backfire" and potentially dangerous category are liquid diets, fasts, appetite suppressants, and weight-loss supplements, such as "metabolism boosters" or "fat burners." Studies show that many people who lose weight and regain it have been following extreme approaches to weight loss, including these liquid-only diets, fasts, and appetite suppressants. Relapsers report that weight loss was far easier than maintenance, probably because they went with a quick-fix approach. Using weight-loss supplements and drugs (particularly ephedra or ma huang) may cause potentially life-threatening side effects. So far, we haven't found a pill that is safe enough to be taken permanently. And once you stop taking them, well, the inevitable happens.

How to Know a Good Diet When You See One

A good diet is one you can follow for life. One that you enjoy. It's a strategy that makes you feel energetic and comfortable. It's a way of living that science has shown will enhance your health and possibly even extend your life.

In my practice, I've found a good diet is one that works with your lifestyle, whether you're a full-time mom or high-powered professional. Studies show weight-loss maintainers follow diets that offer flexibility and choice and that can fit into their lives whether they would rather sit down to a meal at home or eat out in a restaurant every day. They also prefer diets that have lots of variety and offer plenty of fruits, vegetables, whole grains, and fiber. These foods are important for controlling weight because of their low caloric density. You're able to eat a larger amount but you feel full with fewer calories.

Maintainers usually get their protein from lean cuts of meat, poultry, seafood, and vegetarian items such as beans. You can save hundreds of calories a day by eating leaner meats, not to mention the health benefits you receive.

Balance is important too. As mentioned above, maintainers do eat some healthy fats, such as the monounsaturated oils found in canola oil, olives, nuts, and seeds, and the omega-3 fatty acids found in deep-water fish and flaxseed. But fat consumption is kept moderate because it has a very high caloric density. A tablespoon of fat contains 120 calories, the same amount you'll find in 4–6 ounces of fish, 3 cups of fresh strawberries, or a pound of carrots.

Weight-loss maintainers also report eating fewer sweets, which tend to be so calorie dense that it's very difficult to lose weight if there's a substantial amount of them in your daily diet. Just one chocolate bar contains

250 to 300 calories, the same amount found in many frozen meals! Over time, maintainers' taste buds actually change and they begin to enjoy and prefer wholesome, healthy foods. Sweets are not completely eliminated, however. Successful maintainers occasionally treat themselves. They just do it wisely and make sure they enjoy every darn bite!

If your diet is too low in calories or carbohydrates and you're losing weight very quickly—say, more than 2 pounds a week—it can leave you energy-drained and unable to be physically active. If this happens, I advise you to stop whatever diet you're following immediately.

First, if you're too drained to exercise and you're losing weight quickly, you're losing at least 50 percent water and muscle. You may end up being very thin, but also very flabby and unhealthy!

Second, research has shown very clearly that physical activity is probably the most predictive factor in whether or not you keep your weight off once you lose it. So your diet should be getting you primed for new exercise habits, not making them more difficult. When you've lost your weight, your increased physical activity patterns should be in place, so it's smooth sailing from then on.

Interestingly, successful weight-loss maintainers say that keeping weight off is easier than losing it—the opposite experience of re-gainers. It may be that "quick-fix" approaches don't give you enough time to develop the new eating habits you'll need during the maintenance phase of your weight management. I observed this happening in real life when I first started out in private practice.

Many years ago, I worked with people in the Optifast program. It was my job to teach them to change their eating habits after they had lost weight with this doctor-supervised, modified fast. When they came into my office right after having lost all that weight so handily, I have to tell you, they were—how can I put it—*cocky!* It felt so easy to lose. They didn't have to learn any new eating habits or even exercise much to lose the weight.

But then came maintenance, a whole different story. Consciously they knew they would have to eat differently from the way they did before they lost their weight. Unfortunately, most of them weren't psychologically ready to do that. The ease of fasting away the pounds had destroyed their ability to maintain a lower body weight. I'm not saying you have to suffer while losing weight in order to keep it off. But my experience has been that it's best to be working on the habits you'll need to have in place during your maintenance phase.

I finally tried Optifast myself just to experience what my clients were going through. Just like them, a few days after my fast ended, I began bingeing. I gained back the weight I lost and more!

So, the good news is that depriving, depressing diets don't work, and you'll never, ever have to go on one. What my clients tell me every day is they don't have to suffer, that losing weight is easier and more positive than they ever imagined. It's the little things they do every day that add up to lasting results.

Katherine's Diet Primer

I'd like to give you a primer that will help you evaluate any diet you may come across. First, before embarking on any diet, it would be very helpful to answer these questions:

1. Will the diet work for you and your lifestyle? Is it individualized to take into account your personal history, family background, and special nutritional and exercise needs?

Studies demonstrate that for a diet to work and last, it needs to complement you, your personality, and your lifestyle. Successful weight-loss maintainers use a variety of techniques that work for them. Most diet books provide a one-size-fits-all approach: Atkins, Sugar Busters, Pritikin, detox plans, combination diets, and fasts all have one particular plan you must follow. Yet scientific studies prove that one size *doesn't* fit all when it comes to successful weight loss and maintenance.

2. Does the diet advocate a balance and variety of foods?

Variety is the spice of life. If your diet forbids entire food groups, life can become pretty grim. In addition to the nutritional imbalances you would suffer, can you imagine a life permanently devoid of breads, ice cream, or all of your favorite foods? Studies confirm that weight-loss maintainers allow fattening treats into their diets periodically. But most diets forbid them entirely. They don't teach ways of fitting in foods they refer to as "forbidden." Relapsers often give up and gain their weight back because of this "good food" versus "bad food" mentality promoted by so many of these fad diets.

3. Is the diet based on up-to-date, scientifically credible research that demonstrates it will improve your health rather than damage it?

If your diet isn't supported by most of the scientific establishment and peer-reviewed medical journals, I would go back to the drawing board.

Low-carb diets in particular go against everything science has discovered in the past 50 years about what comprises a healthy diet and what kind of diet is most likely to promote long-term weight loss. We know from many, many research studies that consuming animal fats is probably the unhealthiest aspect of the typical American's eating habits, yet low-carb diet plans encourage people to eat unlimited quantities of these fats. The Atkins Diet is the most notorious diet of this type, but others, such as The Zone Diet and Sugar Busters fall into the same category. Studies show that this type of diet puts you at greater risk for heart disease, stroke, and several cancers.

Combination detox/blood-type diets don't have a lot of evidence against them simply because credible scientists haven't done any studies. Perhaps this is because these diets are so obviously silly and unhealthy that no one wants to waste time doing research on them. You don't need to do a controlled, double-blind study on fire to know that it will burn you.

4. Does the diet promote a positive attitude toward food and eating?

Eating is one of our greatest pleasures in life and you don't need to lose or compromise that enjoyment just because you want to lose weight. You can continue to savor great food while shedding unwanted pounds. Eating under a lot of rules and regulations about required or forbidden foods takes all the pleasure out of sitting down to a meal. And what fun is that? Successful weight-loss maintainers use other strategies, such as learning how to cope with life's problems more effectively so they don't eat for emotional reasons. This kind of strategy gives them the ability to take pleasure in every meal.

5. Does the diet promise quick results—a loss of more than 2 pounds per week—that might destabilize your metabolism?

Many diets promise superquick results, but studies show the body can only metabolize about ½ to 1 pound of fat per week. If you're losing faster than that, you may be losing valuable water and muscle, and you're almost sure to be on a regimen that is too rigid to stick with for long. Some diets are so low in calories that they actually lower your body's rate of metabolism, which makes losing weight and maintaining it more and more impossible as time goes by.

6. *Does the diet require exercise or physical activity?*

If there's one thing that scientists broadly agree on, it is that physical activity is necessary for health, healthy weight loss, and lifelong weight maintenance. If you're losing weight without exercise, chances are your calorie intake is too low and studies show you're unlikely to maintain that loss. And if you're not replacing fat with muscle, you're likely to end up with a body that is smaller but no more attractive than the one you're trying to change.

7. *Does the diet require special packaged foods, liquid or herbal supplements, or megadoses of vitamins and minerals?*

Do you see yourself popping fistfuls of pills or sending for food in the mail for the rest of your life? Realistically, diet plans that include prepackaged foods or megadoses of supplements are not approaches to weight loss and maintenance you'll stick with permanently. You're far better off finding a diet that includes real food at every meal—food you can buy at the local supermarket. If you're concerned that you're not getting enough vitamins and minerals in your meals, then take a multivitamin with breakfast every day.

8. *Does the diet have a scientifically established track record of success that has been demonstrated over time?*

Losing weight is not rocket science. Everyone knows that if you simply eat less, you'll lose weight. But keeping the weight off over time— even many years—requires real skills, such as knowing how to plan healthy, balanced meals; knowing how to handle eating out at a restaurant, party, or friend's home; building strategies to cope with boredom and emotional stress; and finding ways to motivate yourself to be physically active every day, now and forever. If a diet doesn't help you acquire these skills, then it won't work over the long term.

9. *Does the diet have unacceptable side effects?*

If you're tired and your health is worsening, this isn't the diet for you. You may not be getting proper nutrition—in fact, you may be literally starving yourself. Remember, you're trying to become thinner and healthier, not emaciated and sickly. If you're using diet supplements, you may be facing yet another health risk: dangerous side effects like increased blood pressure and changes in heart rhythm. These side effects have been known to send people to the hospital, and some have even died.

The High Road to Healthful Weight Loss

Think Yourself Thin is a way to create a personalized, balanced plan that allows you to eat all of your favorite foods. *You* pick the techniques you can fit into your life. If you're constantly traveling, you can't be expected to cook all your meals at home. If you enjoy cooking, you should be able to continue feeding yourself and your family meals everyone enjoys. *Think Yourself Thin* also provides you with a Metabolism Toolbox (see page 461) that lets you calculate your calorie needs based on a tried-and-true scientific formula that has been used by nutritional scientists for decades.

CHAPTER 4

Breaking the Spell
of Childhood

"Like mother, like daughter" is a phrase with deeper meaning than we often appreciate, especially where eating is concerned. I know this from intimate experience. I grew up with a lovely, caring mother who happened to have a weight problem and as a result followed diet after diet, hoping to find the elusive elixir that would finally make her thinner. She seemed ashamed of her body, frustrated by her weight, and unhappy with herself. Her shame and frustration made a big impression on me, and the miseries of being overweight and dieting scared me. I was determined not to go through the same thing.

Being a child, however, didn't give me much power over my destiny. Studies show that daughters of dieting or food-restricting mothers are far more likely to develop eating problems than other girls are. We shouldn't be surprised. How many times do you catch yourself sounding like your mother or your father when interacting with your own children and loved ones? You always swore you would be different from your parents, right? But how often do you hear their words coming out of your own mouth: "You're going to break your neck doing that!" or "A penny saved, a penny earned!" Ugh! Likewise, while I didn't want to repeat my mother's experience with weight problems and dieting, I inevitably did—without even being aware of what was happening.

My own weight problem didn't show up until I was in college, but my eating problems had begun much earlier. As a child, I developed a voracious appetite. Although friends occasionally teased me about it, no one gave my eating a serious second thought because I had always been so thin. What I didn't realize was my appetite led me into a pattern of consuming food that would eventually prove my nemesis. My weight gain problems didn't yet appear because I was very physically active as a child. Those days of carefree eating, however, would soon be over.

A Time of Reckoning

When I went away to college, my physical activity level plummeted. Gone were the days of playing out in the fresh air after school—skating, biking, swimming, and playing ball games. There was no more gym class, gymnastics, dancing, or cheerleading. The numbers on the scale began to creep up and my energy levels began to sag. Sometimes I would find myself completely fatigued before the day even began. My declining physical state was pretty obvious to at least one person—my 75-year-old grandmother. I'll never forget her admonishing me: "You're too young to be so tired all the time!" She was right, of course. I was turning into a slug.

Lack of exercise wasn't the only problem. I also shared my mother's obsession for sweets, which fit right in with our mutual love of baking. Pastry baking was a fun activity we had always done together and from which we had always taken a great deal of pleasure. As a child, I had enjoyed the spoils of our labor a little too much, especially when there were brownies involved. I would always eat more of our homemade brownies than anyone else, even though I'd end up feeling stuffed and miserable. Now, in college, I really went overboard indulging my sweet tooth. I would regularly bake my favorite chocolate chip bars and caramel popcorn, and once I even baked a cheesecake from scratch, which my roommate and I shared every day until it was gone. My weight went up correspondingly. I was my mother's daughter all right.

Ups and Downs of a Journey to Weight Loss

I was also my grandmother's granddaughter, however, and I took her admonishment to heart. I recognized that it was time to turn things around. The only problem was that solving my problem wasn't quite as easy as recognizing it. A couple of years of fits and starts went by before I made real progress. I began my journey by finding ways to increase my physical activity. I decided to be smart about it and actually got college credit for classes in scuba and fencing! On the side, I took classes in yoga and aerobics. I was amazed at the results. My energy returned and I got into shape in no time.

Unfortunately, I hadn't really learned my lesson. Losing weight was too easy! A couple of phys ed classes had put me right back on the road to slenderness. The idea of maintaining my weight loss, however, never occurred to me. Inevitably, I became complacent and stopped exercising. Guess what? My weight shot back up (duh!).

Looking back on it, I don't understand why I didn't just continue exercising regularly. I imagine I thought that shedding excess pounds was like any other problem: you find a solution, and the problem's over with. Unfortunately, controlling my weight wasn't so simply accomplished. I now know, both from experience and from many studies of the subject, that you can't maintain weight loss over the long term unless you are physically active on a regular basis. In those days, however, I was a very different person. I figured that if I was putting on weight again, the physical activity approach hadn't really worked. Besides, just like my mom before me, I hated exercising!

This time I took a different approach: dieting. In fact, I dieted with a vengeance! I started with the Scarsdale Diet, which was basically starvation. Did it work? Yeah, it worked. But did I keep it off? Nah! Instead, the dieting actually seemed to lead to bingeing. I didn't know it then, but that was the beginning of a cycle of dieting and bingeing that would last for a long, long time.

Eating Disorders Are Family Disorders

By now, it may be so obvious to you that I was repeating my mother's misfortunes, but honestly, I didn't have a clue! Putting myself on a diet should have been a big tip-off that something was wrong, but I wasn't open to tip-offs. I wanted to lose weight. Period. Maybe if I had stopped and thought about it or sought help, I could have figured things out and avoided all the ups and downs, but that would have been too easy for Miss Smartypants Katherine.

My experience is typical for people across the country. Study after study shows the importance of parental modeling on a child's eating habits.

One such study, reported in the *American Journal of Clinical Nutrition*, found that mothers who report high levels of out-of-control, uninhibited eating have daughters who eat this way as well. Another study found that today half of all 5-year-old girls know what dieting is. When asked, the girls described dieting in several relevant ways: "you do not eat," "to lose weight," "drink diet soda," "drink a milk shake." The researchers found the girls' exceptional knowledge was easily predicted: If a mother was dieting at the time, her little daughter had a pretty good idea of what dieting meant.

If your mother restricted her own food intake, she probably restricted yours as well. But this strategy backfires. There is a strong tie between parental control and fatness in children. Another study, published in the *American Journal of Clinical Nutrition*, found that the more a mom restricted a particular food, the more attractive that food became to her kids. In other words, restriction actually *enhanced* the kids' preference and made them less able to regulate their food intake.

In the study, if mothers restricted access to high-calorie snack foods, their daughters would overindulge in those foods when they finally gained access—even if they had just eaten lunch and reported they were full. The 4-year-old girls who were studied ate to the tune of about 250 extra calories, a pretty substantial volume for a small child. The researchers also found that this behavior affected self-esteem. After the girls overate, they felt terrible guilt about themselves and their eating and expressed a negative self-image. These are the seeds that sow years of future anguish—and eating disorders.

Sowing the Seeds of Health

Parents don't need to restrict a child's food intake if they bring only healthy foods into their home. Children will eat what is available to them and will learn to prefer healthy foods if they are positively and regularly offered. But there are some hurdles to get over.

Researchers have discovered that you carry an innate love of sweets with you from the moment you're born. By age 4 months, your love for salty food blossoms as well. These preferences can be modified by your experiences, by what you're exposed to, and by your growth, development, and age. If you're mainly exposed to salty and sweet foods as you're growing up, you may find developing a taste for vegetables a difficult challenge. One study, reported in the *Journal of the American Dietetic Association*, confirmed this. The study demonstrated that children will develop a preference for high-calorie food if that is what they're regularly given—and often that's exactly what they're given. Why? Because it's easy to prepare. Parents don't have to work at it, and kids just naturally go for it. Often, high-calorie foods reflect what's in the parents' own diet. Another study found that children who preferred the fattiest foods had the most overweight parents.

Vegetables, on the other hand, are low in calories and are full of life-saving vitamins, minerals, and phytochemicals, but they can be bitter, and most children don't like bitter. It's an acquired taste. Developing it in kids is a tough job for parents, but it can be done. Although children will generally avoid new foods—they have "food neophobia" unless the food is sweet or salty—a parent can help them develop new preferences almost from the moment they're born. In one study of 4- to 6-month-old infants, mothers who introduced a new fruit or vegetable found it took only one feeding to increase the infant's acceptance of the food. The acceptance was also generalized to other similar foods. If an infant had experience with one vegetable, other vegetables were more readily eaten.

As with everything else, of course, the older you get, the harder it is to learn new skills or acquire new tastes. Unlike their younger siblings, when children aged 2 to 5 were given opportunities to taste a new food, it took between 5 and 10 exposures to see an increased preference. But the change was startling. Although the first exposure usually resulted in a very negative reaction, by the time the kids reached their 10th or even 20th try, they were eating the new food—even green beans, which they hated at first—as if it were ice cream! Repeated opportunities to smell and look at new foods also increased acceptance.

Studies show three effective ways in which you can help a child to expand the variety of his or her diet: 1) emphasize that the new foods taste good, 2) provide opportunities to sample good-tasting new foods, and 3) let them see you and other people enjoying new foods.

What is *not* effective? Sternly pointing out that vegetables should be eaten because they're "good for you!"

Cleaning Your Plate and Other Bad Habits

Another childhood factor that may be affecting your eating habits is how you were encouraged to eat and what portion sizes you were given when you were little more than a toddler. At age 3, children eat only what they need, not more, not less. But one study shows that when they get older, around age 5, they become more responsive to external cues to eat and are more likely to overeat if either they're encouraged to do so or they're given larger portion sizes.

Yet another relic from your childhood that can affect your current weight is your relationship with your television set. Did you develop a serious television-watching habit when you were a kid? Researchers have found that the prevalence of obesity among children is directly related to the hours of TV they watch on a daily basis. In fact, they have concluded that TV viewing is a double threat. It not only represents inactivity but is also associated with eating high-calorie foods. The more TV a child watches, the more likely he or she is to consume foods advertised on TV, which tend to be high calorie.

The Younger the Better

Children have an easier time losing weight and keeping it off than adults do, as long as the whole family is involved in the process and you start helping them develop healthful eating habits early. An overweight child's chances of becoming an overweight adult increase as he or she gets older, so an overweight teen is especially vulnerable. If the problem hasn't been solved by then, a teenager has a 70 percent chance of having a serious weight problem in adulthood.

About a third of all adult obesity begins in childhood, according to one study, and obesity that began in childhood tends to be more severe. It is also associated with a greater number of adverse medical and psychological effects. The study also found that if you were an overweight child at 1 to 3 years old, the likelihood that the obesity will persist does not increase significantly. However, if you also had overweight parents, you have a much greater chance of developing adult obesity. Parenting is critical to what you become.

Your History Is Not Your Destiny

Even though you can't change the facts of your childhood, you can change your reactions to them and succeed in your efforts to lose weight. The first step is to think back and try to remember your childhood experiences. Once you face your childhood influences and understand the foundations of your eating habits, you're in the driver's seat. You can start making fundamental changes in the way you think and feel about food and eating. So let's quickly review some general childhood experiences and how they relate to you now.

• If your parents brought high-calorie, unhealthy foods into the house, chances are you have a preference for those.

• If sweet, fatty, or high-calorie foods were available in your home, but restricted, you probably developed an even greater preference for them.

• If you developed an obsession with sweet, fatty, or high-calorie foods, you may now have a problem with overeating, followed by feelings of self-loathing and guilt.

• If your parents didn't love fruits, vegetables, and healthy foods, then you probably have a hard time eating tomatoes, squash, or carrots.

• If your parents didn't encourage physical activity or you weren't physically active as a child, you may very well have a hard time being physically active today.

• If you were encouraged as a child to keep eating even after you were full, if you were often served portions that were too large, or if you ate mostly at restaurants, where large portions are the norm, you may have developed a habit of ignoring your body signals and overeating if there is food sitting in front of you. Classic childhood obesity and eating disorder research found that children have to learn to discriminate hunger cues from other distress cues. If parents are not good at detecting hunger in the child and responding appropriately from other distress cues, the child may become overweight.

If any of these childhood histories pertain to you, you are not alone. Even if your parents were wonderful in many ways, as mine were, but weren't the best role models in the area of eating habits, physical activity, and weight, you could have an uphill battle ahead. It's definitely winnable, but you have to set your mind to it.

Isabel and Jennifer

These finding are clearly reflected in not only my own life, but in the lives of the clients I've had the privilege to work with over the past 20 years. It's with uncanny and sad regularity that the problems my clients currently face can clearly be traced back to the peculiar circumstances of their childhoods.

Isabel

Take Isabel. She started dieting at a very young age. Her large, Italian family was concerned about her weight as she was growing up, but they weren't sure how to handle it. None of them ever experienced a weight problem. On one hand, they encouraged her to eat, on the other hand, she was criticized for being overweight. Her mother would try to keep certain foods away from her. Nothing seemed to work. So, without knowing what else to do, when she was in 5th grade her mother sent her to Weight Watchers, where she lost her first 10 pounds. Of course, it's impossible for children to handle the problem on their own. She gained the weight back quickly. She struggled throughout her childhood and teens and has fought the battle her whole life.

In my practice, I've found that it's harder—though far from impossible—for adults to deal with a weight problem successfully when they experienced the problem as a child. And the studies confirm this. I'm not sure of all the reasons. My guess is that your self-image and personality are formed as a child and your body weight and lifestyle (eating habits, physical activity) become ingrained.

Also, we know based on studies today that families are critical to reversing a child's weight problem. In Isabel's case, she didn't get proper support from her family. Her parents were bringing high-calorie foods into the house, but trying to restrict them from Isabel. They were also encouraging her to eat, eat, eat! They never encouraged her to be physically active. Yet they were criticizing her all the while. Today we know that these approaches simply don't work. In fact, they backfire.

After experiencing such a childhood, dealing with your weight problem as an adult can feel especially depressing. It reminds you of all those difficult times you experienced as a child, all the failures and disappointments. It made you feel separate then and it makes you feel separate now—singled out, different from everyone else, lonely. Those memories and resentments start flooding back with every entry in that darn food diary, with every "no thanks" to your favorite sweets, with every look at the scale.

And these feelings will sabotage your efforts, as they sabotaged Isabel's efforts for many years. Today, however, at age 30, and after several ups and downs, Isabel has successfully lost 50 pounds and is happily at her ideal weight. She is overcoming her childhood resistances to weight loss. She's open to understanding her feelings and wants to make positive changes in her life. This is one of many reasons why I admire her so much. Once we uncovered her childhood resistances, the rest was easy....

At first, Isabel avoided keeping a food diary, even though I asked her to keep it without judgment of any kind and knowing she would receive no criticism from me, and even though she knew studies show keeping a food diary is important for success. She said it made her feel different to pay so much attention to what she was eating. It made her feel bad deep down inside. We discussed her childhood and realized this played a large role in her inability to focus on what she was eating. She had such a negative experience as a child, her automatic response was to avoid and resent the diary. Identifying and facing these feelings completely changed her outlook and her ability to help herself by keeping the diary.

Isabel also had a habit of grabbing snack foods and meals throughout the day, without thinking or planning. I think her love of this kind of eating is related to all the restricting she experienced as a child. Of course, her snack-grabbing and disorganized eating habits also made keeping the diary difficult. But soon, Isabel realized the connection between her ways of eating and her childhood experiences. She was able to understand that she's a different person now, with a new outlook and goals, and that this behavior was undermining what she wanted from her life today.

She realized she needed to become an organized eater in order to beat her weight problem. She began planning better, going to the grocery store once or twice a week to make sure she was stocked up on wholesome tasty foods—including frozen foods—as well as ingredients for recipes she could fix on the weekend and quick meals she could fix at home. Though this didn't have the excitement of eating on a whim, it would be her new grown-up style of eating.

Through the years, Isabel had a hard time regularly exercising because she was never physically active as a child. What's interesting is that every time she stopped exercising she gained weight. So she knew intellectually that regular physical activity would have to become an integral part of her life if she wanted to change her weight. To get herself into the groove and get motivated, she started by working with a trainer and finding exercises that were fun. She even asked her boyfriend to go on walks with her so that they would develop a healthy habit together. Of course, this presented wonderful opportunities to get quality time together and become closer.

Isabel was able to identify the bad eating habits and attitudes formed in childhood that were holding her back. She also appreciates the good habits she formed during those early years. Her family instilled in her a love of all foods—including wholesome fruits, vegetables, and whole grains—which eventually made it easier for her to lose weight. All in all, she has been able to focus on the positive lessons of her childhood, reduce the negative influences, and overcome her weight problem.

Isabel is not alone. Many people have been able to make these wonderful, deeply rewarding changes in their lives. First, identify the habit you know in your heart is preventing your success. Chances are its roots are in childhood. If you find yourself sabotaging goals you have set for yourself, it may help to see your self-destructing behavior as your subconscious communicating. That subconscious often is your childhood anxieties speaking to you, pulling you back to your old fears. Once you discover the basis of those feelings, you can deal with them successfully and conquer them, since they're usually based on irrational feelings and fears which are no longer relevant in your life today.

Jennifer

Jennifer is another client who faced a conflict and transitioned successfully. But only with a very large dose of brave self-reflection.

Jennifer had never been at an ideal weight in her entire life. She'd been overweight as a child and had tried to help herself by dieting a few times during her teen years, but she had always gained the weight back. By the time she was in her twenties she had decided to give up.

Then, at age 34, she came to me for weight-loss counseling. She wanted to give it one last try. This time, using the approaches in this book, she succeeded. She said she loved losing weight this way because it was "easy and somehow 'crept up on me.' It didn't feel like big changes, and since it was mostly self-motivated with choices made by me, it didn't feel like punishment."

Jennifer's job calls for her to travel the world. She's in Paris one week, Hong Kong or Istanbul another. So she lost weight under the most difficult circumstances.

But it wasn't all smooth sailing. At one point she had successfully lost about 60 pounds and had 30 more to go. She came into my office with tears streaming down her face. She said she was "sick of it! Sick of the whole thing...of paying attention to what I'm eating, of having to say no to invitations, of denying myself my favorite foods."

"It's just not fair," she continued. "Everyone else can eat whatever they want or whatever crosses their path." She wanted to "take a break" from losing weight.

Well, needless to say, I was distressed to see her feeling so terrible, and I would have supported any decision she made about her progress. But I also had to ask her to think about where her feelings came from. She remembered that when she was a child her weight problem made her feel different from everyone else. And she admitted that paying attention to her food made her feel different—even today as an adult. It was a very hard feeling to live with.

We discussed the fact that as an adult, she can make decisions to eat anything she wants. But in our rich society, there are consequences to saying yes to every food you're offered.

She also realized from our conversation that she wasn't really so very different from most people. Studies show that more than 6 out of 10 Americans are overweight. That means a majority of people should be "paying attention to" what they eat. Far from being set apart from everyone else, she was actually part of the unhealthy majority!

I wasn't sure where Jennifer was going to end up when she left my office. I was hoping she wouldn't give up, but felt all I could really do was support her in whatever decision she made.

At the next session she surprised me by saying she was more motivated than ever! She spent the week talking to her healthy, fit friends. They confided in her that they don't accept every invitation to eat out, either.

And they make conscious decisions about what they'll eat or not eat. Jennifer realized that feeling apart was a vestige of her childhood and was not based on the reality of her life today. She even came up with this very cute analogy, which she e-mailed me after she left my office:

"I just wanted to thank you for today. It really helped. I have to remember this is like my budget. The universe is grossly unfair in not providing me with unlimited funds (the ability to burn 5,000 calories a day). But this is not fixed by my spending outside my limits (exceeding the calories I burn) and racking up credit card debt. (No, no, I can't go back to plus sizes!) Anyway, I feel much better and quite motivated."

This is another example of how reflecting on your childhood can help you understand why during some vulnerable moments you may actually sabotage your own progress. I wonder what would have happened if we didn't have our talk or if Jennifer wasn't willing to be brave enough to face her feelings and understand the reality of her life today. I'd like to think she would have come to these realizations on her own. I'd also like to think that with a little soul searching, reflection, and honesty with yourself, you will do the same.

CHAPTER 5

Stop the Irrational Monster

Your thoughts and feelings affect your behavior and your success at achieving successful weight loss, or anything in your life. There are a lot of confusing or irrational impulses at work for all of us. Otherwise, how can you explain why we don't always do what's best for us? We're complicated creatures with motivations and impulses we don't always understand. These impulses or feelings, which we may not be conscious of, influence our approach to eating and self-care, among other things. We're all a product of our past and have complex subconscious factors at play which in turn affect our behavior. Many go back to our first days as an infant, others relate to cultural and environmental influences as we were growing up.

In this chapter, I'll explain where your thought patterns come from, how they might be influencing your weight loss success, and how you can harness them and use your reasoning and thinking to help you achieve success—regardless of the environmental or childhood influences you need to overcome.

You can't change your childhood and you can only partially change your environment. Your thinking, on the other hand, is one thing you can consciously seize upon to create a strategy or road map to succeed. It's by controlling and changing thought that you can understand your resistance to essential habits you'll need to develop to be successful.

You may believe your thinking is pretty straightforward. But scientists have been studying thinking since the beginning of civilization. In the twentieth century there were pioneer researchers in the field of "cognition" (thinking) who came up with many compelling theories about how our thinking affects our behavior and how we can change both to lead more fulfilling lives. Many experts believe cognitive therapy is the only therapy most people need; they believe our thought patterns are that significant. In fact, it's largely recognized among obesity experts that cognitive therapy—or learning to change the way you think—is necessary for successful weight loss and maintenance.

Different Thinking, Different Results

Changing the way you think can turn you from a chronic relapser into a successful weight-loss maintainer, because we've seen it happen in major studies. Here are some of the factors that typically separate people who experience weight control success from those who don't.

They face their problems. Studies show that even though both groups, maintainers and relapsers, experience an equal number of negative life events and stressors, relapsers tend to cite those negative life events as reasons behind their regaining weight. The researchers found very specific attitudes and coping strategies separated those who successfully maintained weight loss from those who relapsed. Successful maintainers confronted their problems and dealt with them by using problem-solving skills or stress management techniques. Relapsers, on the other hand, avoided or turned to food in order to forget or escape from their problems.

They set appropriate goals. Weight relapsers set unrealistic weight-loss goals for themselves, which makes them feel unhappy even when they achieve modest improvements. They set themselves up for feelings of failure, which lead to regaining lost weight. Weight-loss maintainers tend to be "patient," make modest goals, are more likely to implement behavioral change, and feel positive about even minor improvements, all of which help them continue and ultimately be successful with their maintenance.

They view themselves more positively. The "self-talk" of weight maintainers and relapsers has been analyzed in many studies. What have we learned? Weight relapsers tend to describe themselves more negatively. They attach their weight to their self-esteem and end up feeling valueless because of their body size. Maintainers, on the other hand, are more likely to be gentle and forgiving of themselves, using phrases to describe themselves such as "out of shape," which is more positive and hopeful, and implies that they need merely to get back into shape.

Stumbling Blocks on the Road to Weight Loss

Understanding and being open to changing the way you think is essential to permanent weight-loss success, according to research and my personal experiences with clients.

A pioneer of cognitive therapy, Aaron Beck, call self-destructive thinking patterns "automatic thoughts" because they're reflexive, they're not usually even noticed, though they are constantly flowing through your mind, and they affect the way you think, feel, and behave. These thoughts create a continual internal dialogue, which the famous researcher and theorist Albert Ellis called "self-talk."

Simply hearing your automatic thoughts is the first step to gaining control over the emotions causing you to resist healthy behavior change. Learning to understand your feelings may seem formidable, but it is doable, and critical for understanding and solving emotional overeating or bingeing.

Take Sarah. She knows that self-monitoring is essential for successful weight loss and maintenance, but she still doesn't keep a food diary or monitor what she eats in any way. Mind you, most people don't enjoy keeping the diary or focusing on every morsel they eat, but they overcome that and do those things anyway. Most grow to realize the importance of keeping a diary and develop a healthy respect for the power of self-monitoring because it works and ultimately is one of the reasons for their success.

Some people, however, can't seem to overcome their dislike enough to do self-monitoring (or physical activity, or any other weight-loss strategy), and unfortunately, they're usually not successful at achieving their goals. So I try to help everyone who has this kind of resistance to do an analysis of how they feel as they keep their food diary to get some clues as to what the resistance could be.

In Sarah's case, she said she just "didn't like it," "it was inconvenient," and she "knew what she was doing." But once we went deeper into how she "felt" keeping a diary, memories of her very unhappy childhood came flooding back. She remembered feeling "left out" by her family members, who wouldn't allow her to eat the same foods they ate. She vividly described being taunted and demeaned by school kids for being fat. These memories had taken root in her unconscious and colored what she was trying to achieve, even though they had nothing to do with her very successful life today. In facing those memories and understanding the roots of her resistance, Sarah was able to begin self-monitoring and solve her weight problem. She realized her feelings were based on irrational fears and beliefs, which were no longer applicable in her life.

Any time you resist making beneficial changes in your life that you think you really want, something deep in your heart or subconscious is probably keeping you from achieving your goals. It's worth it to get to the bottom of it. It helps you grow as a person and get what you want out of life. John, another client who experienced resistance, hated self-monitoring because it made him feel like someone was constantly watching over him, bossing him around. Not paying attention to what he was eating was a form of "rebellion" for him. Rationally, he came to realize that rebellion ended up hurting only himself. After he reminded himself that losing weight was *his* goal—and his alone, since no one was forcing him—he was able to overcome his resistance, self-monitor, and lose weight.

Understand Your Feelings

I was raised to "think positive" and ignore any hurt or negative feelings I might be carrying around. Perhaps you were too. It's not uncommon. Or perhaps you avoid negative feelings simply because they're unpleasant. In either case, you may find that you've been so used to ignoring or escaping from negative or undesirable feelings that you're not even aware that you have them. Instead, you just get this nagging feeling, which you don't quite understand and which may make you want to overeat or binge as an escape from the feeling.

Years ago, the following happened to me: I parked my car in the lot a block away from my office and, feeling very depressed, had an overwhelming desire to run to the corner store, pick up a bag of my favorite cookies, and eat the whole thing. Instead, I stopped and thought about why I had this urge. What was I feeling? I knew I was down in the dumps but didn't quite know the specific reason why. I had just had a disappointing meeting, and deserved to feel let down, but why was I *sooo* low?

Upon further reflection I realized I felt disrespected—humiliated, really—as a result of the other person's behavior in the meeting. And it's true that while the other person wasn't very nice, was insensitive, and I deserved to feel a bit let down, my feeling was an overreaction based on my own personal sensitivities. Who cares if she wasn't nice. I'd never have to see her again! And even if I did, chances are she had a problem that day that had nothing to do with me. She probably had no idea she was rude. In any case, *it didn't really matter!*

As I thought about this, I was able to let go of the cookie temptation. I decided to calmly walk to my office and call a friend instead. I had gotten through the situation unscathed.

Bad Situations Can Lead to Good Choices

People who find themselves in upsetting situations, as I did, tend to react in a very predictable fashion. Only by going off automatic pilot and thinking in new ways can someone hope to cope in a positive way and avoid that bag of cookies. Here's what usually happens:

1. An event occurs. ("I was treated rudely.")
2. You interpret the event. ("I am worthless.")
3. You talk to yourself. ("That jerk!")
4. You get emotional. ("I feel awful.")
5. You decide how to escape. (" I'll get a bag of cookies.")

How do you break the cycle? The secret lies in steps 2 and 3. The way you interpret an event and talk to yourself about it can determine what happens at steps 4 and 5; that is, the way you respond emotionally and what you'll do next.

So how do you change your interpretations? You first have to understand how and why you make interpretations. You make interpretations based on past experiences and beliefs, which are sometimes irrational and can lead to negative self-talk. Psychologist Albert Ellis outlined some typical irrational beliefs:

• You must be loved by everyone, versus *you need to respect yourself.*
• Certain acts are wicked and the people who perform them should be severely punished, versus *certain acts are inappropriate and the people performing them are behaving stupidly.*
• It is horrible when things are not the way you'd like them to be, versus *you need to cope with how things are.*
• Misery is externally caused and forced on you, versus *emotional disturbance is caused by the view you take of conditions.*
• If something is dangerous you must be terribly upset, versus *face what's fearful, render it nondangerous, and if you can't, accept the inevitable.*
• It is easier to avoid than to face life's difficulties, versus *avoiding life's difficulties makes them harder in the long run.*
• You need something other, stronger, or greater than yourself on which to rely, versus *you need to take the risk of thinking and acting independently.*
• You should be thoroughly competent, intelligent, and achieving in all possible respects, versus *you should accept yourself as an imperfect creature.*
• Because something once strongly affected you, it always should, versus *you can learn from your past experiences but not be overly attached to them.*
• You must have perfect control over things, versus *the world is full of chance but you can still enjoy life despite this.*
• Happiness or ideal health and weight can be achieved by inertia and inaction, versus *you are happiest when vitally absorbed in creative pursuits, or when you are devoting yourself to people or projects outside yourself.*

You can clearly see in my story that my initial reaction to the woman's rude behavior was rooted in irrational beliefs: that I had to be loved by everyone—including her; that she was wicked; that it was horrible things did not turn out the way I expected; that I didn't have control over the event; that it was easier to eat cookies than to face the difficulty.

So with all this irrational thinking going on, how on earth was I able to avoid going for the cookies? I was able to stop the behavior because I short-circuited my automatic thinking. Instead of just acting on autopilot, I decided to reinterpret the event ("She was probably having a bad day; she's not so bad"), then changed my self-talk ("Who cares? I'll never have to see her again"), and instead of finding a way to escape, I found a way to cope (I went back to my office to talk with a friend).

Acknowledge and Identify Your Feelings

Jealousy, humiliation, anger, loneliness, and boredom are feelings you'd rather not have, but they are normal emotions and a permanent part of the human condition. There is only one constructive way I know of to deal with these feelings: face them. Once you face how you feel, you'll find a load is lifted from your shoulders.

Who wants to admit to feeling lonely? Shouldn't we all be loved by everyone all the time? Who wants to admit to being angry? Or afraid? Shouldn't we always have perfect control over things? Who wants to admit to feeling embarrassed by a negative incident you caused? Shouldn't you be thoroughly competent, intelligent, and achieving in all possible respects?

Yes, we're back to Albert Ellis. Irrational ideas go hand in hand with denying emotions, and as we've seen before, one prop we often use to help us avoid acknowledging our feelings is food. Ask Douglas.

One afternoon at the office, Douglas was having a very strong sweets craving. Since Douglas knows himself pretty well, he guessed the craving might have something to do with an emotion he wasn't allowing himself to feel. He stopped and thought a minute. That's when he realized that he was upset because his boss was yelling at him.

He then did some reasoning. His true fear was that he would lose his job. This was a fear that was hard to face but was understandable based on past experience. He'd once lost another job because of an angry boss. As he thought about it rationally, however, he realized that he really had nothing to fear in his current situation. His boss was a terrific person and was normally very calm, respectful, and reassuring. It was only around deadline time (now) that her behavior changed. It suddenly dawned on him that she became sharper with everyone during those times, not just with him.

Douglas reminded and reassured himself that her behavior had nothing to do with him personally. Suddenly, his sweets craving disappeared.

Douglas successfully labeled and faced his fear and was then able to reinterpret his feelings and his self-talk to change his behavior and avert a binge.

Change Your Self-Talk

How you talk to yourself has a deep influence on your eating behavior in ways you may not even be aware of, so it's important to pay attention to the dialogue that goes on inside your head. What you choose to say to yourself is influenced by how you've learned to interpret the events around you. The operative word here is *learned*. Since your interpretations of events and your subsequent self-talk are learned, you can also learn *new* ways of interpreting events and talking to yourself.

Once again, this brings us back to the ideas of Albert Ellis. If you base your interpretation of events on irrational thinking, how can your self-talk be anything but irrational and negative? Two ideas in particular seem to plague people with eating problems: The notion that you have to be perfect, and the belief that you need to be loved by everyone.

Being Perfect

Often we make unrealistic promises to ourselves, such as "I'll never eat chocolate again," or "I'm through with junk food," or "I'm going to exercise every day." These belong in the category of "irrational ideas" because they require perfection in our behavior, which is impossible. The fact that you set yourself impossible goals dooms you to failure before you start!

Ellen is a good example. She used to feel so guilty when she "went off her program," that she would completely relapse into old bad habits and gain all of her weight back. Since she left herself no room for even one mistake, she always failed. Fortunately, she has since found that if she allows herself a wonderful dessert or a night out once a week, she is much happier. First, it's a much more realistic goal to say, "I'll do my best to eat healthy most days of the week, but I'll plan a splurge or two and enjoy it." This gave Ellen the flexibility to enjoy herself, not feel guilty, and get right back on the program after her splurge. She was ultimately very successful at losing weight. But it took practice for Ellen to learn not to feel guilty after splurging. The more she successfully went back to healthy eating, the easier it became, the more confidence she felt that she could succeed, and she did.

Remember, life is not black and white. It is mostly a series of gray areas. An all-or-nothing attitude won't get you very far. If you had a flat tire, would you decide you could never drive again, then go ahead and slash the remaining three? That may sound ridiculous, but how is that different from the following statements: "Since I missed exercise this morning, I'm a failure, I can't do it, I might as well give up and not go the rest of the week," or "I had one candy bar. That proves I don't have what it takes. I just blew it. I'm going to throw in the towel."

Instead, what if you said: "If I exercise five out of seven days of the week, I'm a success. Missing one day isn't going to derail my efforts," or "That one candy bar I just ate is not, by itself, enough to make me gain weight. I'll get back on the program immediately."

Needing Love from Everybody

If you find that you're doing things for others that you know will keep you from your own goals, perhaps you believe you must be loved by everyone. If that's the case, self-sabotage may be an issue for you. If you delve deeply enough into your motives, you might find your issue really isn't about meeting the needs of others after all.

Take Rachel, for example. Rachel found it very difficult to cook a light dinner for her and her husband. She was sure he would never accept anything but a huge, soup-to-nuts meal every night. So she continued to make large dinners, which made it difficult for her to control her own intake. Not surprisingly, she couldn't lose weight. When she finally asked her husband what he thought about eating lighter meals, he was happy to make a change. Rachel couldn't believe how easy it was and wondered why it took her so long to ask him. That's when she realized *she* was the one who was hooked on the large, elaborate dinners. It was something leftover from her childhood—the importance of the family gathered around dinner—that she was afraid to change. Of course, what she didn't realize was that eating a heavier or lighter dinner isn't what made the dinner special, it was the people present and the warmth of family conversation.

Elizabeth was another person who seemed to be putting other people's needs in front of her own. She had trouble with her weight every year around Halloween. Why? She wanted to be a great neighbor and give out the best candies to the children. She began planning Halloween weeks ahead of time, which she thought meant buying candy weeks ahead of time. But, inevitably, she was the one who ate the Halloween candy. This happened year after year—as did her subsequent struggles with gaining weight. Elizabeth finally realized she was buying the Halloween candy mostly for herself. It wasn't easy to face that fact as she liked to see herself as a generous person (which she is!). And while it was hard to break the habit the first year after she made that realization, the results—not buying candy until the day of Halloween and giving any leftovers to the last trick-or-treaters—were worth it. No more struggling with uncontrolled eating or weight around Halloween.

In both of these cases, Ellen's and Elizabeth's goals for weight loss were clashing with an inward belief that they weren't quite aware of until, after much failure, they decided to explore. They were sabotaging their own efforts without understanding why.

I believe strongly that you can achieve whatever you want in life. But exploring your feelings to understand how your thinking and feeling may be affecting you is an important step. It's important that you start noticing how you think, what your expectations are, and what kinds of goals you're setting. You can do this by keeping a log of your thoughts and feelings, or talking regularly with a supportive friend or spouse about what's really on your mind. Awareness is the first step. Once you're aware of the way you think, you can begin to change.

Cope Directly with Your Feelings

Coping directly with your feelings is not always easy. Sometimes the thought of drowning your sorrows in a pint of ice cream seems so much simpler than discussing what's really on your mind with your spouse or your boss. Ordering a pizza may seem like a less painful solution than facing your problems of loneliness or boredom.

If you learn to cope directly with your feelings, however, not only will bingeing become a thing of the past, but you will find your life improving in ways you only imagined before. Will it be easy? Of course not! Having a good life, good health, a good weight, all take purposeful work. It's irrational to think that happiness (and ideal health and weight) can be achieved by inertia and inaction. But challenge is a good thing! You are happiest when vitally absorbed in creative pursuits, or when you are devoting yourself to people or projects outside yourself.

Once you have recognized your feelings and allowed yourself to really experience them, it's time to get moving, to do something about them. Here are some suggestions:

When you feel lonely, instead of eating...call a friend or loved one, invite people over for dinner, get a pet, go out for a walk and visit a neighbor. As you make an effort to fill your loneliness and invite people into your life, you'll find your life is full of friends and your loneliness is a thing of the past.

When you feel bored, instead of eating...sign up for a class, join a support group, volunteer for a charity, get involved in your community. If you make an effort to fill your life with creative and interesting pastimes, you'll wonder why you wasted so much time feeling bored.

When you feel angry, instead of eating...think about what is making you angry, and communicate how you feel with your journal, with a supportive friend, or a loved one. As you learn to communicate your feelings, listen to your inner voice nonjudgmentally, hear others, and be heard. You will grow personally and spend more time being happy rather than angry.

When you feel low, instead of eating...cheer yourself up! Do some exercise, listen to your favorite music, browse through some frivolous magazines, read an absorbing novel, call a friend, take the day off, spend more time with your family, or reach out to a professional counselor. As you begin to pull yourself out of the doldrums, you'll realize the effort is worth it.

Stacy is someone who learned firsthand the benefits of getting feelings out into the open. After work one day, Stacy felt so stressed, she wanted to order Chinese take-out and "pig out." But, as luck may have it, she didn't have time because she had to pick up a friend at the airport. During the 45-minute drive home from the airport with her friend, Stacy began talking about her situation at work. As she talked, she began to realize that she felt abused and unappreciated by her boss. Talking about it with her friend was not planned, but lifted a huge burden. When she and her friend got home, they had light dinners and went to bed.

So, you may ask, what happened to the Chinese take-out? When reconstructing what happened in our counseling session, Stacy said talking out her feelings with her friend made her forget about her "pig out."

She said she didn't even realize that she was upset about her boss until she saw her friend's face and the emotions rolled out. Had she not met with her friend, Stacy surmises, she probably would have just felt depressed and "pigged out" without knowing why.

Not only did this talk with her friend help her avoid overeating, it clarified to her how she felt about her boss and her work and that she needed to start looking for another job. She did, and found another one soon after.

As Stacy learned, using food to escape from emotions is not only a temporary way to avoid our emotions, it can keep us from living our life to the fullest.

Resolve Conflicts

Experts say conflicts in life are inevitable. It's not a matter of *if*, but *when* you have them. Success in life is not a matter of how much conflict a person experiences, but how he or she deals with it. For instance, studies show happily married couples have just as much conflict as unhappy or divorced couples, but happily married couples deal with conflict more effectively.

Why? Happy couples are better at communicating feelings, being open to conflicting opinions, and finding solutions without affixing blame. They're also better at "agreeing to disagree" and at coming to compromises. There are whole books written on this subject, so we're barely skimming the surface here.

The experts say what's most important about resolving your conflicts with your spouse, your boss, or your friends is to simply learn the other person's story and then to share your story with him or her, which opens the door to finding a way to satisfy both your needs. It's not always easy, since people are often emotional when they're in conflict. But it can be done without spoiling a relationship if you respect the other person's point of view, share yours, and think like a mediator. That means being able to see that neither of you is right or wrong, you're just different.

Before Mary learned how to deal with conflicts in her life, she would come home from work every evening and go on an eating binge. Through professional guidance, she discovered that her reasons for bingeing had to do with unresolved conflicts with her boss. She decided to take steps to resolve those conflicts, that is, to try to understand her boss better and to express herself better. After a short time, Mary noticed her relationship with her boss improved. They still didn't like each other much, but at least they understood each other better and began respecting each other's points of view. Soon, Mary's bingeing stopped. She realized she had been using the food to escape from her difficult feelings about her boss and her job. She no longer had to escape from the conflict. She faced it and surmounted it.

Reward Yourself For a Job Well Done

Regular, consistently given rewards reinforce a job well done and make your successes repeat themselves.

It's okay to pat yourself on the back when you do something worthwhile that furthers your goal of eating right and getting healthy. You might feel silly saying "You Go, Girl!" or "Way to Go, Buddy!" to yourself when you pass up a plate of brownies, but you deserve it. This form of positive reinforcement works because it ultimately internalizes the value of what you're trying to change or do.

You can even ask a supportive friend or spouse to reward or positively reinforce you. If it makes you feel good for your spouse to notice that you've fixed a wonderfully healthy meal, ask him or her to mention it. If it makes you feel good for your spouse to reward you for going to the gym, tell him or her what you'd like as a reward—a bouquet of flowers? A trip to the masseur? A walk together? Or just a nice comment?

Of course, you don't have to wait for someone else to reward you. Every time you successfully step toward reaching a goal, no matter how small, treat yourself to something nice. It doesn't have to be expensive. It could simply be watching the sunset or allowing yourself a long-distance call to a loved one.

Don't Be Hard on Yourself

Every goal you set for yourself, whether or not you achieve it, gives you an opportunity to learn about yourself. Successes teach us what we need to keep doing, and failures teach us what we need to do differently. It's a win-win situation. But some people have trouble seeing it that way.

Joanna, for example, couldn't see anything positive in her weight-loss efforts. The first things Joanna talked about when she came into my office were all the things that had gone wrong with her weight-loss program during the week since I'd last seen her. "I overate on chocolate," "I couldn't exercise on Tuesday," or "I was stressed this week."

I soon began to realize, however, that even though Joanna focused on what had gone wrong for her, more things had actually gone right. So she overate on chocolate once, but she didn't do that on six out of seven days. So she couldn't exercise on Tuesday, but she exercised every other day but Tuesday. And even though she was stressed this week, she coped beautifully by talking it out with her family. In fact, she largely stuck with the program and lost weight.

As I began pointing out to Joanna all of the things that went right each week, she began to realize that she was doing a pretty good job, and she became proud of herself. You can imagine that this made it easier to keep on doing great stuff!

Whitney's case was different. She could see her positive achievements when they occurred, but she had moments of irrational thinking that undermined her. She had been doing quite well on her program until her son's birthday party, when she had binged on sweets. When reviewing what happened, Whitney recognized she had done a lot of things very well that week, but when she had eaten a piece of cake, she felt so guilty that she had gone ahead and eaten party foods the whole weekend long, so she had no weight loss to report.

In retrospect, Whitney realized irrational thinking was probably responsible for her weekend of bingeing. Instead of just planning on having a piece of birthday cake and enjoying it, she didn't allow any room for mistakes. So after having a piece of cake she felt like she "blew it," and she gave up on her goals for the rest of the week.

The next week, Whitney had another birthday party (she has six children!), and we decided she should definitely enjoy a slice of cake and even splurge for the birthday meal. Since she allowed herself this flexibility, Whitney still lost weight that week.

As you can see, with some close observation and simple analysis of your own behavior, you can spot and change the areas in your thinking that are irrational and lead you away from your weight-loss goals. Once you begin using these tools, you'll be well on your way to thinking yourself thin!

CHAPTER 6

Mind Over the Environment

You may feel at times that your eating is out of control. Perhaps you're at a party and you suddenly realize you've just consumed a meal's worth of very fattening little appetizers. Or you're talking on the phone, standing in your kitchen grabbing snacks from the cabinet and hardly aware you're doing it. Your favorite TV show is on and suddenly you have a big bag of chips in your lap. You're walking through the office and grab M&M's off your secretary's desk or a chocolate bar from the vending machine. You're in a meeting, cookies are offered, and you just can't resist. You're on the way home from work and your car seems to have a mind of its own as you're calling out your order at the fast food drive-through. You do all of these things in part because of your environment.

Your behavior makes you feel depressed or frustrated because you can't figure out why you do what you do and why you don't seem to have "will power." You may already have given up on your weight-management efforts because you don't think you're "disciplined" enough.

I know sometimes it feels as if those of us who want to be trim and healthy are fighting an uphill battle. Well, that isn't just our imagination. We are designed to eat what's available and tons of it. Since the beginning of time, humans have been subjected to regular famines. The people who ate more and stored more body fat were protected. They survived to pass on their genes to generations to come. That means you and me.

The problem is that the tendencies to overeat and store that we've inherited through our genes are backfiring. This is the first time in human history that food has been so abundant—too abundant, some say. Once upon a time, we had to expend lots of energy in hunting or growing and farming our food, but today, with a push of a button or a snap of the fingers you can have the most delicious and fattening food in front of you in a matter of minutes, if not seconds.

To give you some idea of just how much food our culture of abundance provides, consider this: The U.S. agricultural system produces 3,800 calories' worth of food per person per day, which is *double* what most people should be eating. The marketing, availability, flavor, and abundance of all that food, much of it processed and high in calories, make resisting it a challenge for everyone. Hence, the majority of Americans—six out of ten—are overweight or obese.

In order to be in the trim, fit minority, most of us have to think about controlling our eating most of the time, according to researcher James Hill, who has studied thousands of successful weight losers and maintainers for more than a decade through his study called the National Weight Control Registry, which I mentioned earlier in Chapter 1. In fact, all of the most comprehensive studies of people who successfully lose weight and keep it off show that weight management is something you have to be committed to and work toward. It can't be taken for granted. It's a jungle out there. A jungle of edible temptations.

Understand Your Eating Habits

The first challenge you face is identifying the environmental forces at work in your life and seeing how they shape your daily behavior. I have found that even well-intentioned, nutrition-savvy people are overwhelmed by the blizzard of food options that constantly surround them. Eating habits are affected by a wide array of subtle and not-so-subtle influences that work on us 24 hours a day. Among others, these influences include the vending machine down the hall at work, the inviting sign in front of the restaurant around the corner advertising "Buffet Special!" the contents of your refrigerator at home, your enthusiastic mother admonishing, "Eat more, eat more!" and your lack of time to cook healthy foods.

Once you better understand the nutritional minefield out there, see how you are influenced by it, and learn to accept your strengths and weaknesses, you can begin to make changes that will help you feel in control and achieve your goals. It doesn't take "discipline" or "will power" at all. It's simply a matter of knowing thyself. . . and planning accordingly!

I know this from personal experience. I used to work in a medical building in downtown Washington, D. C., and I walked to and from work every day. The problem? There were too many food temptations on the route I took. The solution? I began walking a different route. It may seem simple, but it worked. Some people might think I was weak; that I wasn't able to control myself when I passed by all the bistros and fast food joints—and those people would be right! I was weak. I was often tired and stressed, and it would have felt so great and been so easy to sit down with a drink and a big plate of nachos after work. Or stop in for a double-mocha cappuccino and a raspberry sweet roll in the morning. The temptation was too great for me, I accepted that weakness in myself, and so my solution was to avoid it.

Of course, avoidance isn't always a practical solution. When I moved to Georgetown, a restaurant- and boutique-filled neighborhood in Washington, I found that every time I walked down trendy M Street, I had to stop for an ice cream cone. It was just beyond my control. I swear, the ice cream shop would just jump out at me and say, "come on in and stay a while!" As I thought about why this might be happening, I realized that before I moved Georgetown, I would occasionally come for a visit, and always stopped somewhere to treat myself to an ice cream cone. I had developed a "paired association" between Georgetown and ice cream.

For obvious reasons I knew I had to break this habit. To do so I needed to give the problem some thought, plan ahead, and stack the odds in my favor. Here are some strategies I used that you might find useful:

• **Eat first.** The next time I walked through Georgetown, I ate before going and made sure I wasn't hungry in the least. This, as you may know, is also a good strategy to use before you go shopping for groceries. It'll keep you from buying junk foods on impulse.

• **Bring supplies.** To make the temptation even less overwhelming, I brought along a luscious piece of fruit.

• **Stay out of harm's way.** I decided to visit boutiques or magazine shops instead of restaurants, which would be more inspiring for keeping a slim figure.

These strategies worked for me. I broke my ice cream habit. Was it easy? Not all the time. But the more times I successfully walked through Georgetown without stopping, the better I felt about it, the more positive reinforcement I felt, and the easier it got.

Learning to Take Control

Let's briefly review some of the environmental factors at work in your life, what the experts say, how successful weight losers have conquered their situations, and how you can successfully deal with yours.

A Matter of Taste

Studies show the most accurate predictor of how much of a particular food you'll eat at one sitting is its taste. If something tastes good, you'll eat more of it. At birth, we are naturally drawn to sweets, and by age 4 months, our craving for salty things blossoms as well. Unfortunately, sweet and salty foods tend to be dense in calories, and many of them are fatty. So how do you deal with your built-in preference for them?

Researchers have found that your tastes can change and you can learn to enjoy the flavors in more natural foods. If you surround yourself with more wholesome foods, you'll be more likely to eat them. That is true with children as well as adults. One major study showed it took about 12 weeks for adults to get used to the flavor of lower-fat foods and about 24 weeks to really begin to enjoy them. Interestingly, if they were given fake fats or substitutes, they continued liking fat and the switch was more difficult.

Many successful weight-loss maintainers report that one key to their success was changing their preferences for calorie-dense sweets. A study of maintainers, published in the *American Journal of Clinical Nutrition*, found that "ultimately they did not want to eat as much and that such foods as candy and donuts were no longer appealing because they were too sweet or fatty. They changed their cooking methods to avoid fried foods with extra fat and found themselves able to deemphasize food in their lives."

The important point is that you *can* shape your own food preferences by what you expose yourself to, and this will get easier as you grow, develop, and age. So many of my clients tell me that they begin to appreciate the wonderful flavor of fruits and vegetables when they make an effort to buy beautiful, ripe produce at the grocery store or farmers' market. Of course, it's always ideal to buy directly from the farmer when the food is at peak ripeness and the flavor is most developed.

My client Julie used to grab a candy bar every afternoon—oh, and a sweetened Starbuck's coffee drink every midmorning. Then we analyzed her day and realized the calorie contributions of those sweets was 600 calories daily, which amounts to 1 pound a week! Julie was disappointed at first, but then decided to switch to the natural sweetness of fruit. It's been a few months, but today, she can't imagine eating those sweets on a daily basis again. The most important part is that she is truly enjoying the natural sweetness and flavors of fruit and vegetables. I hear this kind of story from my clients daily.

The key to developing a taste for more wholesome, natural foods such as fruits and vegetables is to surround yourself with them wherever you go—at home, at the office, even in the car. Try new recipes and share them with the people you love. Have wonderful dressings on hand for salads; interesting oils, herbs, and spices for stir-fries. And keep trying new foods. Invite friends over for taste-testing, recipe-testing, or recipe-swapping parties. Get your family involved. I try to keep my own pantry stocked with delicious, healthy foods, and I'm always trying new recipes and pleasing my family and friends with them. There's nothing like sharing good food to inspire a joy for it.

Over time, these are the foods you'll be drawn to for your everyday sustenance and enjoyment. You'll be able to save the sweets for the occasional indulgence and your waistline will be all the smaller for it.

Proximity, Familiarity, and Availability

Science tells us that if there is more food around, our natural tendency is to eat it. And these days there is, to put it mildly, *lots* of food around. The

U.S. Department of Agriculture food surveys show there has been a 500-calorie per person per day increase in available food between 1984 and 2000. That translates to a potential *50-pound weight gain per person per year!* The USDA estimates that the increase comprises 24 percent sugar, 32 percent fat, and 39 percent white flour—the major ingredients in processed high-calorie sweets and snack foods.

Fattening, salty, and sweet foods (remember, the kind we're designed to crave and go for?) saturate our environment. Would you ever have imagined 20 years ago that today every gas station would carry dough-nuts, chips, and pizza? Or that you would have entire floors in your local mall dedicated to food stalls? There's cheap food for sale everywhere and people are grabbing it and eating it everywhere: in cars, while skating or walking down the streets, while shopping, on subways and buses. You can't even watch a movie without hearing the constant crackling of candy wrappers and the "chomp" of popcorn eaters.

Eating in all of these places can lead to changes in your dining habits and associations between food and locations before you even realize it. Remember how I always paired Georgetown and ice cream? A classic Russian study done by a scientist named Pavlov long ago demonstrated how this happens. He had a group of dogs which he fed regularly, and every time he fed them, he would ring a bell. After a while, the dogs got so accustomed to the bell and eating that just hearing the bell would make them salivate. They had developed a "paired association" between being fed and the bell.

We humans are not much different from Pavlov's dogs. If you regularly eat in front of the television, for instance, you may have developed a "paired association" between eating and the TV. If you routinely consume snacks at your desk, you've probably developed a paired association between your desk and snacking. A client of mine, Rachel, once said that every time she sat down to do bills, she got hungry. After further questioning I found that she was doing her bills at her dining room table. And, naturally, there's a paired association between your dining room and eating. Another client, Mike, said that every time he had a stiff deadline, he'd sit in front of his computer with a giant bag of candies. He paired deadline with candies! And he had a daily deadline! Ouch.

So, if you're like many Americans and you eat while you're distracted with doing other things or in places other than a normal "eating place," such as a dining or kitchen table, you may have developed paired associations with eating and many things in your environment. If that's the case, you're at a disadvantage. Your environment, rather than your natural hunger, is controlling when you eat.

Another client, Marcus, realized that his biggest downfall was stopping at a fast food joint on the way home from work and downing a fatty, high-calorie meal. He determined if he could change this habit, he would have his weight problem licked. But the drive home was so tempting, the tasty, fattening food so easily available, it wasn't easy. That is, until he started stocking up on delicious foods so that his refrigerator was nice and full. Once he made this simple change—to stock his refrigerator with easy-to-fix dinner fixings, or to make flavorful batch recipes—it was easy to get all the way home without stopping. The thought of that homemade veal stew waiting for him at home made it easy. So while Marcus couldn't change his route on the way home, he could change his environment in a simple—but quite significant—way, so he could lose the weight, and lower his high cholesterol and blood glucose, to boot!

Obviously, one way to naturally reduce food consumption is to control where you eat. To achieve that, both Rachel and Mike changed the location and activity related to their eating. Rachel decided it would be more helpful not to get an urge to eat every time she sat down to do bills, so she started doing bills at her desk. Mike realized if he was stressed before a deadline, he probably needed to do something to deal with that stress more effectively, so he began deep breathing to help him relax and it worked for him. He no longer ran to grab a bag of candy at deadline time.

One of the differences between Europeans and Americans that may partly explain why Europeans are slimmer is that in France or Italy or Sweden there are set times and places for eating. You don't have food joints on every corner open all the time. People aren't eating while walking down the street or talking on the phone. They're taking time for and savoring their meals. In Europe, most establishments are simply open for lunch and dinner. Period. The food in Europe is also still relatively local and seasonal. That means it's less processed or less highly flavored with salt and sugar. Since the food is in a more natural form, and isn't constantly available, there's less temptation and less partaking.

But we're Americans, and we eat on the go all the time. Sometimes it's just unavoidable. In that case, it's important to have wholesome foods with you wherever you go. If you're driving to the beach, pack them in your car. If you're visiting mom for the holidays, bring baskets of fruit as a gift. Make sure they're high quality, ripe, and delicious, and that you have enough on hand. If you plan to eat three fruits a day, you'll need 21 pieces of fruit for the week—and that's just for you! So plan in advance.

I also recommend that you make things easier on yourself by keeping "difficult" foods out of your house or office or anywhere you spend a lot of time (and for many of us that includes our car!). It's important to remind yourself that you're not shunning sweets because of any moral failure on your part. During the holidays, Beverly found that if she gave away her fattening leftovers from Thanksgiving, she wasn't tempted to eat a Thanksgiving feast day after day after day. In the past, that's what she'd done and gained 5 pounds in a single week. This year, she decided to do things differently. After she enjoyed her Thanksgiving meal, she kept the turkey, made a wonderful turkey soup and turkey sandwiches for several days. She kept the salad and the vegetables. But she gave away the cheese and crackers, the stuffing, the mashed potatoes, the pie, and the ice cream. This way, she enjoyed Thanksgiving day to the fullest, but didn't have to suffer the negative consequences when it was over.

Studies have made it very clear that we humans have a natural tendency to be attracted to fattening foods. So why put yourself through that torture? Learn your strengths and weaknesses, accept them, and stack things up in your favor.

Potent Portion Sizes

Studies show that a major factor that influences how much you eat is simply how much you're served. If you're given a larger amount, you eat a larger amount. If you're served a smaller amount, you eat it and are satisfied.

At age 3 years, portion size won't affect a child. Infants and toddlers still seem to be pretty good at regulating energy intake based on internal feedback. They will eat only until they're satisfied and then stop. But by the age of 5, when given larger portions, they will eat more, even if they're no longer hungry. The older we get, the more easily our behavior is influenced by our environment. In one study, lean young men, who are usually good at regulating their food intake, were given two different portions of macaroni and cheese: 16 ounces and 25 ounces. When they were given 16 ounces, they ate 10 and said they were satisfied. But when they were given 25 ounces, they ate 15. Just because they were given more, they ate 50 percent more calories!

While studies show clearly that to lose weight, you have to take in fewer calories than you burn, the American public seems confused about how serving sizes may influence their weight. In a survey conducted for the American Institute for Cancer Research, 78 percent of adults said just the opposite: that eating certain types of food is more important than eating less food when trying to lose weight. In the same survey, only 1 percent of the respondents answered questions about serving sizes correctly.

It's no surprise. People have no real point of reference, what with "supersize" offerings in every restaurant. In 40 years we've gone from an average 6-ounce serving of Coke (under 100 calories) to the 62-ounce "Big Gulp" (600+ calories). In the 1950s, a fast food hamburger contained about 210 calories. Today, an "extra value" or "supersize" meal will contain 1,300 to 1,500 calories. And have you ever noticed that today's restaurants don't use normal-sized plates? Everyone gets their own huge platter, and they've come to expect it. Otherwise they don't feel they're getting good value for their money. Based on research conducted by the Center for Science in the Public Interest, the average restaurant meal contains about 1,000 calories. And it's not unusual to be faced with 1,500 in one entree. In one popular chain restaurant, a single slice of most of their cakes weighs in at a whopping 1,500 calories! For a single slice!

Not only have meal sizes increased, but snack sizes have, too. You used to be able to buy a small, 1-ounce bag of potato chips—about 150 calories. But today's "small bags," if you look closely, contain 2 ounces and will contain two servings, for about 300 calories. When you compare that against a piece of fruit, the preferred snack of the old days, that's a 240-calorie difference. A new study confirms that Americans are eating more snack foods and it's taking up a larger percentage of their daily intake. Twenty years ago, snacks were about 11 percent of our diet. In 1996, that figure soared to 18 percent. Americans are eating double the amount of high-calorie, processed snack foods than they ate just 20 years ago.

You may think these numbers are small. But an increase in just 100 calories a day produces a weight gain of 10 pounds in a year. If you compare that to the increase in serving sizes everywhere, and at every meal and snack, you can see why the fattening of America has been so swift.

When my clients visit malls, I recommend they avoid the food court entirely. It's best to think ahead of time about what you want for lunch, and then eat before going, come back home to eat, or plan ahead which restaurant you'll visit where you can order something healthy. Best not to get swayed at the last minute by the aromas and visuals.

Make your plan ahead of time and stick with it. At the gas station, don't go into the convenience store with all the pizza, hot dogs, cookies, candies, and chips. If you're on a long trip, pack a cooler with a beautiful lunch of leftover grilled chicken, sandwiches, and fruit. You'll enjoy it so much more and won't be sorry later.

In your favorite restaurant, to avoid eating the huge portions, try ordering an appetizer instead. My client, Debra, does it all the time and says she's completely satisfied. Or share your main course or ask the waiter to wrap half for you to take home. (See Chapter 16: Restaurant Eating Without the Bulge, for lots more tips on dining out.)

Your Life on the Run

Have you ever heard someone joke that when you eat standing up or when you're driving, the calories don't count? Well, believe it or not, that's half true. The calories don't count in your brain, but they count toward your expanding waistline.

In today's culture, people are mindlessly eating everywhere: walking down the street, in-line skating down the street, driving in their car, riding the roller coaster, while working in front of their computer, watching TV and videos. When you eat without paying attention, without sitting down and enjoying your meal, you run the risk of wanting more. And we all know where that leads, since there's no escape from available delicious food.

When you're on the run, you may think you're eating less, but you may actually be consuming more. Why? Because the tendency is to eat more stuff from the vending machine, the fast food joint, or the kiosk on the sidewalk or at the train station, and all that junk food is loaded with calories.

You're also likely to eat in restaurants more. USDA food surveys show that restaurant eating accounts for 34 percent of the calories consumed by the average person. Now, think about that for a moment. What is your restaurateur's priority? Is it serving you healthy meals so you don't feel full when you leave or so that you can live a long and healthy life? *I don't think so!* Restaurant meals are designed to be over-the-top delicious and saturated with tons of high-calorie fat so you'll come back for more. Going to restaurants more simply means you're eating more calories (unless, of course, you're following my *Think Yourself Thin* restaurant tips!).

Time is another crucial element in making food choices. How our time is allocated between work and home can be a driving force in deciding whether to eat convenience foods, snack foods, or healthy foods, and whether you actually sit down to eat or skip regular meals—especially breakfast. The incidence of skipping breakfast in the United States has increased from 14 percent to 25 percent between 1965 and 1991. Today, more Americans are routinely skipping breakfast than ever before.

Why do I mention breakfast? Seventy-eight percent of NWCR subjects, people who have lost an average of 72 pounds and have kept it off for an average of 6 years, report regularly eating breakfast every day of the week. Breakfast eaters also reported more physical activity than non–breakfast eaters. Eating breakfast is a characteristic common to successful weight-loss maintainers and may be a factor in their success.

That's because someone who eats breakfast regularly has a more adequate micronutrient intake and gets a smaller percentage of their calories from fat. These findings are more striking for those individuals whose breakfast includes a ready-to-eat cereal. Studies also show that breakfast skippers eat more calorie-dense food later in the day.

Skipping breakfast affects teens' weight, too. Nutrition researchers studying teens have found a definite relationship between regular breakfast eating and one's body mass index (BMI). The majority of thinner girls (60 percent) eat breakfast. As breakfast eating declines, the BMI increases, so that most of the heavier girls, nearly 80 percent, are failing to eat breakfast regularly.

Frances, a very busy local TV reporter, worked very difficult hours and never seemed to have time to eat. Yet she was overweight and wanted to lose 30 pounds. We made two changes to Frances's life and she lost her weight handily. First, we added breakfast. Since she was rushing out the door at 4 A.M., we came up with a very simple to-go breakfast that fit her lifestyle perfectly. It was a peanut butter sandwich, yogurt, and fruit. She loved it. Everyone at her TV station loved it, tried it, and lost weight, too! Adding the breakfast helped Frances get through her day without cravings. The second thing Frances did was start gourmet batch cooking. Traveling around in her TV van left eating too much up to chance and she didn't have time to cook during the week. So on the weekends, Frances would make two or three batch recipes, say a pasta dish and chicken dish. She brought a little cooler in the van with her stash and had delicious lunches every day. (So did the TV crew, by the way, who got so hooked on her meals that she finally had to show them how to cook them themselves.) Frances protected herself from being in a position where the only choices would be between fast food and fattening food. Frances lost the weight she wanted to, and is now with a national network.

Mass Media

Studies have found that the prevalence of obesity is directly related to all the television viewing we do. Watching TV represents both inactivity and altered patterns of food consumption. Just being so sedentary carries health risks, of course, but what's worse, the more you sit and stare at that box, the more likely you are to consume foods advertised on TV, which in turn are likely to be loaded with calories. The mass media may provide us with a view to another world and give us a broader culture, but they don't offer us a very healthy picture of the food that we could or should eat. In one study, researchers created a food pyramid based on the food products shown on Saturday morning television commercials. The picture wasn't pretty unless you think sweets, fast foods, and snacks should make up a person's diet.

Watching TV has another, far more subtle effect on weight control. On one hand it exposes us to all kinds of messages that tell us to eat tons of delicious high-fat, high-sugar, high-calorie food. But at the same time it puts us under the pressure of a cultural obsession with thinness. This disconnect encourages restrictive deprivation diets, which studies show lead down two very different, but equally unhealthy paths: either weight regain, usually within six months, or dangerous eating disorders.

I've decided to keep television mostly out of my life. I keep it in a separate room on a different floor from the kitchen, dining room, and bedroom. This way, I watch only when there's something specific on that we want to see. And while not always easy, I keep food entirely separate from the television. Even if the news is on and I'm hungry, I'll do one or the other. After dinner, lights go out in the kitchen and that's it for the night.

Social and Family Influences

As we've said, being surrounded by food temptations can have a huge impact on the way you eat, but so can being surrounded by people. One study found that overeating was associated with, among other things, dining with friends, at restaurants and at social events; being very hungry; and having a negative mood. It might sound like these are only occasional situations, but they can set up repetitive patterns. If overeating occurred at the previous meal, say, in a restaurant or out socializing, you are more likely to repeat the overeating, especially if you're in a negative mood.

Now, I'm not saying you have to move to a mountaintop and become a hermit. In fact, if you surround yourself with people who support your efforts at being healthy, or value being healthy and fit themselves, you're more likely to be successful, and not having that kind of support can make you feel pretty discouraged. Remember my client, Jennifer, who almost gave up on her weight-loss goals (after losing 60 pounds) because she felt all alone in her efforts and sacrifices? During the next week when she spoke with healthy, fit friends, she found she wasn't alone at all. They were making the same efforts and sacrifices, they just weren't vocal about it. That discovery helped Jennifer continue in her efforts.

So, if all of your friends are overweight, socialize by going out to restaurants, and don't make an effort to be healthy or fit, you may be facing a challenge, but if they're people who have goals similar to yours and support your efforts, they can be of tremendous help to you. My recommendation is to change your social circle and make new, healthy, fit friends. They're not difficult to find. Just sign up for dance classes, hiking trips, exercise classes, healthy cooking classes, or even seminars at the local university.

As we've seen, the people, places, and things in your world can have a profound effect on the way you eat, but you can have as much an influence on that world as it has on you. It's all a matter of choices. A few simple changes in the way you arrange and think about your environment can pay huge dividends in terms of weight control.

Of course, there's one environmental factor we haven't yet looked at, and it's probably the most important one of all: your family. In the next chapter, we'll see how those people who are nearest and dearest to you can all work together toward a goal of healthful eating for a healthy weight and body.

CHAPTER 7

The New Family Eating Plan

With strong emotional and practical support from our families, it is possible for all of us to live in a balanced, nutritionally sound and healthful way. But without that support—given the temptations and pressures of our culture of abundance—it may be close to impossible to do so. It only makes good sense to view the family environment you create as a very powerful force that can foster powerful early habits, shape daily routines, and mold lifelong expectations.

America's Overweight Families

Let's start out with this simple fact: More Americans are overweight than aren't. Don't believe it? Take a trip to the mall or scan the audience at a movie, concert or sporting event. What do you see? Most recent studies indicate that six out of ten adults are overweight or obese. But what is even more alarming is that the young are following in our footsteps. Nearly a quarter of all children are either overweight or obese, and the number is growing. In fact, since 1968 it has doubled.

While some health care professionals continue to quibble about exactly what constitutes an overweight child, most experts agree that children above the 85th percentile for their age are overweight and those above the 95th percentile are obese. Teens and adults with a body mass index above 25 are overweight, and those whose body mass index is above 30 are obese.

Overweight and obesity affects children of all races and economic backgrounds. However, a disproportionate number of these children come either from low-income Caucasian families, or from all income levels of African American, Mexican American, and Native American families.

Although genetic factors play a role in obesity development, researchers are skeptical that this explains the current problem. They say the environment accentuates genetic predispositions toward weight gain. This makes sense. Since genetics have not altered over the past several centuries, the environment has played the largest role in increasing the rate of obesity among both children and adults.

The problem does not end with childhood. Kids may not grow out of it. Seventy percent of overweight children between the ages of 10 and 13 will become overweight adults. And there will be a steep price to pay. A recent study showed obesity can raise a person's health care costs by as much as 35 percent and medication costs by 75 percent. Obesity exacts a higher toll than smoking or drinking. In fact, obese white men and women can lose 13 and 8 years of life, respectively, and obese black men and women can lose 20 and 5 years, respectively, according to a study recently reported in the *Journal of the American Medical Association*. The years of lost life were higher when the obesity was experienced as a young adult, ages 20 to 30.

Unfortunately, kids don't have to wait for adulthood to experience the same obesity-related health problems as their parents. Type II diabetes, for instance, which is normally diagnosed in overweight, sedentary adults, is becoming increasingly evident in children. A study of children aged 19 and under in Cincinnati showed that prior to 1982, 4 percent of all cases of diabetes diagnosed were type II or non–insulin-dependent. However, by 1996, that rate jumped to 16 percent, a tenfold increase in a little over 10 years. Obesity and inactivity were major risk factors for this diagnosis in children, which occurred at a mean body mass index of 37 (higher than 25 is overweight).

Overweight children are not immune from other adult diseases either. They often show adult-like cardiovascular risk factors, such as elevated triglycerides and LDL cholesterol, along with lowered HDL cholesterol.

These children also suffer from higher rates of hypertension, sleep apnea, liver and gallbladder disease, and even orthopedic complications such as Blount disease, which is characterized by bowed legs.

To make matters worse, experts believe that the social consequences of childhood obesity are just as serious as the physical. Obese children become targets of early and systematic discrimination. By the time they are in their teens, a negative self-image has developed, and increased behavioral and learning difficulties appear, according to Dr. William Dietz from the National Center for Chronic Disease Prevention and Health Promotion of the Centers for Disease Control and Prevention.

The National Longitudinal Survey of Youth, designed to examine the effects of obesity in adolescence on social achievement in early adulthood, found women who were obese in late adolescence and early adulthood achieved fewer years of advanced education, had lower family incomes, lower rates of marriage, and higher rates of poverty. These effects were found only in women, even when controlled for the income and education of the family of origin.

The Hurdles to Good Health

The factors that most influence a child's weight are the parenting the youngster receives and the family environment in which he or she develops. For many reasons, today's parents are less able or available to provide effective nutritional guidance. Often parents are struggling to deal with increased economic pressures. Many households are headed by single women. Or if there are two parents, they both work and have less time to guide their children's lifestyles.

The children end up fending for themselves where food is concerned. Television becomes the child care provider, and a poor one at that. Studies show TV is hazardous to a child's health. Based on a government study of over 4,000 children, obesity rates increased with the hours of TV watching. Rates were highest among children watching 4 or more hours of TV and lowest among children watching less than 1 hour per day. In a recent study, obesity was highest in children who had TVs in their bedrooms. They also watched the tube for the most hours.

A number of factors can explain these findings. The researchers found that calorie intake increased as hours of TV went up—by about 175 calories for children watching 5 hours or more. So now you have a triple-whammy: TV watching being the most sedentary thing you can do (besides sleep) compounded by eating more and exercising less.

Television isn't the only culprit, of course. These days, many families rarely eat meals together, which means children are often left to graze on high-calorie snack foods all afternoon while skipping family dinners and breakfasts—a key risk factor for obesity in children. Remember: Nearly 80 percent of heavier teenage girls fail to eat breakfast regularly, while slimmer girls make a habit of having a morning meal. That's a real shame because studies show clearly that when families prepare and eat meals together, the nutritional quality of those meals is superior.

Of course, grazing on snack foods around the house isn't the only problem. Many of our meals are prepared for us outside of the home, and again, these meals tend to be high in calories and low in nutritive value. Today, take-out food accounts for over 30 percent of a family's food expenditures on a daily, weekly, or annual basis, across all spectrums of socioeconomic class. In fact, fast food restaurants are the most frequent source of food outside the home for teenage boys. They're about even with the school cafeteria for girls.

The Power of Parenthood

Very early in life, children begin to learn about eating habits and foods. The family provides most of the information processed by the child concerning what to eat, the proper time to eat, and when to stop eating. Problems occur when parents give faulty signals, often inadvertently, possibly because they have eating and weight problems of their own, which creates eating and weight problems in their children.

Parents—typically mothers—provide the structure, choose the food, and reinforce certain eating practices through reinforcement and modeling. Their dieting and weight-control experience influences children in ways they may not even be aware of. Parents who eat in response to the external cues, such as the mere presence of tasty foods, often have children who mimic their behavior and end up overeating and overweight. One study has even shown that obese mothers and children eat larger quantities of food in less time than do their thinner counterparts; in other words, they eat faster. Why? The child may simply observe the parent and absorb those lessons. Or he or she might have a genetic predisposition to this behavior, increasing susceptibility to overeating in response to environmental factors—for instance, the presence of tasty foods or the discomfort of strong emotions.

Overeating is not the only behavior children imitate. If they see you dieting, they'll do that too, which at worst can be dangerous for them and at best will affect their weight and eating habits in a negative way. These behaviors start as early as preschool. Researchers recently discovered that 50 percent of 5-year-old girls know what dieting is. And when the scientists look further, they find it's easy to predict which girls are diet-savvy: they're the ones with mothers who are dieting.

Even when their kids don't imitate their eating patterns, parents who have weight problems often try to control or restrict their children's food intake inappropriately. It's ironic, because the very problem these parents are trying to prevent, they actually foster because of their overcontrol, which limits the child's natural abilities for self-control.

When a parent tries to control intake by restricting a food that is available in the home, the food becomes more desirable to a child and can cause her to binge. Next come feelings of remorse and reinforcement of a negative self-image. And even if the strategy works in the short term, having too much control over a child's eating prevents her from being able to appropriately self-regulate.

The ability to self-regulate is extremely important in developing good eating habits. How you reinforce your children can undermine this ability. Encouraging them to "clean the plate," to eat at certain times that don't correspond to their hunger, to eat in response to feelings and emotions, or to expect rewards of sweets and tasty food can habituate them to ignoring the signals of their own body. And remember, you reinforce with your behavior more than with your words. Studies show heavier parents were more likely to exhibit eating unrelated to hunger—in response to the mere presence of tasty foods or emotional factors, and children of these parents tend to exhibit the same eating patterns and to be more overweight.

Studies also demonstrate the strong influence of modeling on food choices. If parents don't eat vegetables, children don't. If parent don't drink milk and drink sodas instead, children replace milk with sodas. Even if parents try to encourage their children to eat healthier than they do, children do not respond by eating healthfully, unless their parents begin to follow their own advice. The children rebel against advice that isn't demonstrated by action. In fact, soda-drinking mothers who encourage their children to drink milk instead of soda have children who drink the most soda.

The Teen Challenge

As children move into their teenage years, parental sway over their behavior diminishes and they are more deeply influenced by peers and broader societal factors. Unfortunately the cultural environment reinforces over-consumption of calorie-dense foods, snacks, and sodas, and doesn't encourage physical activity among adolescents. Even the schools to whom we entrust our children for 6 hours every day rely on selling high-calorie snacks, sweets, and sodas to increase revenues. Teens go the cafeteria and choose from menu options such as calorie-dense burgers, pizza, and fries, all of which compete with the healthful school lunch.

As mentioned in earlier chapters, we all have a natural attraction to tasty, sweet or salty, calorie-dense foods. So when they're around constantly, they're very challenging to resist, especially for kids, who rely on adults to provide healthier choices. Studies today find that children, left to their own devices, will choose calorie-dense, fatty, salty, or sweet foods over nutritious foods, or they'll choose food that is familiar to them. This contradicts earlier research, which suggested children will naturally make healthful decisions on their own. The early study's flaw: all the food the children had to choose from was healthful. If all you provide is healthful food choices, your child will eat healthfully while in your care, and that's what matters most.

In the past 20 years, teens' milk consumption has decreased while soda consumption has increased. Two-thirds of teenage boys are drinking three sodas per day, with two-thirds of girls drinking two sodas per day, according to the USDA. Studies have shown a link between soft drink consumption and obesity in teenagers. And when children drink sodas instead of milk, their bone health is at risk, as the teen years are the most important time for building bones.

As was mentioned before, portion sizes in general have gotten bigger. Yet, with all this "food" around, children are not meeting their daily nutritional requirements. A study reported in the journal *Pediatrics* looking at the food intake of several thousand American youths found that only 1 percent of children meet all dietary guidelines for complete nutrition. Sixteen percent weren't meeting any of them and about half were meeting none or only one. They also found that 45 percent of children's total calorie intake consisted of excess fat and sugar.

According to the USDA, among the 75 percent of kids who say they eat at least one vegetable a day, the most popular vegetable is a potato, usually in the form of a potato chip or a french fry. Next comes tomatoes. When you get to the most nutritious vegetables, such as the dark greens, less than 7 percent of kids touch them.

The Role of Exercise

The overconsumption of food, particularly calorie-dense, nutrient-poor foods, is only a part of the story. Half of all U.S. high school students do not meet basic exercise needs, according to the 1997 Youth Risk Behavior Surveillance study administered by the Centers for Disease Control and Prevention. It also found that substantially fewer girls exercised on a regular basis. Black girls exercised even less than their white counterparts.

The report goes on to say that children have a natural need for more daily physical activity than adults. Elementary school children should be encouraged to accumulate more than 60 minutes and up to several hours a day of age- and developmentally appropriate activity. For adolescents, the guidelines are similar to those for adults. The report recommends that per week, adolescents engage in three or more 20-minute sessions of activities that require moderate to vigorous levels of exertion.

The report emphasizes the importance of variety and that the majority of activity should be in the form of play that is intermittent in nature. It adds that "extended periods of inactivity are inappropriate for children."

Developing Healthful Food Preferences in Children

One of my most vivid memories from childhood is the taste of my grandmother's vine-ripened tomatoes. Every year, she would grow at least 20 tomato plants—and only tomatoes—in her backyard in Columbus, Ohio. They were her favorite vegetable, and became mine too. I'll never forget how soft, plump, sweet, and deep red they were. They were the kind you picked and ate, still warm from the day's sun.

My mother grew a variety of vegetables and herbs in our backyard garden, too. This early exposure gave me an appreciation for fresh vegetables, and how delicious they were when they were perfectly ripe and freshly picked from the garden.

Most children will grow to love vegetables. But for most, they are an acquired taste. Studies show that children avoid new foods—they have "food neophobia"—unless the foods are sweet or salty—which is the preference of all infants until aged 6 months. After 6 months of age, food preferences are learned mainly via the child's experiences with food and eating. Therefore, early experience and learning can reduce the fear of new foods and create a love for wholesome foods like vegetables, which are so important for their health and weight, now and in the future.

In a study of 4- to 6-month-old infants, when mothers introduced a new fruit or vegetable it only took one feeding to increase the infant's acceptance of that food, and the acceptance was generalized to other similar foods. If an infant had experience with one vegetable, other vegetables were more readily eaten.

As a child gets older, it may take more exposures for a new food to be accepted. In one study, when children ages 2 to 5 years were given opportunities to taste a new food, they took between five and ten exposures to start showing an increased preference. Repeated opportunities to smell and look at new food tended to increase acceptance. Children's dislike of certain vegetables began to change when they had opportunities to observe peers and parents selecting, eating, and enjoying those vegetables. But it may take up to twenty exposures to the foods for a child to actually come to prefer them.

By the way, saying something is "good for you" is doomed to fail. Children (and adults, too) have to be convinced the food is going to taste good before they'll try it. What works is positively and consistently offerings foods which you, the parent, are obviously enjoying as well.

To Help Your Child, Help Yourself

My mother's weight and eating problems led to my having the same problems, and studies verify that this is a common outcome. The likelihood of your child being overweight is higher if you are overweight. But we also know there are ways to counteract this effect.

Since your goal is to help your child avoid your eating and weight problems, start by avoiding rigid dieting or complaining about your body in front of your child. Your approach should be first to work on yourself by learning new, healthful eating and physical activity habits that are designed to be a natural part of your life, last a lifetime, and are healthful enough for your whole family to adopt along with you.

Teaching Your Children to Listen to Their Body Signals

We know that children, if given a large range of healthful foods to choose from, have the natural ability to self-regulate the amount of food and calories eaten. They can do this in the short term during a meal, but also in the long term. They can naturally adjust what they're eating over a 24-hour period, depending on the caloric density of what they've consumed.

At age 3, children naturally eat what their bodies need. No more, no less. But by the age of 5, according to studies, children will begin to respond to environmental cues to eat rather than their internal cue of hunger. I've spent plenty of time talking about how that can go wrong. But it can go right, too. You can help your child keep his natural inclination to eat in accordance with his body signals and his body's needs.

A study recently published in the journal *Pediatrics* showed that even when parents are overweight and overeat and their children are already beginning to mimic the problem, the kids can learn how to stop overeating by learning to pay attention to signals from their own bodies.

The children in the study who ate when they were not hungry were found to have parents who were overweight and reported overeating—that is, eating when not hungry, as a result of emotions, or simply because of the presence of tasty foods. Through 6 weeks of one-on-one teaching, these children learned to stop eating when they weren't hungry. Through skits, the children were taught about hunger (rumbling in the stomach), eating to fullness (stomach extension, satisfaction), and the signals associated with overeating (stomach distension and discomfort). They watched the video "Winnie the Pooh and the Honey Jar." Next, the researchers used doll play to teach about hunger and fullness. The dolls had stomachs that contained varying degrees of salt to represent 1) a stomach that was empty, 2) a stomach that was a little full, and 3) a stomach that was very full. When the children ate, they were asked to choose the doll stomach that was closest to how their stomachs felt. This was done several times after the children ate their daily snacks to assess how they felt.

The study found that the children who were unable to appropriately adjust their calorie intake before the intervention were successfully able to do so after the 6 weeks of lessons. The lessons successfully overcame the effect of the parent's eating style and weight status.

What to Do When a Child Is Overweight

Whether or not a child's parents are overweight, there are certain approaches you should *never* take with an overweight child. Never put your child on a diet, never tell him he is overweight, never restrict his access to any foods in your house. Don't single him out or treat him differently than anyone else in your family. These reactions backfire and make what may be a temporary phase of chubbiness a serious weight problem.

The solution to your child's weight problem is to make subtle changes your child won't notice: change *your* eating habits (even thin people can benefit by making more healthful choices), slowly change what's available in the home so that only healthful food is around (except for the occasional Sunday night dessert offered to everyone), and make eating a positive experience. For a child to lose weight, he or she must have the entire family's participation; everyone needs to change a little bit and there have to be some compromises.

It's important to help your children at as early an age as possible, since obesity in children as young as 3 can be an important predictor of a lifelong problem. Your efforts will be most effective if started while your child is still in preschool, as that's the time when children are learning many other good health and safety habits, such as wearing seat belts, putting on sunscreen, and washing their hands.

But regardless of age, working with any child can be successful. Studies have found that children who change their eating habits and achieve healthful weight are more likely to achieve permanent results than adults. So odds are your loving intervention will prove fruitful. And studies show it's easier than you might imagine.

My client Lisa was thinking about sending her overweight child to a nutritionist because his pediatrician said he was overweight. I suggested she wait to see what happened after she changed her own eating habits. Lisa was overweight herself and she loved to cook; she particularly loved to bake sweets for herself and her children. Every day it seemed, there was some sort of fresh baked good around the house in which she and her children would regularly partake. Lisa and I realized she needed to eat more fruits and vegetables and fewer sweets if she and her son were going to be successful at weight loss. So she began slowly integrating more fruits and vegetables into the whole family's life.

So instead of only baking together, she and the children would have fun making fruit salads and vegetables and dip. They found creative and delicious ways to eat fruit and vegetables—dipped in peanut butter, rolled in Rice Krispies. Before you know it, the children were eating and preferring more fruits and vegetables. They didn't seem to miss the sweets at all. It may seem simple, but the problem was solved. Her son never had to go on a diet.

Where Setting Limits on Food Is Appropriate

Never bring foods home that have to be restricted or limited. Not only is it cruel to tell a child he can't eat foods he sees other people enjoying, it's counterproductive (and something he'll never forget as long as he lives). Studies show very clearly that when foods are restricted but the child knows they're in the house or in the environment, it creates a situation where that restricted food is desired above all others. Children will actually binge on those foods when they're finally given the chance to eat them—if they sneak them when no one's looking, or if they're at school or a friend's house and the food is available in unlimited quantities.

I recommend limiting restaurant and take-out meals because of their huge portions and excess fat and calories. You can also limit the spending money children bring to school with them. After all, how much money does a child need to bring to school?

Give incentives to your children by teaching them how much money they can save and what they can buy with it. If they don't spend their money on fast food, they can have a lot of money left over each month to buy more desirable things. If the child does choose a fast food lunch one day per week, lighten up the dinner meal that evening as a compromise. He'll probably be feeling less hungry anyway.

Physical Activity

It's up to families and caregivers to encourage children to be physically active. Most children are very receptive to going on walks, hiking or swimming, or simply shooting some hoops with Mom or Dad. With strong family connections, these activities are more likely to be perceived as positive and valuable to the child, and those values can be carried over into adulthood.

Exercise is a time commitment and will take away from other things, so the family needs to prioritize it. Make physical activity part of family fun: take bike rides or hikes, or walk around a zoo or park, for example. It's important also to integrate physical activity regularly into everyday family routines. For example, make a rule that family members must avoid the elevator for going up less than three flights, or must park in the most remote parking place in the lot when visiting the mall. Send your child outside to play for at least an hour (make sure he's supervised!) before he sits down to do homework or play at the computer.

At school, if there are no physical education classes, try to find out what activities your child likes and help him or her pursue them. Anything from team sports to in-line skating will do. If there's no safe place to play outside, buy an exercise video. Have him or her walk to school—with a group of friends for added safety. As parents, it's important to set an example you want your children to follow, so review your own behavior. If you spend all your free time sitting on the sofa watching television, make some changes in your lifestyle.

Healthful Nutrition Equals Healthful Weight

The studies show responsibility for eating should be shared between parent and child. The child should not be restricted from eating what is in his environment. He should decide when to eat and how much to eat based on his body signals. But it's the parents' role to control the environment, to make sure that only healthful, wholesome foods are available from which your child can choose at regular, scheduled times throughout the day that normally correspond to his hunger levels.

Above all, your major priority: Make healthful food delicious!

Nutrition experts concur on the importance of eating a wide variety of foods to receive all of the essential nutrients, since no one food contains all the vitamins, minerals, phytochemicals, and fiber you need. They recommend balance and moderation, and that each day and at each meal you choose appropriate amounts to get the calories your body needs. (The *Think Yourself Thin* menu plans will help. See page 469.)

You've seen the Food Guide Pyramid. It's a simple guideline to help you decide what you and your family should eat. The general rule of thumb is take a lot from the bottom, less from the middle, and a little from the top (according to The American Academy of Pediatrics "Guide to Your Child's Nutrition").

The Food Guide Pyramid is a great visual and largely a helpful tool to help you make nutritious choices for you and your family. But nutrition experts today have found the pyramid could be improved by being more current with the latest scientific findings. I recommend you use the pyramid combined with the following information so that it is more up to date with the latest knowledge we have about optimal nutrition.

You can start teaching your children these principles as early as preschool.

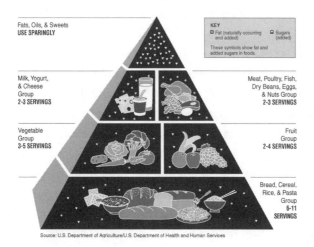

Food Guide Pyramid
A Guide to Daily Food Choices

Fats, Oils, & Sweets
USE SPARINGLY

KEY
□ Fat (naturally occurring and added)   □ Sugars (added)
These symbols show fat and added sugars in foods.

Milk, Yogurt, & Cheese Group
2-3 SERVINGS

Meat, Poultry, Fish, Dry Beans, Eggs, & Nuts Group
2-3 SERVINGS

Vegetable Group
3-5 SERVINGS

Fruit Group
2-4 SERVINGS

Bread, Cereal, Rice, & Pasta Group
6-11 SERVINGS

Source: U.S. Department of Agriculture/U.S. Department of Health and Human Services

Grains

Unlike refined grains, whole grains include all the healthful parts of a grain. Their role in human health is so important that the federal government has authorized manufacturers of whole grains to make the following health claim: "Diets rich in whole grain foods and other plant foods, that are low in total fat, saturated fat, and cholesterol, may reduce the risk of heart disease and certain cancers." The latest edition of the USDA's Dietary Guidelines for Americans says: "Choose a variety of grains, especially whole grains."

Whole grains are rich in fiber, but also in B vitamins and trace minerals such as zinc for the immune system, iron for transport of oxygen, and copper for healthy blood vessels, heart tissue, and bones. Today, all grains are fortified with folic acid, an important nutrient that reduces the risk of birth defects.

A grain consists of three parts: 1) the bran, which contains fiber, B vitamins, protein, and trace minerals; 2) the germ, which contains B vitamins, vitamin E, trace minerals, and phytochemicals; and 3) the endosperm, which mostly contains starch. When a grain is refined to create white flour, for instance, the only thing left is the endosperm. All the fiber, vitamins, minerals, and phytochemicals found in the bran and germ are removed. This is a shame, since whole grains are not only better for you, but taste better. Whole grains have a nutty flavor. If you've ever bought wheat germ you can attest to its nutty, crunchy qualities.

Emerging science has found that people who eat whole grains have less diabetes, fewer heart attacks, and may even reduce their risk for cancers.

You have a choice between grains made with processed white flour or grains kept whole. I recommend you use whole grains as much as possible, like whole wheat bread, whole wheat pasta, brown rice, and whole grain cereals. Look for foods that list a whole grain as the first ingredient, since ingredients are listed in order of predominance.

Grains are a good source of carbohydrate, contain some protein, and have B vitamins, which are important for a healthful nervous system, and vitamin K, which is good for blood clotting and bone metabolism. If unprocessed, grains will also be a terrific source of fiber. In fact, grains are usually the largest source of fiber in a person's diet. Fiber is important for keeping regular, preventing many chronic diseases, and feeling full. Your child's fiber needs, from all sources including fruits and vegetables, should equal his age plus 5. So for a 4-year-old, that's 9 grams of fiber daily. An adult's fiber needs are 25 grams for women and 38 grams for men.

Vegetables and Fruits

Most children or adults don't eat enough vegetables and fruits. They contain essential vitamins, minerals, fiber, and phytochemicals (the chemicals found in plants) that enhance life and prevent disease.

More than 200 studies of various research designs have revealed a strong association between diets high in vegetables and fruits (5 to 9 4-ounce servings—or about 4 cups—daily) and a lower risk for cancer. This is why the National Cancer Institute recommends a minimum of five servings of fruits and vegetables daily. The American Heart Association is also getting into the act. Its latest guidelines place more emphasis on eating fruits, vegetables, and whole grains, rather than on restricting fat because of fruits' and vegetables' influence on the prevention of heart disease and high blood pressure. Many other health organizations, as well as the USDA, are getting on the bandwagon and recommending a plant-based diet as protective against chronic diseases.

The research is clear and compelling. We've known the positive statistics for decades. (Of course, our grandmothers knew them before the scientists did . . . and Thomas Jefferson before that!) But scientists are just beginning to understand *why* fruits and vegetables prevent disease so effectively.

Apparently, each fruit and vegetable is a little factory of nutrients and chemicals—called phytochemicals—with potent powers of healing. An apple alone contains more than 150 beneficial, disease-fighting chemicals. And these are substances you can't get from a pill. They act synergistically in the foods so the whole is greater than the sum of its parts. While an apple has only 6 mg of vitamin C, it has 1,500 mg of vitamin C antioxidant activity because of the interaction of the vitamin C and the other nutrients in the apple.

Research has found that when some substances are added together, they boost each other and produce more than a double effect. This may explain why studies on supplements have failed to show the same health-enhancing and cancer-preventive effects as a diet high in vegetables and fruits—the whole foods.

The phytochemicals in fruits and vegetables have antioxidant effects, stimulate the immune system, enhance cancer-fighting enzymes, influence hormone metabolism positively, and even have antibacterial and antiviral effect. Phytochemicals are the compounds found in plants. By definition, all plants contain them. The term technically includes vitamins, minerals, and fibers. But in the common usage, it has come to refer to all the other compounds in plants that our bodies have evolved uses for. Many of these compounds are potent antioxidants. Others are anti-inflammatories, and still others stimulate the body's detoxification enzymes. You get them in sufficient quantities by eating the 5 to 9 daily servings of fruits and vegetables that the USDA recommends. All fruits and vegetables contain them, but the greatest concentration of beneficial phytochemicals is generally found in the most intensely colorful fruits and vegetables. (Notable exceptions would be onions, garlic, and cauliflower.)

While eating a variety of fruits and vegetables is recommended for maximum health, there are some we call the "superstars," which you should try to eat daily.

The Broccoli Family

People who regularly consume Brussels sprouts, cabbage, and broccoli have reduced incidence of certain cancers, especially cancer of the colon. They actually provide potent anticancer enzymes in the body.

Tomatoes

Men who consumed 10 or more servings of tomato products a week had a 35 percent decrease in risk of prostate cancer relative to those who consumed 1.5 servings or fewer per week. This is largely attributed to "lycopene" in the tomatoes, which is also in other red fruits such as watermelon, pink grapefruit, and guava. Lycopene is a potent scavenger of gene-damaging free radicals. Men with lycopene levels in the top 20 percent had a 46 percent decrease in risk of heart attack compared to those in the bottom 20 percent.

Dark Green Leafy Veggies (kale, spinach, collard greens, and turnip greens)

People who consumed spinach or collard greens 2 to 4 times per week had a 46 percent decrease in the risk of age-related macular degeneration (the leading cause of preventable blindness) compared to those who consumed these vegetables less than once per month. This is attributed to the phytochemical "lutein" in the carotenoid family. Absorption of carotenoids in your body is increased by cooking and by the presence of fat. So cook in a little healthy olive or canola oil!

Garlic

The Iowa Women's Study found the risk of getting colon cancer was decreased by 32 percent in a realistic periodic consumption of garlic. This is largely attributed the the "allinase" found in garlic. Allinase is preserved in foods if garlic is crushed and allowed to stand for 10 minutes before it is cooked. This result should also be found in other *Allium* family foods: onions, leeks, chives, and scallions.

Berries and Red and Purple Grapes

Red and purple fruits and vegetables such as red and blue grapes, blueberries, blackberries, cherries, strawberries, beets, eggplant (skin), red cabbage, red peppers, plums, and red apples are loaded with powerful antioxidants called "anthocyanins." They delay cellular aging and prevent formation of blood clots. In tests at Tufts University in Boston, blue foods quenched more free radicals than any other foods. Blueberries and blackberries were "clear winners" among fresh fruits. (For more informatioin, I recommend *The Color Code*, by J.A. Joseph, D.A. Nadeau, and A. Underwood [Hyperion, 2002].)

High-Protein Foods

To stay healthy, children need a steady supply of protein throughout the day, every day. Proteins are needed by the body for many different functions. They are used to make necessary hormones and enzymes. They're also essential to the immune system and in body repair and disease prevention. And of course, they're the essential building blocks of muscle tissue.

Protein is important for immunity and everyday functioning. It is the major component of all of your body's cells and is needed for the production of hormones, enzymes, and transport carriers. It is important in the metabolism of hormones, vitamins, and other important molecules in the body. The building blocks of proteins are called amino acids and there are nine essential amino acids. The composition of the various amino acids in foods qualifies the protein as high quality and as complete or incomplete proteins.

High-quality complete proteins, which provide all nine indispensable amino acids, are found in animal products, such as meat, poultry, fish, eggs, milk, cheese, and yogurt, and in soy beans. Plant foods contain incomplete proteins and are deficient in one or more of the indispensable amino acids. They need to be "matched" at your meals in order to provide all nine essential amino acids in the required amounts.

The types of protein foods I recommend are extra lean red meats (95 percent lean), game, poultry, seafood, or vegetarian sources such as beans and tofu. This is because fatty meats are too high in saturated fat to consume in large quantities.

Most women should get at least 54 grams—or up to double that amount, per day. Men should get at least 72 grams a day or up to double that amount.

Here's a quick list of protein amounts available in some foods:

7 grams per ounce of meat, fish, chicken, cheese (the leaner, the more protein)

8 grams per 8 ounces milk/yogurt

3 grams per 1/2 cup cooked or 1 ounce dry (1 slice bread) grain

2 grams per 1/2 cup cooked or 1 cup raw vegetables

12 grams per 1 cup cooked beans or tofu

6 grams per large egg (1 large egg white = 3.4 grams)

Dairy

Dairy products are the best source of calcium and also contain plenty of protein, vitamin D, vitamin A, and riboflavin. For children who are less than 2 years old, fat should make up half of the diet, so it's important to stick with breast milk or whole cow's milk. Children 2 years and older should be switched to lower-fat dairy products because of the high levels of saturated fat in whole dairy products. Dairy products are especially important for growing children because of their high concentration of nutrients, particularly calcium, which is necessary for building teeth and bone.

Fats

Fat is a hot but confusing topic. We know that certain fats are related to chronic diseases, but we also know that other fats promote health. The story of fat and health is more complex than even the top scientists once believed. Nutrition is an evolving science. It's important to stay abreast of the science so that you can do the best for yourself and your family.

To many people, the term "healthy fat" seems like an oxymoron. Evolving science is finding that there is a minimum level of fat you must eat to maintain health, but the type of fat you choose is crucial.

Fat is an essential nutrient, one you cannot live without. Without enough fat, children stop growing, skin deteriorates, and vitamin deficiencies flourish. Fat is a carrier of the fat-soluble vitamins A, D, E, and K, and phytochemicals in the vitamin A family such as carotenoids, which are essential for optimal health. Fat also aids in the digestion and absorption of important disease-fighting phytochemicals.

New research indicates that nuts, high in monounsaturated fats and omega-3 fats, are potent preventers of heart attack. Researchers found most of the valuable nutrients are fat-soluble and found in the fat of the nut. Other beneficial monounsaturated fats are in olive oil and canola oil. Research shows that monounsaturated and polyunsaturated fats are important for keeping good cholesterol levels (HDL) high—they're the good guys that "scavenge" the bad guys (LDLs) that clog your arteries, causing heart disease.

Two specific fatty acids are essential in the diet because the human body doesn't produce them. One essential fatty acid is "linoleic acid," which is known as an "omega-6 fatty acid." Without linoleic acid, you can experience symptoms such as a scaly rash and reduced growth. Linoleic acid may promote heart health by lowering bad cholesterol (LDL) and is found in vegetable oils such as soybean, corn, and safflower.

The other essential fatty acid is alpha-linolenic acid, also known as "omega-3 fatty acid." Without enough omega-3 in your diet, symptoms include neurological abnormalities and poor growth. Omega-3s may be beneficial in preventing coronary heart disease, arrhythmias, and thrombosis. They're thought to reduce blood pressure, triglycerides (blood fat), blood clotting, and inflammation—all critical functions in preventing heart disease and heart attack. New evidence suggests omega-3s may also have powerful effects preventing depression, and even Alzheimer's disease and dementia in older people. They may promote eye health and improve immunity and arthritis.

Omega-3s are found in fatty fish, nuts and seeds, particularly walnuts, soybean oil, canola oil, and flaxseed oils. Some animal fat may contain more omega-3s if their feed supplies it. Grass-fed, purslane-fed animals have higher levels of omega-3s in their tissues and eggs. If fish is grain-fed or fed in a way that deviates from normal, as in some farmed fish, it's unclear whether their flesh contains the same levels of omega-3s found in wild fatty fish from cold waters. This proves the point beautifully that you are what you eat—and so are fish and other animals!

Unhealthy Fats and Your Risk for Disease

The National Academy of Sciences has stated that Americans should eat as little as possible cholesterol, saturated fat, and trans fat, while still consuming a nutritionally adequate diet. This is because these are naturally synthesized in the body, are not essential nutrients and have no known beneficial role in human health, but also because of their role in increasing LDL. If people follow these guidelines, they'd be eating very little processed foods, fatty meats, and high-fat dairy products—a major improvement in most peoples' diets.

Saturated fat and trans fat seem to be major culprits when it comes to disease. Saturated fat is naturally hard at room temperature and mainly found in animal fats, but also in some vegetable fats such as palm and coconut oils and cocoa butter. You can reduce your saturated fat intake by choosing leaner meats, trimming away visible animal fat, and eating smaller portions of these foods. You can also choose fat-free or low-fat dairy products. You can replace butter with vegetable oils. All these choices can be made without reducing your intake of essential nutrients.

When cultures who traditionally eat a plant-based diet (predominantly fruits, vegetables, whole grains, and legumes), such as Asians, Mexicans and Africans, move to the United States and switch to our high meat and saturated-fat diet, their rates of obesity, diabetes, heart disease, and breast and prostate cancer (among other things) soar.

Trans fat is largely man-made and is formed when oils are put through the chemical process of "hydrogenation" to make them hard at room temperature. This is the case with margarines, vegetable shortening, and many fast and processed foods. Examples are cakes, pastries, doughnuts and french fries.

I've found that if you reduce your level of saturated fat, trans fat, and calories and get to an ideal body weight, that's the most effective way to reduce your blood cholesterol and your risk for coronary artery disease. If saturated fats are low enough in the diet, you could reduce your total cholesterol by 50 to 100 points within 6 weeks. But keep in mind that it's important to maintain your healthy fat intake at 20 percent to 35 percent of your total calories and to keep physically active so that your good cholesterol (HDL) will remain high.

Dietary Fat and Weight Loss

Fats are very concentrated calorie source. That's why eating a "relatively" low fat diet is important to lose weight. You'll benefit so much from thoughtfully managing your fat intake.

Fat's caloric density is high so it's especially important when energy needs are high, such as in infancy, illness, or high-level athletics. Of course, this can backfire if you're trying to watch your weight. It's important to be aware of the amount of fat you're eating for this reason. But be sure to read your food labels because "low fat" does not always mean "low calorie!"

Balance and Variety

The keys to good health and enjoyment of food are balance and variety. There are no "good" or "bad" foods, just good or bad diets. Even having sweets, fast food, or restaurant meals is fine-occasionally. It's when they dominate your life that you run into trouble. Each meal should be balanced with ingredients from each food group. A dinner for children should consist of mostly whole grain, then vegetables and/or fruit, then lean protein, and last, fat. See the *Think Yourself Thin* Menu Plans on page 469 for a wide variety of balanced menu ideas at different calorie levels, which should help you if you have questions about how to balance various groups of foods.

Involve Your Children

Children naturally love food; they love to play with food, they love to cook and help out in the kitchen. If children are taught how to prepare food, they'll be much more likely to eat and enjoy it. When children feel satisfied with healthful food and they've helped to prepare it, they develop a better connection to it.

One way to help your children enjoy vegetables is by making a game out of preparing the salad: How many colors can we get in the bowl? How many textures? The crunchy broccoli flowerets, the leafy spinach, the soft tomato. How many flavors? A sweet peach, a pungent pepper, a tart dressing.

Studies show if you can create a familiarity and connection between your children and healthful foods, your child will naturally evolve to love and prefer healthful foods. Planting vegetable gardens at home, at school, or in a community plot gives children a sense of ownership. Or simply go to a local farm and pick something. Your children (and spouse) will eagerly come home with the cabbage they picked and try to find some way to include it in that night's meal—in a tart coleslaw, a stir-fried Chinese meal, or cabbage soup. You'll have a cabbage lover in no time.

The more exposure a child has to a food, the more he will prefer it. A landmark study showing photos of children's facial reactions to different foods illustrated this concept beautifully. Of course, every child who tasted something sweet reacted with pleasure and gusto. But the first time a child was offered a green bean, well, hateful, disgusting looks were the norm. But after the 20th time that child was offered the green bean, you couldn't tell the difference between the sweet and the green bean by the way that child enjoyed it!

Unfortunately, many parents give up after the first try. I can't say I blame them, judging by the terrible initial response they're likely to get. But if you continue to offer a food consistently, patiently, and positively, even a resisting child will eventually come around, especially if you're eating and enjoying the food as well.

The Times Your Child Should Eat

Studies show children who are thinner have more structured meal times. It's not a good idea to allow your child to graze on food all afternoon. There is a time and a place for eating. As your child understands his body signals, you can schedule regular meal and snack times for him.

For instance, you may find he is always hungry when home from school. Instead of handing him a bag of chips for him to eat in front of the TV or computer, have him sit at the dining table to eat a nourishing snack. (It's important that you set boundaries about eating for everyone in the family. Eating should be done at the dining table without distractions. You either eat OR play OR do your homework OR watch TV.) When he is no longer hungry and the eating is over, he can do his other activities. Of course, if he doesn't want to sit down to eat, perhaps he isn't hungry. Recognize that as a body signal, and don't push food on him.

You can also develop behavioral associations between eating and other activities. The ideal is for hunger to be the only stimulus for eating. For this to happen, eating should be enjoyed and savored as a sole activity, not accompanied by distractions, which can start to become cues for eating.

Spouses and Significant Others

Many adults report that their weight gain began when they got married. Married life changes your daily routine, so you may be eating heavier meals in the evenings or you may have a busier life with more restaurant meals and less physical activity. Your spouse may have different tastes in food that you've begun to incorporate into your own diet. Often a woman will start eating more food when she's dining with a man, almost as if she's trying to keep up with him. She forgets that the man is larger, more muscular, and has much higher calorie needs. Or a new wife or husband might feel the need to cook elaborate meals every night or go out to fancy restaurants more often as a treat. These kinds of changes can pack on the pounds very quickly.

The same consideration you give to children should be given to your spouse or significant other. No coercing, policing, restricting, or putting anyone on a diet. It's important to simply model healthful behavior and become positively involved in healthier food and physical activity choices. In my experience, a spouse's support—or lack thereof—can make or break a weight-loss program, or any behavior change program, for that matter.

If you have the weight problem

First, ask your spouse to help you in any way you think would make a positive difference for you. It's probably not a great idea to ask him to police your food intake—that gets old fast. And only you can make those kinds of decisions for yourself. I've found it's best to simply ask for positive reinforcement. If you're making special efforts to cook healthful foods or to make it to the gym, ask for little rewards: simple compliments, pats on the back, gifts of pretty lingerie, or even vacations.

Ask your spouse to be physically active with you. Going on a long walk every weekend (or several times a week) is a way to reacquaint yourself with your loved one, to catch up on the weeks' or days' activities. You'll probably get more attention and have more conversation than you do out on a dinner date!

If your spouse is interested, get your spouse involved in new and healthful foods you'd like to try. If your spouse brings food into the house you find tempting or difficult to resist, see if you can find an alternative everyone can be happy with. Instead of a quart of ice cream, perhaps you can switch to individually wrapped low-calorie ice cream bars.

Ask him to accompany you to the farmers' market, a local farm or orchard, or somewhere you both can pick out beautiful, fresh produce. Get him involved in the cooking decisions, if this interests him. Ask if there are any special healthful recipes he'd enjoy. If he does the cooking, you both can explore new recipes until you find a new healthful repertoire you both find satisfying.

I find spouses are more than happy to be a part of any healthful evolution their loved one wants to make, especially if they're rewarded constantly and complimented for being supportive (that's right, compliment *them* for complimenting *you!*). There's nothing like attention and praise for keeping the ball rolling in the right direction. It works with man, woman, child, and beast alike!

If your spouse has the weight problem

Ask your spouse how you can help him and respect what he has to say. And remember, no policing, coercing, or restricting. It doesn't work with children, and it most certainly doesn't work with adults. I know it's challenging. It's difficult to see a loved one suffer, especially when you know his health is at risk. But in the end, you can't want the weight loss more than he does. You can do just so much on his behalf. The rest is up to him.

Creating an environment where only healthful foods are available in the home may be helpful. I find spouses really appreciate someone who helps create a healthful home, a home where it's easy and positive to eat healthfully, and not a drag on anyone.

Keep mealtimes fun, ask your spouse if he'd like to help plan new menus. Be willing to take the time to try new recipes until you have a whole new repertoire of tried-and-true healthful ones. You can even create new traditions for your family. For example, at Thanksgiving, change all those creamed vegetables to stir-fried or grilled.

You can also help create healthful routines, such as encouraging eating together at regular meals, but avoiding late-night snacking. Encourage regular physical activity by offering to be his exercise partner. You could both wake up early in the morning together to exercise, take walks together, go the gym together, and take exercise classes together.

Besides being helpful and reinforcing, part of what you're doing is subtly modeling behavior you'd like your spouse to have. Making healthy changes in your own lifestyle will rub off on your husband without him even realizing it. The next thing you know, your husband will be losing weight faster than you are (although you may hate that part).

The Lucky 13: Essential Steps for Healthful Family Eating

1. Model the lifestyle you'd like your spouse and children to copy.
2. Involve the whole family in food selection and cooking.
3. Present wholesome, healthful food in a positive way.
4. Make dinner time focused family time, making conversation and having eye contact with your family members with no distractions, no phone or TV.
5. Make an effort to reduce TV watching in general for everyone in the family.
6. Substitute TV watching for physical activities, playing games, reading, telling stories, and interacting with family members or friends.
7. Start a garden. Even if all you have is a windowsill, you can plant herbs like rosemary or basil.
8. Give everyone in the family some way to contribute toward dinner.
9. If a child doesn't like a food, don't start making several dishes to please them. They will eat if they get hungry.
10. If a child does something unusual at the table or refuses to eat, don't make a scene, as this will encourage repetition. Go on as if nothing hap-

pened and sooner or later, everything will be back to normal.

11. Structure meal and snack times so there is very little need for grazing or grabbing unplanned foods.

12. Structure meals and snacks so that they are eaten sitting down at a dining table without distractions and with a good amount of time to enjoy the food.

13. Avoid reinforcing, rewarding, restricting, cajoling, or punishing with food at any time, but particularly at the dinner table.

Part II

Weight-Loss Plans That Work for You

CHAPTER 8

Really Simple Strategies for Everyone

Especially appropriate for: *Disorganized Eaters, Emotional Eaters, Entertainers and Socializers, Frequent Travelers, Everyone Else!*

One thing that I've learned in my many years of practice is that there isn't a single diet plan or weight-loss strategy that works for everyone. I almost go crazy when best-selling diet books or weight-loss gurus (who really ought to know better) promise success for anyone who follows this plan or eats only these foods. If only life were so simple!

Anyone who has struggled with weight gain knows that there is a multitude of overlapping factors that play a role. Some of them—cravings for sweets, for example—are constant, or pretty close to it. Others change as our lives change. A 19-year-old who's off to college for the first time will gain weight for entirely different reasons than a senior executive at a bank. Alcohol consumption, going out to restaurants, physical activity (or the lack of it), time pressures—these are just a few of the individual reasons that people gain weight. I suspect there are hundreds, if not thousands, more.

It's true that many of those with weight problems can be grouped into a few very broad categories—those who don't shop regularly or plan efficiently, for example, or those who socialize or travel a great deal. When I first meet with clients, I try to get a sense of their overall life patterns because this makes it easier to devise effective strategies that will fit many, if not all, of their needs.

But I fully recognize that the reasons we gain weight are endlessly varied. You may recognize parts of yourself in later sections of this book, but I wouldn't presume for an instant that you only need more organization in your life, or you only need to control emotional eating. By all means, pay attention to those tips. They'll help you lose weight, I promise! But I'd hate to see anyone focus too much attention on a few weight-loss strategies when there are so many to choose among.

No matter what you think is the "main" reason that you've gained weight, don't skip this section! Some of the following tips can be used every day; others will apply only to certain occasions—when you're talking on the phone, for example, or settling into a booth at the neighborhood greasy spoon.

I haven't put these strategies in any particular order, for the simple reason that they're all effective. In addition, the tips in this chapter and throughout the book vary a great deal in what they ask of you. Most of the suggestions are incredibly easy to incorporate into your life. Going vinaigrette instead of "creamy" on your salads, using oil instead of butter in cooking, going "surf" instead of "turf" in restaurants—these are all very easy changes to make. And yet they still amount to lots of pounds lost.

Other tips require a bit more dedication. Getting a dog and walking it religiously is more of a life change, but one most of my clients relish. Taking up yoga or changing your environment takes a bit more time and thought, as does keeping a food diary or even editing your shopping habits. But even these changes won't be hard if you follow my advice. Whether they're right for you—at this particular time or on any particular day—you'll have to decide for yourself. Try a few of these approaches. If they're not right for you, give them up and try some different ones.

Everyone gains weight for different reasons—and everyone needs different approaches to lose it and keep it off.

Good luck—and good eating!

#1. The Sundae Solution

Now it's official: You can eat a chocolate sundae every afternoon and still lose weight.

One of my clients, Jennie, almost always snacks in the afternoon. She views these snacks as "rewards" for getting through another day of drudgery. Of course, these same snacks contribute to her weight problem.

My advice to her (and I'm pretty proud of it): Have a chocolate sundae every day.

I know this sounds strange, but here's why it helps. The chocolate syrup that you pour over ice cream isn't exactly lean, but that's okay because underneath the chocolate—the sundae part—is fresh fruit instead of ice cream. Fruit is a lot better for you than ice cream, and the chocolate provides a slightly sinful incentive to make the switch seem worthwhile.

Almost any fruit works with chocolate syrup—strawberries, bananas, peaches, take your pick. Apart from the fact that a fruit sundae is deliciously fresh tasting and low in saturated fat and calories, it makes a great substitute for other snacks that really load on the calories.

BOTTOM LINE: Lose 9–35 pounds

A tablespoon of regular chocolate syrup has about 50 calories. Pour it over fruit, and your total is about 110 to 160 calories. Compare that to the usual snacks—a candy bar, for example, has about 250 calories, and an ice cream cone has about 500—and you can see why substituting the fruit sundae can lead to impressive amounts of weight loss. Make the switch every day, and you can count on losing 9–35 pounds in a year.

#2. Set Your Alarm

People who only exercise when they're in the mood generally don't exercise very much. The solution: Put exercise on your calendar—or set an alarm that tells you when to slip on your sweats.

Disorganized eaters tend to be intense. They work too hard, whether their work is running an office or managing a family. They focus on work so much that they find it hard to stop for meals, let alone for regular exercise.

The only way to exercise regularly is to make it an integral part of your day. But first, you have to remember it. I advise people to give themselves reminders that they can't ignore.

Maybe you're the sort who religiously keeps a calendar or a "to do" list. If so, write in an exercise session. Allow for at least 15 minutes, preferably at the same time every day. Give it the same priority that you would any other "must do" event in the day.

Don't keep a calendar? In that case, set an alarm clock, or an alarm radio tuned to an upbeat music station. Have it turn on when it's time for your daily exercise. Set the volume loud so you can't miss it.

BOTTOM LINE: Lose 6–14 pounds

Even a modest amount of exercise—say, walking 5 times a week for 15 minutes each time—burns a lot more calories than slaving away at the office. If you do nothing else but walk most days of the week, you can count on losing at least 10 pounds a year.

#3. Walk the Dog

I'm not kidding. There's no easier way to get rid of fatty leftovers than to activate your canine disposal unit. Besides, dogs need walks, and so do you!

Let me tell you about Peter, a client of mine who lives in a beautiful condominium. Peter is single and has a reasonable amount of free time, but he could never work up the motivation to work out.

Recognizing that he had to get some exercise, and being fully aware of his own lethargic habits, Peter decided to get a four-legged personal trainer. He figured that having a dog would force him out of the house at least a few times a day.

So he visited the animal shelter, where he fell in love with Bitze, a cocker spaniel. Sure enough, Bitze insisted on going for walks several times a day. The two of them took long strolls along the Potomac River. The exercise felt good, and simply playing with Bitze helped Peter unwind at the end of the day.

Here's a bonus. Scientists have been looking at the links between pets and (human) health. People who spend time with their dogs, for example, can have dramatic reductions in blood pressure.

BOTTOM LINE: Lose 46–89 pounds

Peter burned about 5 calories per minute walking slowly or 9.5 calories per minute during his more brisk walks with Bitze. All told, he spent 90 minutes walking each day. As a result, he burned about 450-855 calories every day! Amazing what man's best friend can do.

#4. Do the Bed Stretch

When your body feels alert, you tend to eat less.
When you're physically tired or lethargic, on the other
hand, it's easy to turn to food for an artificial boost.

No one I know really enjoys stretching, but once you've done it, the surge
in energy can be remarkable. One stretch I really like is the "bed stretch."
You don't need workout clothes or tennis shoes to do it. As the name suggests, you don't even have to get out of bed to do it, although you may be
more comfortable lying on a carpet or rug.

Lie on your back with your arms straight over your head and your legs
straight. Fully stretch your arms and legs in opposite directions for 5 seconds, relax, then do it again. Imagine that you're making a "snow angel."
That's all there is to it!

This stretch uses most of your large muscle groups, including muscles
in the shoulders, arms, hands, feet, and ankles. If you do it every day, your
body will feel stronger and more energized. The better you feel physically, the less likely you'll be to depend on food for an energy boost.

BOTTOM LINE: Lose 7 pounds

How much will stretching affect your weight? Well, if feeling better overall helps you turn down a before-bed snack, you can count
on saving about 150 calories right there. If you stretch—and avoid
snacks—3 nights a week, you can count on losing at least 7 pounds.
Stretch more, lose more!

#5. Pour Another Glass

You already know you should be drinking lots of water rather than soft drinks. Here are the real reasons it's so effective.

All of those people walking around with their very own sip bottles—is anyone really that thirsty? Let's forget the trendiness for a moment: Water really is the perfect beverage when you're trying to lose weight.

I advise almost everyone to drink at least 8 full glasses of water daily. It takes up room in the stomach and may act as a natural appetite suppressant. It helps the muscles maintain good tone, and it also inhibits skin sagging that often follows weight loss. Most importantly, your body needs water to metabolize fat!

To get in the habit of drinking water regularly, go ahead and join the crowd. Stock up on one-quart plastic containers and keep them with you all the time—at work, in the car, next to your bed, and so on.

Place bottles of water in front of the refrigerator, a none-too-subtle reminder of what to reach for first.

If your tap water isn't exactly tasty, consider buying bottled spring water. Add sliced lemon, lime, or cucumber to your water. The delicious pure taste will give you yet another incentive to drink more.

BOTTOM LINE: Lose 17–22 pounds

If you are drinking a sweetened, calorie-rich soft drink every day, substituting water will add up to a lot of lost calories.

#6. Baked, Not Fried

The next time you're in a supermarket, read the label on the back of your favorite potato chips. Shocking!

The average 7-ounce serving of traditional potato chips has 1,050 calories. That's potentially more than you'd get in a healthful, three-course dinner!

I'm not suggesting giving up chips (heaven forbid). But I do recommend switching to baked chips. A 7-ounce serving has about 840 calories. It's still not lean, but it's a lot better than the fried kind. Plus, you're giving up a lot of the dangerous fat that's used in frying.

You may find that baked chips are just as tasty as the fried ones—or you may want to add a little bit of salt to bump up the taste. (If you have high blood pressure and have been told to avoid sodium, forget the extra salt.) Or serve them with nonfat salsa: You don't even notice the difference in the chips.

BOTTOM LINE: Lose 3 pounds

Let's assume you eat one bag of chips a week. Switching to baked chips could save you 10,920 calories over the course of a year. Do you enjoy chips every day? The switch will save you 76,650 calories. Now for the clincher: For every bag of baked chips that you substitute for the fried kind, you'll be giving up 5 tablespoons of pure lard. That means that approximately 70 grams of fat won't be calling your arteries "home."

Hey! Pass the chips!

#7. Think Positive Thoughts

The ways you talk to yourself influence how hopeful you are about your goals and your life. Want to lose weight? Think good thoughts!

In the past, whenever something exciting was on my horizon, I would immediately start worrying about things that could go wrong. Take this book. It's one of the most exciting things that has ever happened to me, but my self-talk went something like this: "If my book is successful, I may get unwanted attention and be criticized."

What does this have to do with weight loss? Everything! If your self-talk is negative, you'll almost certainly find yourself turning to food for comfort. You'll be less likely to stick with a weight-loss program, and you'll get discouraged easily. My self-destructive self-talk caused me to procrastinate for ten years before I finally finished this book.

With a combination of professional guidance and self-exploration, I gradually became aware of my thought patterns and the ways in which they were affecting—and harming—my life. Ask yourself if you often have trouble achieving the things you want most out of life. Is it possible that you're subconsciously talking yourself out of them?

CREATING NEW THOUGHTS
Begin by listening to every little thought, day dream, or fantasy that you have—nothing is insignificant. When you find yourself making a negative statement or having a negative vision, explore why it may be happening.

Do you have irrational fears left over from childhood? If so, replace them with realistic goals. Suppose, for example, that your inner voice tells you to eat everything on your plate when you go to a restaurant—you paid for it, after all. A more positive dialogue might go something like this: "Most of what I'm paying for is convenience and ambiance. The actual cost of the food itself is relatively minor. I'm only going to eat what I want."

Here's another example. You might say to yourself, "I'm going to follow this program 100 percent or not at all." Wow, those are high expectations! Here's a more realistic thought: "I'd like to be perfect, but I'm human. Striving for perfection only sets me up for failure. Each of these changes helps, so I'm going to start with what I can do, and add extra steps when I'm ready."

BOTTOM LINE: Lose 20–30 pounds

Suppose that turning negative thoughts into positive ones allows you to exercise 30 minutes a day—exercise you might not be getting otherwise. All by itself, this could help you lose 20–30 pounds in a year. Positive thoughts make it easier to eat more healthful meals. Count on saving 100 calories at every meal or 300 calories at dinner.

#8. Pedal While You Prattle

If you spend more than a few minutes on the phone at a time, you're probably wasting a golden opportunity to lose weight.

Some telephone conversations require total concentration, but most are social chitchat. You can easily be doing something besides putting your feet up. My advice: Get that exercise bike spinning while catching up on your friends' latest dating fiascoes!

Even people who want to exercise don't always get around to it because it takes extra time. Well, here's the time. If the conversation is at all interesting, you'll probably forget that your legs are spinning beneath you.

It helps to get a cordless phone or even a headphone. And if you're going to be making a number of calls yourself, you might want to write the telephone numbers on Post-It notes and stick them on the bike. You can make all your calls without having to quit pedaling and look up a number!

BOTTOM LINE: Lose 10–42 pounds

Just how much weight can you lose while you're pedaling? Let's look at some numbers. Pedaling at 10 miles an hour (a relatively slow pace, easy to maintain while talking) for 25 minutes will burn 100 calories. A faster pace of 17 miles an hour for 15 minutes also burns 100 calories.

Modest phone talkers (say, 15 minutes a day) can lose up to 10 pounds a year this way. If you chat for 30 minutes to an hour daily, you could lose as much as 42 pounds.

Get spinning!

#9. Eat More Salads

Why would I suggest that you add something to your evening meal when you're trying to lose weight? Because salads are in a class by themselves.

Green salads are among the healthiest foods you can eat. They have no artery-clogging fat and almost no calories (assuming you don't drench them in full-fat, creamy Thousand Island dressing). Just as important, they're high in fiber, which satisfies the appetite and makes you less likely to fill up on other, high-caloric foods. This is one reason I advise people to eat a salad at the beginning of a meal, not at the end.

I have nothing against iceberg lettuce, apart from the fact that it's low in fiber and virtually devoid of taste and texture. The best salads are made with other, more exciting greens, such as spinach, arugula, and so on. Throw in some vegetables for additional crunch, color, and flavor, as well as important nutrients.

Obviously, a salad is only as healthful as the topping. You'll definitely want to use a reduced-calorie dressing—and skip the fatty croutons, too.

Helpful: Put the dressing on the side of the plate or in a small bowl. Dip your fork in the dressing, then grab some greens. You'll get the same taste while limiting the calories.

BOTTOM LINE: Lose 20 pounds

I've found, and studies confirm, that people who enjoy a salad every lunch and dinner wind up saving about 200 calories a day, simply because they're eating less of other, more fattening foods.

#10. Substitute Oil for Butter

Regrettably, cooking oils and butter have the same amount of calories. Merely replacing one with the other won't help you lose weight—but you'll be a heck of a lot healthier.

Butter is full of saturated fat, the kind that clogs up your arteries. Oils, on the other hand, contain monounsaturated and polyunsaturated fats—the ones that help lower cholesterol and reduce the risk of heart disease. Olive, canola, soy, and nut oils are among the best choices.

What about margarine? Nope. It's full of trans fats, which are just as bad for your heart as the saturated fat in butter. However, there are a few brands of margarine that contain no saturated or trans fats. These are acceptable.

Even though I started out by saying you can't lose weight by switching from butter to oils, that's not entirely true. If you give up butter entirely and use full-flavored oils in moderation, you'll find yourself cutting out quite a few calories.

Rather than smearing bread with butter, for example, dip it lightly in a dish of measured-out olive oil. Sprinkle on some pepper or salt, if you like. The flavor goes a long way, so you don't have to use very much at all.

BOTTOM LINE: Lose 12 pounds

If switching from butter to oil causes you to use less fat—say, one less tablespoon a day—you could potentially lose up to 12 pounds a year.

#11. Eat More Slowly

I often explain to my clients that eating too quickly contributes to weight gain. But they still have trouble slowing down, so it's probably worth repeating.

Some studies indicate that it takes at least 20 minutes for your brain to get the signal that you've had enough to eat. Let's assume that you gobble down a complete meal in 10 minutes. Your brain won't realize that you've had enough to eat—or, more likely, that you're stuffed—until it's too late.

I'm not a big believer in that ancient advice that advocates chewing each bite 20, 30, or even 40 times. That's a little fussy for my taste. Just try to slow down.

How can you tell if you're eating too quickly? Well, if you often find yourself feeling uncomfortably full when you leave the table, that's a good sign. It means you're putting more food in your stomach than it needs—and you're doing it so quickly that your brain doesn't have time to respond.

Next time, take the time to enjoy and savor each bite. Start by taking a few deep breaths and relaxing before eating. You may want to put your fork down between bites. Chew the food thoroughly (without counting), swallow it, and relax for a moment. Then pick up your fork again.

BOTTOM LINE: Lose 10 pounds

People who eat more slowly invariably eat a little less. Every time you use this method at dinner, you can count on saving at least 100 calories.

#12. Hold the Tuna Salad

Millions of dieters think of tuna salad as the ultimate lean food that will help them lose weight. Bad news: It doesn't work.

In fact, you're probably better off eating a lean roast beef sandwich. Virtually every tuna salad you get in a deli or restaurant is prepared with lots of high-fat and high-calorie mayonnaise—and I mean high! The tuna was probably packed in oil. A sandwich made with turkey breast or lean roast beef, and without mayo, will dish up 200 fewer calories.

If you're making your own tuna salad, of course, you can enjoy tuna and cut the calories at the same time. If you substitute light mayo for the full-fat kind, you'll save 100 calories. Or just use less regular mayo. Using water-packed tuna instead of oil-packed will save you another 100 calories.

The other advantage of homemade is that you can add all the fixings you really enjoy, such as pickles, onions, celery, carrots, capers, or even curry powder. The more highly seasoned ingredients you use, the less you'll notice the "missing" fat and calories.

BOTTOM LINE: Lose 3–6 pounds

Let's assume that you eat a tuna salad once a week. Substituting a homemade tuna salad or a turkey breast or lean roast beef sandwich will save you about 10,400 calories over the course of a year. If you're a real tuna lover who eats it more often, these simple substitutions can add up to some impressive weight loss!

#13. Say "No" to Pushers

To be fair, food pushers aren't bad people at heart. Your mom, your spouse, your friends—they just want to please you. But you have to be firm.

We all know people who aren't satisfied until they convince us—beg us— to eat more, more, more. Their misguided entreaties are hard to resist, if only because we want to be polite.

The challenge is to say no in ways that work. After all, the food pusher is convinced that he's looking after your best interests.

I advise my clients to take a positive approach. Sample the proffered food, but tell your host, "This is delicious. I'd love to have more, but I'm wonderfully satisfied and can't take another bite." Positive, yet firm.

No matter what, don't hide behind the excuse that you're on a diet. This fails in three ways: 1) It gives the food pusher a double signal—that you really want it, but feel that you have to refuse; 2) it is sometimes taken as an insult, as though you're saying that the food isn't good enough for your refined tastes; 3) it may bring up guilty feelings in the pusher, that he or she shold be "watching it," too. All of which challenge the pusher to seduce you.

BOTTOM LINE: Lose 7 pounds

If you manage to resist a food pusher once a week, and decide not to have that 500-calorie dessert, you can easily lose 7 pounds in a year. The pushier your friends, the more weight you'll lose!

#14. Choose "Surf"

Nearly every restaurant offers a "surf" or "turf" special, or a combination of the two. Guess which one I recommend?

The numbers tell the story:

- 6-ounce slab of prime rib: 600 calories
- 6-ounce sirloin: 450 calories
- 6-ounce salmon: 400 calories
- 6-ounce tuna steak: 250 to 300 calories

Even though these are among the fattiest fish imaginable, they still have a lot fewer calories than red meat. They're also loaded with omega-3 fatty acids, which are good for your health, unlike the artery-clogging saturated fat in meat.

Stick with seafood as much as possible. A restaurant meal will always end up being richer than a meal at home, so it's worth cutting calories where you can. This means avoiding fried fish, of course; even blackened can be greasy. Stick to grilled, poached, or steamed fish.

BOTTOM LINE: Lose 4–18 pounds

Choosing salmon over prime rib could save 200 calories; a leaner fish (snapper, for example) will save you even more. For those hard-core meat eaters, switching to fish 6 out of 7 days can result in a weight loss of 18 pounds.

#15. Tighten a Muscle

Actually, you have to tighten more than one, but that's the whole point: A technique called progressive relaxation has been proven to lower stress—and that, of course, lowers calorie intake at the same time.

This easy procedure is among the best ways to lower physical and emotional stress. It relaxes your muscles and reduces your pulse rate, blood pressure, perspiration, and breathing rate. It physically relaxes your entire body, and people who do it regularly experience less of the negative side effects of stress overall.

We've already talked about the ways in which stress contributes to weight gain. Let's face it, we live in a world where stress is omnipresent. Unfortunately, food is equally abundant. Put the two together, and you're going to see a lot of eating that has more to do with frustration and anxiety than with actual physical hunger.

It's not a coincidence that we all tend to gain weight during those times when life is most stressful—during transitions at work, for example, or in the course of divorces or other difficult life events, particularly events we can't control. "Comfort food" makes us feel better temporarily, but the consequences can stick around for years.

Even if the stress in your life hasn't risen off the charts, all sorts of "negative" emotions—boredom, for example—promote the kind of mindless eating that quickly packs on the pounds.

I often recommend progressive relaxation for those with "type A" personalities. They tend to get bored with inactive forms of stress reduction, such as deep breathing (they respond, "Yeah, right!"). With progressive relaxation, you're actively tensing and relaxing the muscles, so it feels as though something is actually happening. Which, in fact, it is.

HOW TO DO IT

Progressive relaxation is a technique in which you tense, then relax, every muscle in your body, starting at the very tips of the toes and working all the way up to the head.

People generally find that it's easier to practice this technique when they're lying down, but you don't have to. Once you get good at it, you can practice it when you're sitting or even standing.

The muscle groups you want to work include the feet, legs, buttocks, abdomen, lower back, chest, shoulders, neck, face, and forehead.

Tense each group of muscles for about 5 seconds. Relax for a moment, take a breath, then move on to the next muscle group. Make sure your breathing is slow and steady throughout.

Mmmmm—it feels good! And you'll like the way you feel afterward, too.

BOTTOM LINE: Lose 19 pounds

Some people find that doing progressive relaxation daily makes it much easier to avoid afternoon or nightly snacks. Think about it: Passing on just one plate of nachos could save you 1,300 calories! So would avoiding your 185-calorie nightly snack.

#16. Eat, Then Shop

I define temptation as pushing a shopping cart down the ice cream aisle when you haven't eaten for 6 hours.

Think of supermarkets as goodie factories for adults. When you're trying to lose weight, nothing is more hazardous than shopping when you're hungry. Foods that would never catch your eye when you're in your right mind will suddenly look very appealing.

I've witnessed this first hand. If I haven't eaten before I go shopping, I find myself tasting every piping-hot sample that's offered. Even the checkout line isn't safe. Some wicked candy bar is sure to leap off the shelf and into the pile of groceries. I suspect that they have Mexican jumping beans in them just for this purpose!

It's hard to say exactly how much of a difference eating before shopping will make. One of my clients, Lisa, said she probably consumed more than 300 calories in free tastings when she shopped on an empty stomach. Another client would get cravings—and buy all the ingredients for—coconut cake. Yet another routinely polished off bags of chips before she checked out.

Do yourself a favor. Eat, then shop.

BOTTOM LINE: Lose 9 pounds

My guess is that if you go shopping twice a week, and if you manage to eat before leaving home, you can count on saving yourself at least 300 calories each trip.

#17. Add the Whipped Cream

Regular ice cream has 350 calories per cup. Fancy ice cream weighs in at 500 calories per cup. So quit eating ice cream, already!

Sorry, I don't mean to sound harsh. But there are so many delicious desserts out there that won't blow your entire day's diet in a single shot. You don't have to have ice cream, at least not every day.

Try this instead. Buy some sweet cherries. Remove the pits and stems, and top them with a nice spoonful of whipped cream. It's delicious, and it's about as low-cal as you can ask for.

Let's take a look at the cherries. A quarter pound has 80 calories. A quarter cup of whipped cream—the pressurized kind you spray out of a can—has about 40 calories. Total caloric load: 120 calories. Compare that to the ice cream I mentioned earlier—or to whatever other sinful richness you have in mind—and the logic is inescapable.

I'm not insisting on cherries, by the way. Maybe your fruit of choice is a juicy pear. A crisp autumn apple. A bowl of berries. Have any of them. Have them all!

BOTTOM LINE: Lose 3–16 pounds

Depending on how often you make this switch, you can make significant strides in your weight loss. Suppose that you eat cherries and whipped cream instead of your usual ice cream once a week. That alone will account for 3–6 pounds of weight loss. Make the switch more often and you'll lose even more.

#18. Take Up Yoga

Forget any lingering impressions of Eastern mysticism. Yoga today is as American as apple pie—and a lot healthier.

A few years ago, yoga seemed pretty exotic. Guys with long beards practiced yoga. College students with lava lamps and beads were into yoga. If my memory serves, the Beatles practiced yoga. Sure, it was good exercise, but it just seemed so . . . weird.

Hey, things have changed. Yoga has entered the American mainstream, and you'll find classes at YMCAs, community centers, and neighborhood recreation centers. Kids do yoga at school. Grandmothers do it at senior centers. Yoga is truly everywhere.

Yoga does have a long and complex tradition of mystical teachings, but that's not the way it's usually taught today. The yoga you're likely to encounter will consist of simple, gentle movements and stretching combined with deep diaphragmatic breathing. The exercises provide quite a workout, and the deep breathing is actually a form of meditation.

There's no question that yoga is one of the best forms of stress control. And, as I keep saying throughout this book, controlling stress is one of the best ways to control appetite and weight gain.

If the idea of controlling stress and losing weight isn't enough to get you to sign up for a yoga class, here are some of the other benefits. It increases muscle and joint flexibility and strength. It improves range of motion and digestion. It helps relieve back pain and headaches. It can even lower blood pressure in some people.

MY STORY

I wasn't very successful when I tried to learn relaxation techniques. I was uptight to begin with, and I always found my mind going a mile a minute when I was supposed to be "mindlessly" communing with the universe. Oh, and I was a total failure at diaphragmatic breathing. I was raised by a military man, whose mantra was, "Stomach in, chest out"—the opposite of diaphragmatic breathing.

Nothing worked until I tried yoga. And then it clicked. Ever since, yoga has been one of the greatest discoveries of my life. After a session of yoga, I find myself more even-tempered, rational, thoughtful, confident, and in control—of my life as well as my eating.

Anyone can perform yoga because the movements can be personalized to individual needs and limits. You can do it sitting, standing, or lying down. You can practice it for 15 minutes or 2 hours. It's all up to you.

BOTTOM LINE: Lose 13 pounds

Let's assume that you do a 15-minute yoga routine every evening. It's very likely to help you avoid your usual snacks of pretzels or whatever—and that can save you about 150 calories a night, 6 out of 7 nights.

#19. Less Creamy, More Oily

I'm talking about salads, of course. Forget those creamy dressings. Go with vinaigrette: It's easy to make (or buy) and it has only a fraction of the calories.

The main reason I tell people to switch to oil-and-vinegar-based dressings is that they contain very little of the saturated fat that's found in traditional bleu cheese or other creamy dressings. Saturated fat is the stuff that's converted into cholesterol in the blood and increases the risk of heart disease and stroke.

To be entirely honest, you won't save an amazing amount of calories when you switch to vinaigrettes—but you will save some. Bleu cheese or creamy dressing has 60–80 calories per tablespoon, for example, compared to 50 in a vinaigrette, and about 40 in a "light" reduced-calorie vinaigrette.

Plus, vinaigrettes are wonderfully tangy and refreshing. You can buy them ready-made, but they're a snap to make at home: Try Dan Puzo's Red Wine Vinaigrette on page 449. It's 45 calories per tablespoon and delicious! If you keep the vinaigrette in the refrigerator, it will stay fresh for more than a month.

BOTTOM LINE: Lose 13 pounds

Most people use at least four tablespoons of dressing on their salad. If you switch from a creamy dressing to vinaigrette, plan on saving 120 calories for every salad. Eat salads every day, and you could save 43,800 calories in a year!

#20. Minesweep for Calorie Bombs

Losing weight is not about discipline or willpower. It's about controlling your environment. Period.

We all have different strengths and weaknesses, which must be considered when you're cutting calories or making any other healthful lifestyle changes.

Let's talk about me, Katherine Tallmadge. One of my main weaknesses is chocolate. I can't stop with one piece. That's simply not "normal" for me. I'll occasionally indulge my passion with a Dove bar or a piece of chocolate, but I've learned never to bring home a full box. It will be gone in a day or two, max.

I'm no better with chips. I have no self-control, and I know it. So I'll occasionally buy a 1-ounce bag. But a big bag? Never!

One of my strengths (finally, something positive!) is that I love fruits and vegetables. I stock up on these all the time.

You have to recognize your own "mines." I advise everyone to minesweep the kitchen for those calorie bombs that can explode your weight. Have a hard time resisting ice cream? Then get rid of the half-gallon. Candy bars your pitfall? Toss out the leftover bags from Halloween.

BOTTOM LINE: Lose 10–29 pounds

Minesweeping your kitchen periodically to get rid of things you shouldn't have in the house in the first place will save a tremendous amount of calories over time. Add the things that you like and should be eating, and you'll do even better.

#21. Beware the Burger Blast

Nearly everyone loves a good, juicy hamburger. Are you one of them? No problem.

Hamburgers are almost an institution in this country. I'm not one to criticize food choices (within reason), but the national fixation on hamburgers—and the frequency with which we enjoy them—definitely ranks among the main causes of weight gain.

Take Harry. One of my clients, he was all but addicted to burgers. He ate them for lunch at least twice a week, and burger dinners weren't unusual. Since the meat used in hamburgers ranges from fatty to fattier, he found himself getting a burger tummy.

No, I didn't advise Harry to quit eating hamburgers. He liked them too much, and I knew that a total prohibition would be counterproductive. All-or-nothing approaches, I've found, generally result in "nothing."

We came up with a more realistic plan. Harry was permitted—no, encouraged—to have burgers periodically, say, once a week. The rest of the time, he had to find other sandwiches that he enjoyed, but were much less likely to add inches to his waist.

LEANER CHOICES

What's a good burger substitute? Check out the deli department at the supermarket. You'll find all sorts of sandwich fixings that are full flavored as well as lean. To put this in perspective, half a pound of grilled hamburger meat has about 800 calories. The same amount of lean roast beef has half this amount.

Grilled chicken breast is an even better choice, with about 280 calories in half a pound. By substituting chicken for hamburger, you'll save 520 calories.

Of course, I'm only counting the calories in the meats themselves. Because switching to lean means results in such dramatic calorie reductions, you can be liberal in your choices of toppings. Want mayonnaise? Why not? A tablespoon of regular mayonnaise has 100 calories. You've saved so many calories by switching meats, you can afford the extra plea-sure. Low-fat mayo has about half as many calories as regular. But by making the meat substitute, I can enjoy regular mayo without guilt.

Most sandwich add-ons don't have enough calories to worry about. Go ahead and load your sandwich with onion, lettuce, tomato, whatever you like. Just to keep it healthy, put it all between slices of whole-grain bread rather than the traditional white kind.

BOTTOM LINE: Lose 6–16 pounds

If you're in the habit of eating a hamburger or cheeseburger every week, and you make one of these meat substitutions weekly, you'll save enough calories over a year to drop 6 to 8 pounds. Serious hamburger hounds who make the switch 3 times a week will lose a whole lot more.

#22. Take Center Stage

Exercise can be a solitary affair, and some people get too bored to keep it up. So make it a group affair—and make yourself the center of the group.

My friend Walsh joined an aerobics class full of women. He's the only man, which means he gets a lot of attention and reinforcement.

My mother began exercising for the first time in her life when a women-only gym opened in her area. She feels more comfortable when there aren't men around, and she gets a lot of attention from the trainers. She feels special at the gym, which is why she keeps going back.

I like company, too. Every Saturday, I take a walk with my good friend Tito. I look forward to these 5-mile walks through Rock Creek Park, and I go regardless of the weather. Walking with a friend makes the time go by pleasantly; it's sort of like a date, but without the romantic complications.

Speaking of romance, walking, rather than eating, is a great way to get to know someone. This is how I got to know Jack, my significant other. Talk about feeling special!

BOTTOM LINE: Lose 12 pounds

People who get extra attention when they exercise are more likely to keep it up. Let's assume, conservatively, that these good feelings motivate you to exercise 2 hours a week. You could lose as much as 12 pounds in a year!

#23. The Dilution Solution

Have you noticed how big the soft drinks at convenience stores have gotten? Apart from the inevitable bathroom consequences, there's a huge amount of calories in those paper cups.

Linda, a good friend, discovered this the hard way. Every day on her way to work, she would stop at the corner convenience store and tank up with a 32-ounce soda. She likes cold beverages, and she definitely likes caffeine. What she didn't appreciate, in retrospect, was the additional pounds she was putting on.

I'm always telling people to drink more water because it takes up room in the stomach and helps control appetite, especially if it's bubbly. It also has a lot fewer calories (none, actually) than sodas or other sweet beverages. Linda wasn't about to give up sodas, but she figured there had to be a way to get more water into the equation.

Here's what she started doing: Every time she bought a soda, she would cram the cup with ice, as much as it would hold. She figured that by the time the ice melted, she was drinking at least as much water as soda. Psychologically, however, she was satisfied because her morning ritual didn't change. Physically, she's now a slim size 8.

That's what I call creative thinking!

BOTTOM LINE: Lose 18 pounds

Let's assume that Linda cut her soda intake in half. That would mean that she was consuming 240 fewer calories every day she went to the office. That's better than you'll do by swearing off some sweet desserts!

#24. Muffin Madness

They look healthy. They even taste healthy. But commercial muffins are little more than concentrated fat.

Are you sitting down? Good, because the numbers I'm about to recite will take your breath away. Just one plump muffin—the super-sized kind sold today at supermarkets bakeries, and take-out shops—can set you back 600 calories. Eat one every day, and you'll consume about 219,000 calories a year. Yikes!

Low-fat muffins are much better. Even though a large one contains about 400 calories, that's a 200-calorie savings over the regular ones. I know, they don't taste quite as rich, but since you're eating them on the run anyway, you'll probably never notice!

Okay, you noticed. Why not make the muffin better by eating it with fruit? You can still do it on the run as long as you use whole fruit: take a bite of muffin, bite of fruit, bite of muffin. . . .

Eventually, of course, you may want to give up the muffin altogether. It's a very high-calorie snack. That's a good idea. Even a low-fat muffin can put on some pounds, but fruit has no calories worth worrying about, and it's loaded with fiber and other important nutrients.

BOTTOM LINE: Lose 21–52 pounds

Switch from a fatty muffin to a low-fat muffin every day, and you can count on losing more than 20 pounds in a year. Give up muffins and switch to fruit, and you'll lose a lot—and I mean a lot—more.

#25. Cook with Spray

One of my clients thought he was making dietary progress by switching from butter to margarine. Fact: All he was doing was swapping a batch of unhealthy natural chemicals for unhealthy manufactured chemicals. He certainly wasn't losing weight.

Butter, except in small amounts as an occasional treat, is among the unhealthiest ingredients in the kitchen. Most margarine isn't any better, and even cooking oils, which have little saturated fat, are essentially concentrated calories.

You can't cook without oil of some kind. Butter and other oils sear the surfaces of foods and lock in juices and flavors. They also prevent sticking.

Fortunately, there is a compromise: vegetable oil spray.

Oil sprays such as PAM take the place of butter, margarine, and cooking oils when you're sautéing or frying foods. But because they're in a spray form, you're able to control with great precision the amount that goes in the pan. If you use pans with nonstick coatings, all it takes is a quick spritz.

I admit, oil spray doesn't lend foods anywhere near the same richness that you get with butter or margarine. But if you're using fresh, full-flavored ingredients to begin with, who needs the extra flavor?

BOTTOM LINE: Lose 10–31 pounds

Each tablespoon of butter or margarine has 100 calories. Substitute a vegetable oil spray for one tablespoon, and you could lose as much as 10 pounds a year. The more you substitute, the more you lose!

#26. The "Whole" Story

Only 7 percent of Americans get the recommended kinds or amounts of disease-preventing, health-giving grains. Make sure you're in that 7 percent!

I always advise people to choose foods that are made with whole grains, rather than refined grains such as white flour. Whole grains contain essential basic nutrients, along with antioxidants that help prevent disease. Whole grains are probably the best single source of fiber. Fiber promotes weight loss by making you feel full on fewer calories. A high-fiber breakfast is almost guaranteed to curtail your hunger throughout the day.

The antioxidants in whole grains work together with fiber and other compounds to lower your risk for cancers, heart disease, and diabetes—by 30 to 40 percent, according to recent studies. In addition, the fiber in grains contributes to digestive health by keeping you regular.

Convinced? Good! Now, here's some advice. When buying bread, pasta, cereals, or even crackers, check the ingredients on the nutrition label. Whole wheat, whole oats, or whole something-or-other should be listed first. Use brown basmati rice or wild rice to increase your fiber. And look for bulgur—it's simply broken-up whole wheat, and it's loaded with fiber. Use it instead of couscous or white rice, which have little nutritional value.

BOTTOM LINE: Lose 21 pounds

If you eat a serving of whole grain at each meal, and if it keeps you from eating an extra slice of bread or that extra half cup of pasta, you'll save 100 calories at lunch and dinner—that's 200 calories a day!

#27. Eat More Pizza

Did you know that Native Americans taught the Pilgrims how to prepare a slice of flame-seared pizza on an oyster shell—and that's why the Pilgrims praised God on the first Thanksgiving?

Okay, enough silly historical revisionism. You get my drift. You can't get more American than pizza. And you can't get much healthier food, as long as you exercise some control over your choices.

Two slices of a cheese-only pizza from Domino's, assuming it's the 12-inch variety, will set you back 375 calories. An entire individually sized cheese pizza, with a thin crust, has 1,100 calories.

Even better are the frozen pizzas you make at home, either in the oven or in the microwave. (I recommend oven-baked because it has a crispier crust, and only takes a few minutes longer.) Check the calories on the box. Chances are, they'll total about 600. Even if you eat the whole thing yourself, you're getting a reasonably healthy meal.

Let's forget weight loss for a minute and talk about pizza sauce. All of those tomatoes in the sauce are loaded with lycopene, an antioxidant nutrient that has been shown to reduce the risk of prostate cancer in men and of heart disease. And since most men classify pizza as one of the main food groups, they're getting excellent protection!

BOTTOM LINE: Lose 3–6 pounds
Pretend it's Friday night and you're enjoying a homemade or frozen pizza instead of the usual greasy carryout. You'll save anywhere from 200 to 400 calories!

#28. Shop at the Farmers' Market

I'll never forget those tomatoes. They were soft, plump, sweet, and deep red—the kind you only get fresh from the vine.

One of my favorite childhood memories is the taste of my grandmother's vine-ripened tomatoes. Every year, she grew at least 20 tomato plants— and only tomatoes—in her backyard in Columbus, Ohio. They were her favorite vegetable, and they became mine too.

It's funny how childhood experiences stay with us. Today, when I shop at a nearby farmers' market, I still revel in those feelings. Physically I am in downtown Washington, D.C., but mentally and emotionally I am picking my grandmother's tomatoes in Columbus!

Enough nostalgia. In my practice, I often instruct clients to visit farmers' markets in their neighborhoods. This has nothing to do with warm and fuzzy; it's because I've found that they lose weight even when they don't make any other changes.

Here's what happens. You go to the farmers' market and stock up on beautiful produce. The more fresh and delicious produce you eat, the less junk you consume, and the more weight you lose.

BOTTOM LINE: Lose 36 pounds

Fresh produce from a farmers' market will make you hungry for a salad every day. Adding salads or vegetable soup to your daily meals will help you cut back on other, more fattening foods. Those delicious fresh fruits do the same thing. You'll lose an impressive amount of weight—and that's without dieting!

#29. Steal a TV

One of my clients, Debbie, was furious when she discovered that her television had been stolen when she was on vacation. But a few weeks later came the unexpected surprise: She was losing weight.

I've heard variations of this story before, and it makes a certain amount of sense.

Watching television doesn't require a tremendous amount of concentration, so we often do other things at the same time—eating being one of the main ones.

Most of us enjoy nibbling chips, popcorn, candies, or other snacks while we're watching TV. Because our minds are on the television, we're not really paying attention to how our bodies are feeling, which means we often consume more calories than we need.

Try something creative. Make a pact with a friend: "I'll 'steal' your TV if you 'steal' mine. We'll donate both of the 'stolen' TVs to Goodwill."

Once the TV is out of the house or in a "TV room" away from where you eat, you'll almost automatically snack less. Plus, think about all the free time you'll have. You won't have any choice but to find more creative things to do, and the more creative and busy you are, the less vulnerable you'll be to food cravings.

BOTTOM LINE: Lose 27 pounds

I sometimes advise people to think of TV as the equivalent of having a 19-inch brownie in the house. If you give it up, you're going to give up calories at the same time—probably about 300 a night.

#30. Lose with Tailoring

Baggy clothes get more and more attractive when you've gained extra weight. They're comfortable, and they also hide what's happening with your body. Can you say "denial"?

Nearly everyone I know has a closetful of out-sized clothing—skirts, blouses, and pants that are a few sizes larger than they used to be. I understand the temptation to let out your clothes or buy larger sizes when you've gained extra weight, but it's the wrong thing to do.

It's all about psychology. "Fat" clothes can make you feel fat. They're also a sign that you've accepted being heavy.

Do just the opposite. Even when you're home alone, wear clothes that fit well. Forget the baggy robe or sweat pants. Wear a form-fitting leotard or fitted pants. You'll feel good when you wear good clothes, you'll also be reminded to think slim, and you'll be less likely to overeat if it feels uncomfortable (or worse—if it shows!). Any reminder to consume fewer calories can be helpful when you're trying to shed pounds.

BOTTOM LINE: Lose 9 pounds

Suppose that wearing fitting clothes around the house reminds you of your long-term fitness goals and keeps you from eating from a 300-calorie snack on the weekends. You're going to lose weight!

#31. Splurge on Expensive Delicacies

One of my clients, Sally, loves hearts of palm. She rarely buys those little cans, however, because they're frighteningly expensive. Then she had a revelation.

Hearts of palm are very low in calories. True, a single can may cost more than a full meal, but Sally figured that the high cost would be more than offset by the calorie savings and improved health.

Here's what she did. She started buying hearts of palm and keeping them on her shelf. Why? Because she loves adding them to salads. She realized that if she could enjoy hearts of palm every night, she would eat salads every night, and that in turn would help her control her weight. That's good value for the money!

Maybe you have a passion for shrimp, kiwi fruit, or crab meat. Don't worry about the cost (remember, you're not using huge amounts). Think about all of the delicious, nutritious meals you'll be able to make. If having a special food in the house helps you eat more of the foods you know are good for you, the cost is justified.

And the cost, incidentally, will be lower than you think. When you're eating more healthful foods, you'll naturally buy fewer junk foods, and when you're at a healthy weight, you have half the medical costs. So you'll actually be saving money.

BOTTOM LINE: Lose 20 pounds

I mentioned earlier that adding a salad to your lunch and dinner can save you 200 calories. If adding your favorite delicacy helps you eat those salads, you could lose 20 pounds!

#32. Join Martha Stewart

You probably have a hobby that you'd like to take up, but can never find the time. Well, make the time! Hobbies are a lot of fun, and they can help you lose weight.

Sewing gives me great pleasure. I do it in the evenings after work, and it helps me forget about the day's frustrations and worries. Plus, I get to create beautiful things I can wear. What could be better for a clotheshorse like me?

I regularly take classes from an expert sewer. This past year, I learned how to make perfectly fitting pants for the first time. I now have three basic pants patterns: pleated baggy pants, flat front straight-legged pants, and casual drawstring pants, all in a variety of fabrics.

Sewing is obviously my thing. What's yours? You may enjoy making window treatments, place settings, or holiday presents. Maybe you've always thought about collecting coins, painting, or playing the piano. My friend Linda started piano lessons at age 40, and it's enriched her life.

Hobbies are a wonderful way to relax and unwind. They keep your mind and hands busy—and out of the pantry or refrigerator all of those times when you're feeling tired or a little bored.

BOTTOM LINE: Lose 9 pounds

I've never done the math, but I suspect that my hobby has saved me hundreds of thousands of calories over the years. I figure that if I sew 2 evenings a week, and avoid the snacks I would have had otherwise, I can save 600 calories.

#33. Reduce Noise Pollution

Have you noticed that the sounds of work have gotten louder? Instead of the whisking of a rake, we're bombarded with the blast of leaf blowers. When's the last time you heard the tsk-tsk of a push mower? Sure, power tools are easy to use—and that's precisely the problem.

A quick equation: If you clear your yard with a leaf blower, you'll burn about 4 calories a minute. Use a rake, you'll burn 6 calories. Doesn't sound like much? Well, consider this.

Jobs done with traditional tools take longer than those done with power tools. This means you're going to get more exercise no matter what. Let's assume that you mow your lawn 10 times during the summer (and have to remove the clippings), and you rake leaves twice during the fall. I don't know how big your yard is, but we'll further assume that your total calorie expenditure with the leaf blower is about 60, while plying the rake burns 80 calories.

Guess what? That's enough to lose a pound right there. If you have a lot of trees, a wide expanse of grass, and you're particular about the way your yard looks, you're going to lose impressive amounts of weight.

BOTTOM LINE: Lose 5 pounds

Hand tools don't require gas or much in the way of maintenance, and they're great for your health. And they're a heck of a lot quieter than power tools, which will make your neighbors very happy! Lose 5 pounds for every season you rake by hand.

#34. March for a Cause

Many health and political organizations sponsor marches to raise money as well as awareness. It's a chance to make your voice heard—and get some exercise at the same time.

A client of mine lost her mother to breast cancer, and decided to get involved. To honor her mother and help raise money for breast cancer research, she signed up for a 3-day, 60-mile walk.

Walking 60 miles, if you haven't done it lately, is a heck of a lot of exercise. At the very least, it requires a few weeks (and preferably months) of training. And that's what my client Renee did. She took a lot of shorter walks in order to get in shape for the big event. By the time the march rolled around, she had already lost 30 pounds.

Since then, she has gotten involved in a number of other causes, and marching has become her way of speaking out. She appreciates the exercise, especially because she's helping herself and others at the same time. As a bonus, getting involved in causes has increased her sense of confidence and self-worth, and this in turn has encouraged her to lose weight and look her best.

BOTTOM LINE: Lose 60 pounds

Getting involved in community and national causes is a great way to pump extra meaning into your life. And if you walk 40–50 miles a week, you can expect to lose about 60 pounds.

#35. The Amazing Sandwich

Lunch should supply important nutrients, be reasonably low in calories, and keep your energy high all afternoon. The humble sandwich does all three.

I love sandwiches, salads, and soups for lunch. I feel particularly good, and am most productive, on afternoons when I haven't overeaten. At the same time, I need to eat enough so that I won't have cravings a few hours later.

The easiest way to meet these goals is to make a sandwich—assuming, of course, you have the fixings on hand. The next time you go shopping, pick up a loaf of whole-wheat bread, a jar of mayonnaise ("lite," if you prefer), sliced reduced-fat cheese, and several luncheon meats. Today's stores have lean versions of everything: lean bologna, turkey bologna, extra-lean ham—all kinds of lean. I've found that half a pound of cheese and a pound and a half of luncheon meats is enough to make a sandwich every day of the week.

A good sandwich also needs produce. I might buy 14 tomatoes at the farmers' market, so I can have 2 tomatoes each day for lunch. I'll also pick up bags of greens for green salads. (Out of season, I buy greens at the grocery store.) For salad dressing, I'll buy a bottle of "lite" whatever, or I'll make my own vinaigrette at home.

BOTTOM LINE: Lose 21 pounds

When I have all the necessary ingredients and prepare my own lunch, it saves me at least 200 calories daily. As an added bonus, I feel alert all afternoon because I haven't overeaten.

#36. Hit the Ground Running

No one believes me when I tell them that they can burn 600 calories before going to work or before even waking up! They look even more surprised when I explain that it's the best way to do it.

Everyone knows they should exercise. Some people even want to exercise. But it's virtually impossible to do once you've embarked on the daily routine of carpooling children, getting through the workday, or running from class to class. Let's be honest: Even on those days when you plan to exercise, you'll often find a way to cancel it.

Try this: Wake up in the morning. Yawn. Roll out of bed, go to the bathroom, have a drink of water, and slip on some exercise clothes. Don't check e-mail or phone messages. Start moving. Now! Right away! Exercising first thing in the morning is one of the best things you'll ever do for yourself. And before you know it, it's over with before you're even awake!

Here are some of the reasons. (1) Showering after your exercise session will relax and awaken you at the same time. (2) Morning exercise is like taking an energy pill. You'll drink less coffee, which means your entire day will go better—and you won't experience that afternoon dip in your attention span. (3) You'll know that you've done it! Exercise is out of the way, so you don't have to wonder when you're going to fit it in. You'll be able to spend the rest of the day concentrating on all the other things you want to do.

A SUCCESS STORY
Dan, one of my clients, is an adviser to corporations around the world. Once his day starts, he's at the mercy of his clients, who include secretaries of state and members of the president's cabinet. Dan loves his job. He loves it so much that he would much rather please his clients than take care of himself.

From long experience, Dan has learned that he has to exercise first thing in the morning. If he doesn't, it will never happen.

Without fail, he gets on a treadmill for 30 minutes every morning before he goes to the office. Three times a week, he meets with a personal trainer—early in the morning, of course.

Oh, one more thing. Dan did something radical in the business world: He adopted a no-breakfast-meetings policy. What has this intransigence cost him? Well, he's still in demand—and he's lost 20 pounds in the few months since he started!

BOTTOM LINE: Lose 28–42 pounds

All it takes is 30 minutes in the morning: Just walking briskly will burn up to 28 pounds in a year. Jogging on a treadmill will burn even more. Another great thing about morning exercise: You do it at the best time of day, without midday heat to contend with.

#37. Lead a Snake Dance

You can lose an amazing amount of weight just by having more fun in your life—especially when you're having that fun on company time.

Let me tell you about Jay. A computer whiz (and a client), Jay used to sit on his butt all day in front of his monitor. Largely because of his lack of activity for at least 8 hours a day, Jay found himself registering 250 pounds on the scale.

My solution: I advised Jay to become the founding member of the "Tour d'office." Every hour on the hour throughout the day, Jay starts a brisk, 5-minute walk down the office corridors. He invites everyone to follow him, and they wind through the halls doing a snake dance.

It's not the type of thing that seems like exercise, but it is—very good exercise, I might add. See if you can do something similar without interrupting work too much. Snake through the halls. Dance around the cafeteria or in the parking lot. Bring along a portable CD player and blast Caribbean rhythms to spur everyone on.

Other ideas: Take pictures of all the fun and post them on the office bulletin board; set up (non-food) rewards for the people who participate consistently; and get the boss involved (good luck!).

BOTTOM LINE: Lose 24 pounds

If you follow Jay's plan and move at a brisk pace, you'll find yourself burning about 8 calories per minute; 40 calories in 5 minutes; 320 calories each work day; and 83,000 calories a year!

#38. Buy Better Dairy

Milk and other dairy foods are incredibly nutritious. Too bad they're also fattening—unless you choose wisely.

Many of my clients won't touch dairy foods because they don't want the extra calories. I gently try to set them straight. Dairy products are by far the best source of calcium, the mineral that protects against osteoporosis. Traditional dairy products are high in saturated and artery-clogging fat. But things have changed. If your goal is to lose weight, there are many fantastic dairy products that will help you do it.

Suppose you switch from whole milk to 2 percent: you'll save 20 calories per serving. Switch from 2 percent to skim: another 20 calories saved. Low- or reduced-fat cheeses can save you 30 to 50 calories per ounce, depending on the type you buy. And substituting low-fat yogurt for whole yogurt saves at least 50 calories per cup.

Even if you are lactose-intolerant, you should be able to drink half a cup of milk 4 times a day without symptoms. Lactase-fortified milk can help. You can add lactase tablets to milk before drinking it. Or you can have milk, cheese, or yogurt made with soy, which doesn't cause discomfort.

Important: When buying soy products, check the label to make sure they're calcium fortified. Each serving should provide a third of the daily calcium requirement, just as dairy products do.

BOTTOM LINE: Lose 16 pounds

Substitute 3 daily servings of low-fat dairy food for the full-fat kind, and you'll cut out about 150 calories daily.

#39. Say "Hi" to Your Feet

Believe it or not, your feet should do more than keep a footstool company in front of the TV. In the primitive days of yore, they were actually used for locomotion!

Americans don't walk very much anymore. We're also heavier than ever before. Hmm...I wonder if there's a connection?

Robert, one of my clients, is a case in point. He wasn't much of a walker, and he was having a heck of a time losing weight. Then the elevator at his office went on the blink. He started walking up the stairs out of necessity.

One thing led to another. He kept taking the stairs even when the elevator was repaired, and he walked at other times, as well. Did he lose weight? Yes—and he did it with almost no effort and without dieting.

To reacquaint yourself with your feet, you could follow Robert's example and use stairs instead of elevators. Or climb the stairs part of the way, then take the elevator the rest.

Another tip: When you drive to work, park at the far reaches of the parking lot and walk the rest of the way. It won't add up to heavy exercise, but it will make a difference.

BOTTOM LINE: Lose 11–22 pounds

Climbing stairs consumes, on average, 15 calories per minute. Let's say you do it for 10 minutes each work day. In a year's time you'll lose 11 pounds. Climb those same stairs for another 10 minutes at your lunch break and you'll lose at least twice that much. In just minutes.

#40. Win with Gadgets

Basic kitchen tools are important. But to lose weight, there's no substitute for good kitchen gadgets.

I'm not talking about lemon zesters and in-the-shell egg beaters—those intriguing utensils that people buy, use once, then lose at the bottom of a kitchen drawer. I'm talking about gadgets that reduce fat consumption, control calories, and make batch cooking a dream.

What you have to have:

• Two nonstick 8" or 10" sauté pans. You'll use a lot less fat with nonstick coatings.
• 2-quart and 3-quart sauce pans.
• A heavy-duty stockpot—perfect for large batch recipes.
• A food scale to help you get a handle on proper serving sizes.
• Plastic containers that are freezer- and microwave-safe. Get large as well as portion-sized containers.
• Baggies for leftovers, cut-up fruits and vegetables, and for taking lunch to the office. Get pint, quart, and half-gallon sizes

BOTTOM LINE: Lose 12–52 pounds

If you make every recipe in nonstick utensils, and use one less table-spoon of oil a day, you'll save 120 calories—and lose up to 12 pounds—in a year. Packing a container with a healthy lunch will save you 400 calories a day, compared to what you'd consume if you splurged in a restaurant. That healthy fruit snack in a baggie? It has about 150 fewer calories than many high-fat snacks. As for portion control, count on saving 250 calories daily because you won't over-estimate the amount you need to eat. We all tend to be overly generous to ourselves that way!

#41. Breathe Deeply

Before you eat anything, take your food to the table.
Sit down, close your eyes, and take three or four
deep breaths to relax your mind and body.

Do this with *every* morsel of food you consume, whether it's a peanut or
a slice of pot roast—or even the tasting that you do when you're cooking.
Hey, what's wrong with slowing down? I'm not suggesting "do not eat."
All I'm saying is that you should take the time to sit down and really get
to know that you are eating, and what you are eating.

Step back in time for a moment. When you were an infant, and later
as a child, you knew when you were hungry, when you were not hungry,
and when you were satisfied after being hungry. You ate and stopped eating appropriately in response to those signals. No matter how delicious a
food was, or how much you loved it, if you weren't hungry, your mother
could not get you to eat it. If you don't believe me, ask her!

As the years went by, you (along with every other human adult on the
planet) began to eat in response to external signals. For example:

• **Time of day:** "Hey, it's dinner time" or "You can't eat now, it's not time."
• **The presence of food:** "Look at that delicious pie! Let's have some!"
• **Pleasing a loved one:** "I made your favorite key lime pie, honey, have
a piece."
• **Parental reinforcement:** "If you're good, you'll get some caramels!"
• **Anger:** "You can't have any, you've been bad!"
• **Feelings:** "Have some ice cream, you'll feel better."

All of these are reasons for eating—and none have anything to do with
hunger!

Learning to listen to your body's *real* hunger signals all over again is
one of the keys to long-term weight maintenance. It takes practice and
attention, but awareness is the first step. Once you master eating in
response to your body's signals, your body will fall back into its natural
healthy shape, and stay there forever.

▌BOTTOM LINE: Lose 17 pounds

One of my clients, Michael, is a big eater. When he started to practice "mindful" eating, he was amazed to discover that he was often perfectly content to leave food on his plate. In other words, he was satisfied with less than he was before. If you eat out a lot in restaurants, where portions are extra large, mindful eating can make an impressive difference. If, for example, being deeply aware of your body and the food in front of you causes you to eat two fewer slices of bread than usual, you'll save 160 calories. That really adds up!

#42. More Snacking, Fewer Calories

Bet you never heard that before. But it's true: People who snack between meals find it easier to lose weight because they actually take in fewer calories.

"Snack" is a loaded word. In our society, it has come to mean something "extra," or at least fattening. That's not the way to think of it. Snacks give you calories when you need them. Snacks keep you satisfied, so you're less likely to experience runaway hunger or emotional cravings.

Snacks have to be planned, of course. Otherwise, you'll find yourself stuck with whatever's available, even if that means foraging in your coworker's desk.

My favorite snack is fresh fruit. It gives you a sweet fix and it makes you feel full, but not too full. If fruit alone doesn't satisfy your hunger, try garnishing it. Smear a tablespoon of peanut butter on your crunchy apple—yum! The peanut butter only adds 90 calories, and they are 90 satisfying and healthy calories. Or have a handful (a small one) of nuts along with the apple.

Other options: Have an ounce of cheese with your fruit. Or, if you're really hungry, some yogurt. Midday snacks reduce the amount or dinner you'll need, so you're more likely to eat light at night, which is important for weight loss.

BOTTOM LINE: Lose 19–26 pounds

If your healthy snack keeps you from your usual vending machine pick-me-up, you'll save about 250 calories right there. Do it every day, and you'll lose a lot of weight in a hurry.

#43. Turn on Your VCR

Your mother, your hairdresser, and your shrink have all told you to get at least 8 hours of sleep a night. So why aren't you doing it—especially now that you're trying to lose weight? Maybe it's time to enlist the help of your VCR.

I had never thought about VCRs as a tool for weight loss until I talked to Robert, an unusually discerning client who had struggled for a long time to keep his weight under control.

At some point, Robert began to pay attention to his nightly routine. He discovered an interesting pattern. By 10 o'clock at night, he was usually yawning and ready for bed, yet he stayed up until after midnight. Why? Because he was a Letterman freak. He couldn't bear to hit the sheets until he'd laughed at David's latest stupid pet tricks.

Upon further reflection, Robert realized that these Letterman comedy routines would be just as funny the next day. That's when his dust-gathering VCR came to the rescue. He began setting the VCR to tape that night's show. Once the machine was set, Robert went to bed. The next evening, right after dinner, he'd relax by watching the previous night's show. By 9:30 he was ready to reset the VCR once again.

ROBERT'S INVENTORY OF BENEFITS
We still haven't talked about why using a VCR in general, or taping Letterman in particular, helped Robert lose weight. Here are some of the reasons:

• Robert was now getting to bed early enough to pack in his eight hours of sleep. That made him more alert the next day—and the more alert he felt, the less likely he was to turn to snacks for "artificial" energy.
• Robert's late-night sessions with Letterman invariably involved munching. Getting his "late-night" TV fix right after dinner, when his stomach was already satisfied, meant fewer empty calories later on.
• Early to bed, early to rise. Robert found that he now had enough time

in the mornings to exercise and eat a healthful breakfast. Big-time calorie savings, there.

• For some clients, THIS IS IT! If you get enough sleep, exercise 30 minutes in the morning, eat a big breakfast and lighten up in the evenings, that's enough to lose all the weight you want and feel great forever. Just ask Vivien and Dan and Michael and Jay and . . . etc., etc.

BOTTOM LINE: Lose 16–66 pounds

Just cutting out late-night snacking saved Robert 150 calories a night. A healthy breakfast—and less snacking later—added up to more saved calories, and his newfound exercise routines also did their part. To break it down, Robert stood to lose 16 pounds by not snacking at night, 20 pounds from the exercise, and another 30 pounds by preparing his own breakfast, which prevented him from indulging in the 200-calorie midmorning doughnut and from attacking lunch and saving at least 100 calories there. Love that Letterman!

#44. Listen When You Chew

Actually, you don't have to go that far. But you should focus your entire attention on your food. Enjoy and savor every bite.

Too often, our meals are overwhelmed by distractions. The TV in the background. Music on the stereo. The newspaper propped against a cereal box. Add internal distractions, such as work worries, and the food itself gets scant attention.

Why is this a problem? Because when you eat on autopilot, when your mind is somewhere else, you don't enjoy your food very much. More important, "mindless" eating generally turns into overeating. When eating doesn't provide psychological satisfaction, you'll crave more food than your body actually needs.

Eating a delicious meal deserves your entire attention. After all, you're feeding your body, and what's more important than that? So turn off the electronic gizmos. Think about what you're eating: the taste, texture, aroma, and so on. If you're dining with someone, put your fork down when you want to talk. Pick it up again when you're ready to pay attention to the food.

This is especially important at work. Get away from your desk if you can—and if you can't, at least don't talk on the phone or work while you eat.

BOTTOM LINE: Lose 21 pounds

Once you start focusing your attention on the food in front of you, you'll almost automatically eat a little less. In fact, even if you leave only a few extra bites on your plate, it could add up to a savings of 200 or more calories daily.

#45. Walk Somewhere...Anywhere

When we were infants, we couldn't wait to get off our knees and start walking. Now that we're adults, it's a different part of our bodies that we have to get off of.

Does your derriere get more of a workout than your legs? That's a real problem if you're trying to lose weight.

The solution isn't hard-core exercise (sigh of relief). All you really have to do is get walking. Long, brisk walks are good, but so are strolls and ambles. Walking the dog. Going to the mailbox. Any kind of walking will help you burn calories and lose weight.

Where you walk is up to you, but make it someplace pleasant that will contribute to your motivation. If you have to drive to get to your starting point, at least that's putting the buggy to good use! You'll walk a lot more if the place you like to walk is easy to get to.

Helpful: Buy an inexpensive pedometer at a sporting goods store. You'll have an accurate record of how far you're walking, which is great for motivation. Wear comfortable walking shoes, as well as layers of clothing to take off as you get warm, or put back on when you're cooling off.

BOTTOM LINE: Lose 6-14 pounds

Walking briskly for 1 mile 3 times a week, will add up to about 21,060 calories burned in a year. Do it every day, and you'll lose impressive amounts of weight in a hurry!

#46. Write It and Lose It

The food diary is the main tool for self-examination of your eating habits.

Socrates told us that the road to wisdom is to know ourselves. This is never more true than in your eating habits.

It is important that you begin observing objectively what you eat and the way you eat, for this is the cornerstone of your program: your own observations.

That's what Frank discovered. Frank, a 39-year-old defense department employee, lost 2 pounds during a week in which he was simply keeping a diary. He swore he ate normally, just as usual—and even ate everything he wanted. The same thing happened with Deborah. She was shocked (pleasantly!) when she stepped on the scale and found she'd lost 4 pounds. And Miriam, a 50-year-old writer, found that keeping the diary helped stop her weight from spiraling upward, where it had been going for several weeks, if not months.

The reason: Just paying attention was enough to make a difference! The diary, called a self-monitoring device in behavior modification lingo, plays three important roles.

First, if it is kept at the time of eating or within 15 minutes, it can change behavior as behavior occurs—and without your even realizing it or trying to change. For instance, Ella, a wife, mother of two, and government lawyer, found that she was consuming most of her day's calories—almost subconsciously—while cooking dinner. This was happening so automatically that she didn't even know she was doing it until she began writing it down. Of course, having to write down every little item while she was trying to cook became tiresome, so her desire to eat decreased. Also, just the realization that she was, in effect, eating two dinners every night gave her impetus to change.

Debra C., on the other hand, found that without even thinking about it, she grabbed M&Ms from a coworker's candy bowl every time she walked by. This, of course, began adding up after the eighth or tenth time! And because she was grabbing the candies on the go, she wasn't even tasting or enjoying them. Her heightened awareness began to inhibit the behavior.

Peter H. found he didn't even know he was eating or how much, since others always prepared his food—until he began observing, asking questions, and started seeing it written down in black and white.

The diary allows you to differentiate between unconscious eating and savoring what you really enjoy. All of these people are successes. They may not have been perfect, nor have lost weight, but they kept the diary at the time of eating and learned about themselves and their eating habits. And none of them realized they had made changes until we looked over their week's diary in detail.

Research shows this way of changing is more likely to succeed long term: that is, observing your behaviors and making decisions about changes to make. I am simply your guide, helping you discover and learn, whereas *you* are the creator and owner of your own success.

The second function of the food diary is simply learning. At the end of each day, week or month, you can look back and analyze for yourself what style of eating works for you.

This brings us to the third function of the diary, which is helping you individualize your weight-loss program so that it fits into your lifestyle and is something you enjoy living with. Now, isn't this the only way to do things?

Individualizing your plan is critical to your long-term success because nothing can last unless it is enjoyable and works into your lifestyle. Through keeping the diary consistently, you can find that perfect "middle ground" for you. You will be able to eat in a way which you enjoy and can live with, but which also achieves your weight and health goals.

BOTTOM LINE: Lose 23 pounds

If keeping the diary enhances your attentiveness and helps you eat less here or there or even think twice about that vending machine candy bar, you could save 220 calories per day.

CHAPTER 9

How to Help Your (Unsuspecting) Husband Lose Weight

Especially appropriate for: *Commuting Dads, Stressed Executives, Monday-Morning Quarterbacks.*

Jack, my significant other, is pretty straightforward about food: He sees it, he eats it—quickly and uncritically. Now, this characteristic is good and it's bad. It's good because anything I fix him, he loves. It's bad because if I'm not the one fixing his food, there's no telling what he's inhaling.

The more you can set a good example for your family, including your husband, the more likely he is to eat and prefer whatever you make available. Though you can't have total control, this chapter will give you ideas about ways you can help your husband—without nagging.

It's important you don't have food in the house unless everyone has free access to it. So fill your home with healthy, wholesome foods everyone can enjoy.

WALK THE WALK
Model the eating habits you want your husband to adopt. Criticizing and controlling doesn't work. But if your offer is to "do as I do, not as I say,"

155

your husband will have respect for your help and advice.

Above all, don't force the situation. In the end, your husband will lose weight only if he wants to. All you can do is your best, which means keeping your own and your husband's environment as healthy as possible. Here are some ways to do that.

#47. Make Exercise Dates

I'm not suggesting you stop enjoying restaurants. But instead of making eating out your primary entertainment, find other ways to be together on a date.

When Jack and I first met, I wanted to establish some healthy routines, so instead of relying on dinner out as our major activity together, I suggested we take walks. Jack loves to walk—and talk—and so he loved the idea. We really got to know each other during those long strolls together and still try to get in at least one long walk a week.

My client Isabel decided to walk regularly with her husband, and she says she enjoys those times together more than any other. When you're walking, it's just the two of you and no distractions. You can discuss your day at work, your week ahead, or just enjoy nature.

Walking, of course, isn't your only option. There are so many fun physical activities you can do together. Go bowling, skating, dancing, tour a zoo or a museum, golf together, go swimming or biking together. The important point here is to link healthy, pleasurable physical activities with quality time together. It won't even seem like you're exercising—because you're not! You're having fun together, communicating and burning calories while you're at it.

BOTTOM LINE: Lose 9 pounds

With just one long (4-mile) walk a week, your man can burn 500–600 calories. That's a weight loss of 9 pounds in one year.

#48. A Breakfast Bar Is Not Enough!

Undereating is the main cause of overeating. Men particularly need to start their day with a large, wholesome breakfast.

In today's fast-paced world, it seems as if we're always running a few minutes late. Your husband is probably inclined to rush out the door for work without having had a solid breakfast. This is *not* a great way to start the day, particularly if weight loss is the goal.

Men have high calorie needs and high metabolic needs. They're just plain bigger and need more food. Yet breakfast is the most common meal for them to skimp on.

Skimping at breakfast means he'll start craving soon after arriving at the office. It means he'll be grabbing the office doughnuts or cookies whenever they're passed around and probably become a frequent visitor at the vending machine, searching for junk food. It means he'll be ordering burgers and fries or greasy Chinese for lunch. When he's hungry, he just can't help it!

As we've seen, studies confirm that weight loss maintainers eat breakfast. That's why it's important he get a nice, big breakfast every morning—one you provide him or teach him to provide for himself.

Most men need at least 700 calories at breakfast to start their day. To find out your man's calorie needs, go to the "Metabolism Toolbox" on page 461. Once you determine his daily calorie needs for weight loss, divide that number by three, and you have the recommended calorie levels for each of his daily meals.

Be sure and provide a breakfast that matches his preferences. If he's in a hurry and likes a simple, cold-cereal breakfast, that's great. Or if he enjoys a hot bowl of oatmeal, the sky's the limit as to the options. But make sure he gets enough, and be sure to include nuts or a healthy fat and protein of some kind, because it'll make him feel full longer.

To make life easier for him, have cereal and a measured amount of nuts on the kitchen counter so all he has to do is pour the milk and grab the fruit. Or, try the "to go" breakfast, which is a simple peanut butter sandwich, yogurt, and fruit, all of which he can grab and eat at the office (hopefully *not* in his car!).

Another important reason for him to eat a good breakfast: fiber. Men should eat at least 38 grams a day, according to the latest guidelines by the National Academy of Sciences' Food and Nutrition Board. It's possible to get that amount if he's eating a high-fiber breakfast, but nearly impossible without one.

BOTTOM LINE: Lose 20 pounds

Provide your man with a healthy breakfast and save the doughnut calories. He can lose 20 pounds in a year this way.

#49. Send Him to Work with Terrific Snacks

Men love healthy food as much as anyone else. If they don't eat it, the problem is usually access. So the key is to make sure he has healthy foods that are easily accessible, but make sure they're delicious things he'll enjoy. If it's there, he'll eat it!

Unfortunately in most work environments there is no shortage of unhealthy, high-calorie eating options lurking around every corner. Vending machines with their candy bars and chips; bakery shops with their super-sized cookies, muffins, and bagels; secretaries with bowls and plates loaded with cookies, doughnuts, and candies; and fast food establishments on nearly every block. Experts say we live in an obesegenic society—a society that actually promotes obesity—because we're inundated with so much tempting food.

A good way to help keep your husband from succumbing to these temptations is to send him off to work with healthy snacks that will sustain him throughout the day and help him turn away from the omnipresent candy bars and salted chips.

Due to my encouragement, Jack has gotten into the habit of bringing at least three pieces of fruit with him each day to the office. And I don't even have to remind him anymore. Of course, that means we have to buy 21 servings of fruit every Sunday at the farmers' market, just for Jack! But he's gotten so that he loves picking out his fruit for the week. (Yes, it's taken several years to get to this point.)

I like to mix high-volume, filling, low-calorie foods, like fruits or vegetables, with calorie-dense, lean proteins or healthy fats, which will help him feel full longer. Remember that healthy balance helps you eat just the right amount of calories to make you feel satisfied.

Some snack ideas:

• One ounce of his favorite nuts (160–180 calories) with a piece of fruit (60) and some yogurt (100–200)

- One ounce of crackers (100) or a sliced apple (60) and a tablespoon of peanut butter (90)
- fruit salad (100) mixed with nuts (160)
- yogurt (100–200), wheat germ (50), and fruit (60)

BOTTOM LINE: Lose 30 pounds

A healthy snack containing 200–300 calories beats the super-sized cookie (600) or microwave popcorn every time. Help him lose 30 pounds in a year.

#50. Send Him Off with His Favorite Lunch

Pressed for time and opting for convenience, your man is likely to purchase a lunch that would break your heart—and expand his waistline.

Probably one of the greatest challenges people face in keeping their weight down is the lunch they have during the work day. Sometimes they even skip lunch—a situation hazardous to self-control later.

But take heart, there is one very reasonably healthy, cost- and time-saving option: bringing a lunch to work (how retro, you say?). In a perfect world, he'll prepare his own lunch, which includes tasty and healthy batch leftovers or sandwiches made with lean meats. You may have to get him started down this road by packing a lunch or two for him and showing him what a reasonable and delicious alternative this is to his time-consuming, expensive, and high-calorie take-out or restaurant meals at work.

If he has access to a microwave and you've made a gourmet batch meal on the weekend (see Recipes starting on page 401), simply pack a plastic container full of one of his favorite dishes, like Tallmadge's White Beans with Garlic and Basil. If your man enjoys meat, throw in some healthy, spicy sausage. For balance, simply add a fruit or vegetable. And, voilá! A fabulous lunch for your loved one.

Of course, everyone loves a great sandwich and this is a perfect alternative to something that has to be heated up. Choose a whole-grain, high-fiber bread so it's full of flavor and adds to his fullness. Next, choose a lean luncheon meat. Today's grocery store deli sections have a huge number of choices to choose from. Pick up some extra-lean ham or roast beef, fresh turkey, or chicken. You can even buy extra-lean pastrami and corned beef. Today's reduced-fat cheeses are full of flavor. Add a tablespoon—or two—of his favorite mayonnaise (I've found a delicious canola mayo)—depending on his calorie needs. And don't forget the tomato, lettuce, onion, and pickle!

If you want to try something new, try some spicy soy cheese or vegetarian hot dogs or meats on his sandwich.

To balance out the lunch, in a plastic container, pack a salad with a light vinaigrette (depending on his calorie needs) or even a serving of soup in a thermos. Pack the sandwich in an insulated bag with an ice pack to keep it nice and fresh. It may be a good idea to separate the veggies from the sandwich to prevent the bread from getting soggy.

Today, we're at the office for most of our waking lives. I'm sure your man is no exception. That means it'll be worth it to help him surround himself with delicious, healthy, and wholesome foods that are easy to grab and fill him up—but not out!

BOTTOM LINE: Lose 22–50 pounds

By taking his lunch to the office, at about 700 calories, he'll save at least 300 to 800 calories by not buying a burger and fries or greasy Chinese meal. If he does this five days a week, he can lose 22 to 50 pounds in one year.

#51. Healthy, Light Dinners

The next time your special guy comes home looking tired and hungry, offer to cook him a burger, but make it a turkey or veggie burger. And instead of a huge serving of fries, give him a heaping salad.

The dinner meal is very significant for weight loss. Eating heavily in the evenings is the culprit behind many people's weight problems. There are a variety of factors contributing to evening being a very vulnerable time for overeating. If you haven't eaten properly during the day—at least two thirds of your day's calories before dinner—you're likely to be ravenous. And a ravenous person is not a rational person—the mouth becomes a Hoover (need I say more?). So many people tell me that if they don't eat well during the day, nothing seems to satisfy that deep sense of hunger that develops during the late afternoon. They have trouble stopping once they've started eating in the evening.

Evening is a time when people need to release pressure from the day. And if you don't have the stress management skills to deal with this pressure effectively, the first things you turn to are food and drink. This is why *Think Yourself Thin* is full of stress management strategies—so you can lead a healthier life by coping with your stresses appropriately rather than with food, drink, and excess calories.

Another potential evening pitfall is the activity you choose after dinner. Lately, it's become the American pastime to zone out in front of the TV. For many, this involves mindless munching on high-calorie snacks. *Think Yourself Thin* is full of ideas for you and your family to reduce TV watching and increase life-inspiring and life-enhancing activities—even if all you do is sleep! (Sleeping is better than overeating, and if your body tells you that you need to sleep, then maybe that's what you should be doing!)

So, after your man has eaten his healthy breakfast, lunch, and snacks for the day (comprising two-thirds of his calorie needs) and has spent some time changing clothes and relaxing at home after work, he'll be satisfied and happy with a delicious, light dinner.

One of the least understood truths of food and nutrition is that high-quality meals are also very tasty. As you prepare your evening meals, I recommend you try to make a renewed commitment to preparing delicious, fresh, healthy, and light dinners for your man and your family (or encourage him and your children to cook).

Your family will come to love and look forward to these dinners every evening. They'll come to recognize that heavy, bloat-promoting meals don't taste as good or feel as good. Lighter, healthier meals actually increase energy and increase the evening's enjoyment.

So many of my clients were worried that their husbands needed a heavy meal at night, but when they made the switch to lighter dinners, they were just as happy. You'll see: As long as the food tastes good, you present it in a positive way, and they can see you enjoying it too, your whole family will embrace any meals you choose to offer.

Everyone likes burgers, but sometimes people don't realize that turkey burgers and veggie burgers are every bit as delicious as ground beef packed with artery-clogging saturated fat and calories. Helping introduce this simple substitution into his life will be something he will appreciate.

Think Yourself Thin is full of simple, gourmet batch recipes so you can do most of your cooking on the weekends, and plan for the week ahead.

BOTTOM LINE: Lose 30 pounds

Save hundreds of calories by serving a light dinner. If your light dinner replaces one greasy take-out meal daily, count on saving at least 300 calories—and losing 30 pounds a year.

#52. Fill Your Home with Healthy Snacks and Desserts

My male clients tell me that the biggest influencing factor on what they eat is what's nearby. So stock up on apples, bananas, grapes, and other fruits to have at hand around the house.

Most people love to eat fresh vegetables with dips. On the weekend, clean and chop vegetables and make a healthy dip using fat-free sour cream, yogurt, or a dip such as hummus. If he loves nuts, divide them into 1-ounce portions and keep them in plastic baggies in the fridge.

I emphasize fruits and vegetables because they're so filling for so few calories. They also contain substances that are vital for health. Each fruit and vegetable is a little factory of nutrients and chemicals—called phyto-chemicals—with potent powers of healing. An apple alone contains more than 150 beneficial, disease-fighting chemicals. And these are substances you can't get from a pill. They act synergistically in the foods, so the whole is greater than the sum of its parts. While an apple has only 6 mg of vita-min C, it has 1,500 mg of vitamin C antioxidant activity because of the interaction of the vitamin C and the other nutrients in the apple.

The phytochemicals in fruits and vegetables have antioxidant effects, stimulate the immune system, enhance cancer-fighting enzymes, and even have antibacterial and antiviral effects.

All fruits and vegetables are terrific sources of nutrients, but some are superstars. In fruit, berries and purple grapes get the highest ratings. The greatest concentration of beneficial phytochemicals is generally found in the most colorful fruits and vegetables.

BOTTOM LINE: Lose 30 pounds

When nutrient-dense, low-calorie fruit and vegetable snacks replace calorie-dense nutrient-void junk food, save at least 100 calories per snack. If you eat three snacks a day, lose 30 pounds in a year.

#53. Negotiate Ground Rules for Eating

Sure, watching TV together can be fun and relaxing, and make for great quality time, but when you pair it with snacking it's a sure-fire way to pack on pounds.

Let me suggest that you discuss with your man some mutually agreed-upon practices about eating. This important subject is often neglected in households and unhealthy practices and habits often emerge if left to chance.

I have found people do better when eating is practiced mindfully. (See Tip #146.) Every bite is enjoyed and savored and there are no distractions when eating meals and snacks.

Your husband may balk at this at first—especially if he's used to noshing in front of the TV—but I've found that over time everyone in the family benefits from this style of eating. It strikes me as no coincidence that the emergence of the TV dinner has coincided with greater girth. Eating in front of the television is, by definition, a mindless activity that piles on calories without benefit.

Couple eating with other activities and you set up a situation where that activity can become a "trigger" to eat. This wreaks havoc with your body's natural need for you to eat in response to its internal cue, hunger.

It's also a good idea to serve food individually in the kitchen rather than "family style." You can serve reasonable portions, and the temptation of more food at the table doesn't influence how much food is eaten. This way, your husband is more likely to eat in response to his body signal. If he's still hungry after finishing his plate, he can get seconds. But my client, Lois, asks her man to wait 20 minutes so that he can be sure he's still hungry, because it may take that long for your meal to register in your brain.

BOTTOM LINE: Lose 30 pounds

Helping your husband adopt mindful eating could save at least 300 calories of night-time snacking. He could lose 30 pounds in a year.

#54. Stealthy Healthy Super Bowl Party

Most guys I know love to watch football. Left to their own devices, the food of choice may be chips, pretzels, or other junk food. Here's a way to go on the defense and tackle those calorie-laden snacks.

Pizza, subs, sausages—they're all popular sports-watching snacks. It's what's easy—and guys are used to it. But I've found that when you serve healthy, tasty alternatives, they're just as happy. So why not serve a plate of fresh fruit such as apple slices, grapes, and pineapple? How about a tray of fresh crudités: carrots, cucumbers, red peppers with a nice dip made with fat-free sour cream or a hummus-style dip?

My experience is that guys are pleasantly surprised at how delicious and enjoyable healthy foods are and they won't groan the next morning when they hop on the scale. I've also had men tell me how much more they enjoyed the party because they didn't feel bloated and uncomfortably stuffed.

More options are Barbara's Oven-Fried Chicken (see Tip #69), Tallmadge's Chile Non Carne (page 418) served with baked chips, or even Patrick O'Connell's Grilled Salmon (page 445).

BOTTOM LINE: Lose 15 pounds

Every Sunday, save your husband 1,000 calories by serving healthy party foods to him and his friends. He could lose 15 pounds in a year.

#55. Teach Him to Cook

You'd be surprised at how many guys really want to learn how to cook. So show him some of your low-cal chef's secrets—just be sure the fire extinguisher is handy!

Let's face it, a lot of modern guys just don't know how to cook. Born and bred on microwave or restaurant food, they've never felt the need to roll up their sleeves, step up to the stove, and prepare a meal. Admittedly, this experience can be something of a shock for the uninitiated, so take a little time and teach your man how to put together some basic meals that are easy and convenient, and include his favorite foods. Let him decide what he would enjoy learning.

When I first met Jack, he didn't know how to boil water. His kitchen cabinets and refrigerator were literally empty, except for beer and ketchup. He exclusively ate take-out food, fast food, and frozen meals. So I knew I had to start small. To begin, I taught Jack how to prepare a simple burrito so he would be less inclined to swing by the Chinese take-out on the way home. He simply dumps canned black beans into a flour tortilla, adds reduced-fat cheese, places the whole thing in the microwave, and voilà! A home-cooked meal. Add chopped tomatoes and peppers and you have a balanced lunch or dinner appropriate for his caloric needs.

Your man may have more intermediate cooking skills. My client Gary, who knew some cooking basics, was encouraged by his wife to cook one meal a week. He would choose a healthy stew, soup, or salad—like Tallmadge's White Beans or Chile Non Carne, and it also became his packed lunch the next day.

My client Louis was even more adventurous. A busy architect, once a week he cooked a fancy—but healthy—gourmet meal for his family. To make it more fun, he asked his sons what they would like to make and once they chose a Rabbit Stew from a healthy French cookbook. He was so pleased—and so was his family—that he could cook such a delicious and unique meal, which was also calorie-controlled and healthy.

No matter what his skill level, your husband will embrace cooking, I guarantee it. I'm so amazed that Jack, as inexperienced as he was in the kitchen, has come to love fixing meals for himself and me—as simple as they are. As a result, he achieved his weight goal.

BOTTOM LINE: Lose 30 pounds

Help your man participate in the kitchen so he can save hundreds of calories per meal. Lose 30 pounds in a year.

#56. The Cookout or Tailgate Party

Ssshhhh. Don't tell the guys, but you can actually turn that pre-football tailgate party your husband throws into a healthful event. Best of all, the food will be so delicious, he'll never suspect he's doing something that's good for him.

The secret is in the grilling. If he's the kind of guy who brings a portable grill or hibachi to the parking lot, he can cook up some chicken or salmon that's to die for! (See the grilled salmon recipe on page 445.) Even burgers can be a healthy choice if they're not made with meat that's dripping with fat. Make burgers leaner by choosing round steak and having the butcher grind it. Or he can grill filet mignon steaks or a tenderloin roast for a feast that's fit for a line-backer. For a down-under treat, he can put some shrimp on the barbie.

If you want to be really creative, make shish kebabs for him to take along, using lean meats such as chicken, pork tenderloin, and beef tenderloin. Any meat can be marinated in teriyaki sauce or another favorite marinade.

Everyone loves grilled veggies: Spray a little olive oil over veggies, salt and pepper to taste, and grill. Or pre-prepare his veggies at home. Slice them up; put them in a container; add olive oil, salt, and pepper; shake the mixture up; and he's good to go. Great, tasty choices include sliced mushrooms, sliced peppers, and sliced zucchini.

He can also snack on pretzels or fruit (Yes! Real men eat fruit!) cut up and ready to eat. And if he absolutely insists on bringing beer along (light beer is a better choice), send plenty of diet sodas, sparkling water, and slices of lime with him to dilute the effects of the alcohol.

BOTTOM LINE: Lose 15 pounds

If your man saves 1,000 calories every weekend, he could lose 15 pounds a year.

#57. Stretch Out with Yoga

A few calming moments of yoga eases tension, and can also ease your man's ravenous after-work appetite.

After a long, stressful day at work, most of us are inclined to relieve our stress by inhaling a quick meal, grabbing a beer or glass of wine, and plopping in front of the TV out of sheer exhaustion. There is another way.

When your man gets home from the office, why not do some real relaxation? Nothing beats a nice evening stroll, a backyard chat against the backdrop of relaxing music, a hot shower, or a few yoga stretching exercises for calming the nerves, forgetting work worries, and letting you and your man really enjoy your evening.

Yoga is one form of exercise that's actually quite relaxing. You may get a little resistance at first, which is why it would be most effective if you did it yourself and invited him along. Put on some soothing music and encourage him to change into something comfortable as soon as he arrives home. Ask him to join you to do a few stretches. Give him a refreshing glass of water or an herbal tea if he's thirsty.

Do the yoga stretches and deep breathing for at least 15 minutes and you may find his appetite is reduced and he'll be happy to wait for your light, healthy dinner.

BOTTOM LINE: Lose 50 pounds

Helping your man establish a relaxation ritual after work—or any time it's needed —will calm his mind, soothe his soul, and tame his appetite, saving him at least 500 calories in snacks and booze. He may lose 50 pounds in a year.

#58. Shed the Car, Shed Some Pounds

Stow that Subaru in the garage, give him bus and train schedules, and get him out there! An invigorating walk to work or to a bus-stop or train depot can energize him for the day, and work off excess pounds.

I once worked with a middle-aged man who was trim, vibrant, and full of energy, but insisted he never exercised. This struck me as unusual. As I probed further, he mentioned casually that he walked to work every day. Turns out, this was no ordinary walk. He set his schedule so that he left home an hour before he was due at the office and walked 4 miles to work every morning.

Not all of us can walk to work easily. But a lot more of us can do more walking than we sometimes realize. If your husband doesn't get regular exercise but enjoys walking, encourage him to walk all or some of the way to work. I have clients, for instance, who get off the bus or subway early so that they have a mile left to walk.

I've even had clients who moved closer to work so that they could walk. This, they felt, was an immense improvement in their quality of life—and it freed them from commuter hassles.

BOTTOM LINE: Lose 10 pounds

Walking just 1 extra mile a day can lead to a 10-pound weight loss in a year. Walk more, lose more.

#59. Recreational Day Trips or Spa Weekends

What better way to spend a Saturday afternoon than strolling along a beach, hiking through a park, canoeing down a river, or even climbing a gentle mountainside? Little will he suspect that he's working off that extra slice of pizza!

One of the best ways to clear your head, enjoy yourself, and re-energize your spirit is to get out of town on the weekend and challenge yourself a little physically. For most of us, these kinds of fun recreational activities are easily accessible and inexpensive, but are far too often overlooked.

The next time you find yourself and your man stretched before the TV watching a movie you've seen three times before, head outdoors, get some fresh air, and get moving. Your man won't even know he's exercising.

BOTTOM LINE: Lose 15 pounds

A weekend of physical activity could burn 1,000 calories easy. Your man could lose 15 pounds if he does it just once every weekend.

#60. Serve Soup as an Appetizer—Every Night!

I'm firmly convinced that soup is one of the under-rated foods out there. Everyone loves it and it is the perfect way to begin almost every evening meal. Not only is soup delicious, it is also very filling and relatively light on calories.

Studies show that when water is incorporated into your foods—such as with a soup—people naturally eat about 100 fewer calories per meal. So using soup as an appetizer is a sneaky way to help you and your husband consume less without even knowing it.

Making soup a part of your evening (or lunch) meal or having a hearty, main-course soup for your entree will be a welcome addition and will fill you up with fewer calories. (see Soups Recipes on page 424).

BOTTOM LINE: Lose 10–20 pounds

Eat 100 fewer calories at dinner by adding soup and lose 10 pounds in a year. Do it at both meals and lose 20.

#61. Sneak Veggies into Dinners

Carrots, cucumbers, and cauliflower can be your allies in serving up low-calorie and filling dinner meals. Find out his favorites and sneak them into salads and side dishes.

My client, Jim, likes to affectionately call his wife "wonderfully, tactfully devious!" and he loves it. He says she's always helping him eat more fruits and veggies by fixing his favorites and incorporating them into his meals. He appreciates her efforts because he never developed a taste for vegetables or fruits growing up but is now, finally—at the age of 40—learning slowly but surely to love them.

I have several clients who insist they don't like vegetables, but every time they eat them, they love them. I've found the best thing to do is to gently and subtly introduce vegetables into meals. Your man will love it even if he doesn't expect to. There's always a way to cook it so that he'll like it. The key is to be patient and try lots of different techniques.

Grilling vegetables is a favorite of most people. If you don't have a grill, you can roast them in the oven. Simply cut them into large chunks or slices, spray or brush them slightly with olive oil, add a little salt and pepper, and they're ready for the grill. You'll want them soft in the middle and crunchy on the outside, so cooking time is generally 15–30 minutes, depending on the veggie.

Study after study shows weight loss maintainers eat vegetables! It's a fact: When serving vegetables at a meal, people naturally eat about 100 fewer calories because vegetables fill you up, yet have very few calories.

BOTTOM LINE: Lose 10–20 pounds

Sneak vegetables into your husband's dinner and he'll save 100 calories a night. Do it at lunch, too, and he'll save another 100. He can lose 10–20 pounds simply by adding vegetables to his meals!

#62. Fitness Gifts: Easy Exercise Equipment

While it's true us gals like chocolate and flowers for Valentine's Day, I think we can show our affection to our men by giving them simple gifts that will keep those love handles under control.

When next Valentine's Day or your man's birthday or other significant event rolls around, why not give him a membership to the local health club, an appointment with a personal trainer, or some exercise equipment? Many of today's trainers use simple but effective exercise equipment such as medicine balls, light weights, and elastic bands that offer wonderfully exhilarating and productive workouts. These are all easy to handle and don't take up much space in the house.

Give him a few sessions with a trainer, a good book, or videotape on using the equipment, and he'll be hooked.

That'll be important because as we age, we lose muscle, and muscle is critical for health and metabolism. Muscle loss is the main reason we gain weight as we age; our bodies need fewer calories because we have less muscle to burn calories. Working out with weights not only burns calories but builds muscle, so in the long run, he'll actually be burning more calories while doing nothing!

BOTTOM LINE: Lose 4–5 pounds

Even if all he does is work out two times a week for 15 minutes, he'll burn at least 300 to 400 calories extra per week. That'll help him lose 4–5 pounds.

#63. Subscribe to Fitness and Health Magazines

Most everyone likes to browse through magazines to kill a little spare time. To help his "spare tire," get a subscription to a workout or exercise magazine—even an "extreme sports" one—and leave it lying around in plain sight!

For those men wondering what they can do to work out, there is an enormous amount of practical information available. But the quality of advice can vary, so do a little research and browsing yourself, then select a magazine that would be most useful and inspirational to your man.

Some men find fitness and sports magazines very inspiring. It brings them back to a time when they were younger, in shape, and more alive. It may remind them that they can have all of those things again—if they participate in a little physical activity.

These magazines also may give him hope that it's not too late. There are plenty of success stories he can look up to and model himself after.

BOTTOM LINE: Lose 15–20 pounds

A fitness magazine may be just the gift to keep your man motivated and interested in getting—and staying—physically fit. If that inspires him to exercise just 15 minutes a day, he can lose 15–20 pounds in a year.

#64. It Takes Two to Tango

Take classes together—dancing, tennis, pottery, heck, even join a bowling league!

Several years ago, I asked Jack to take me to a Viennese Ball in Washington, D.C., and suggested that we take advantage of dance classes offered by the Austrian Embassy. We participated in a fun and lively 8-week course that helped us do a passable basic waltz at the ball. But it also got us out and physically active together. It was great exercise and great fun.

The next year, we took tango lessons at the Argentine Embassy. It didn't really matter how good we were at dancing (we weren't). What mattered was that it was a lot of fun. We also met other like-minded people.

The point is, exercise doesn't have to be drudgery. You can simply dance your way to fitness. Every city has dance classes of some kind. You might need to invest in some steel-toed shoes for protection and be wary of gangly guys with sharp elbows. My client Renee actually got a black eye from her (very loving and mortified) husband while dancing. But they became thinner!

Of course, if dancing isn't your thing, take a tennis class together—or golf. Anything will do. Trust me, you'll feel like kids again. Your man won't even know he's exercising.

BOTTOM LINE: Lose 7 pounds

Going to a dance or tennis class with your husband will help him burn at least 500 calories a night. Do it once a week and he could lose 7 pounds over a year.

#65. Teach Him "Plate Geography"

Help your guy learn how to judge a healthy meal by noticing how much of what's where on his plate. A man will never ask for directions, but show him a map and he'll be on the right road!

A sensitive but important area to broach with your man is some of the basic facts of sensible nutrition and eating. If you're careful to be respectful and kind, your man will appreciate your knowledge of such things as: How much meat should compose a serving? What should your plate of food look like?

And your man isn't the only one confused about portion size. A survey by the American Institute for Cancer Research showed most people have no idea what proper serving sizes are. Another study showed most people underestimate what they eat by twenty percent.

Show your man how to divide his plate up (half veggies, a quarter protein, a quarter starch), and various clever ways to measure food portions (meat the size of a deck of cards, or the size of your palm, or no bigger than a fist, etc.) Determine his calorie needs, then check out the *Think Yourself Thin* menu plans for some ideas to make this even easier.

BOTTOM LINE: Lose 40 pounds

By teaching your man proper portions, he'll be able to serve himself perfectly balanced meals and he could save 400 calories a day. That's 40 pounds in a year.

#66. Dads Are People, Too

Coaching a team, being more involved in neighborhood or school activities, helping friends with yard work, or just walking the dog, Dads can stay fit just by being a local hero.

Dads are an important part of the family and neighborhood, but sometimes work responsibilities may make it difficult for them to participate and they can feel left out. Encourage your man to coach a local team or even play with his friends in healthy ways, such as joining golf leagues, bowling clubs or a Sierra Club canoe trip.

Let him know that regular physical activity isn't an optional thing to be taken care of only when everything else has been done, but is an essential feature of his daily life.

BOTTOM LINE: Lose 7 pounds

If your man gets out just once a week to do yard work or coach a team, he could easily burn an extra 500 calories a week.

CHAPTER 10

The Plan for Moms

Especially appropriate for: *Working Moms, Time-Crunched Executives, Den Mothers, Harried Homemakers*

Moms are people too. And as a mom, you have very special needs. You're responsible not only for yourself, but also for the health and well-being of your loved ones—which can mean stress, worries, time constraints, and lots of compromises.

You try to cook healthful, delicious meals, but sometimes they're not appreciated. You'd like to have more time for creative pursuits, but they're difficult to fit in. You spend half your time acting as chauffeur to your children, when you could be benefiting from walking, relaxing, or even pursuing a creative hobby or job.

When you're trying to lose weight, others in the family want to be supportive but may not know how to do that for you. In the past, your idea of dieting may have been to separate yourself from your family, to eat differently.

But this is a new approach. I've mentioned the importance of eating as a family. *Everyone* in the family should have access to the same healthful, wholesome foods—whether they're trying to lose weight or not. There's no need for anyone to be separated from the family. In fact, it's detrimental.

So here are some tips on how you can make weight loss fun, how you can not only lose weight, but improve the habits of your children at the same time, and how you can make time for things that are important to you.

#67. Change Family Rewards

Yes, food is love. But consider changing your own and your family's reward systems in order to make weight loss easy for yourself—and to prevent the same habit from developing in your children.

When you've had a hard day at work or feel you need a reward for doing a good job, what's the first thing that comes to mind? If it's a cold beer, a glass of wine, crackers and cheese, or some other type of high-calorie food or drink, chances are it's not only your reward, but the reward you use for your family, too. But we know that using food as a reward can make weight loss difficult. Let me tell you what my client Lois did.

Lois realized that if she continued using food as a reward, she would never solve her weight problem. She also realized that her children would learn the same habits and suffer the same weight problem she has (they already did). But she didn't want to deny her children food rewards she thought they loved. She decided to initiate a change. They convened a family meeting and voted on what they felt great rewards would be for, say, doing well at school or playing well at a game or getting through a tough situation.

Lois was surprised to find that two thirds of the rewards her children chose had nothing to do with food. Talk about a dose of reality! Lois decided this was a good sign. Though she was raised with food as a reward and still felt that drive to eat whenever she deserved a pat on the back, she knew it was something she needed to change in order to lose weight. Her family's making the decision for her gave her the opportunity to make that change.

BOTTOM LINE: Lose 30 pounds

Change your reward from food to fun family games and save a least 300 calories a night—that's 30 pounds in a year!

#68. Do the Stealthy Snack Switch

That old saying "Out of Sight, Out of Mind" really works! Keep low-cal snacks around and your family *will* eat them. If they're hungry, they won't even notice they're not noshing on nacho chips.

My client Brittany grew up in a home full of chips, cookies, and candies. While she didn't have a weight problem as a child—as she was very physically active—she has one now. And she has a terrible time resisting, you guessed it, chips, cookies, and candies. What we're exposed to as children tends to stay with us for life.

But Brittany knew that in order to lose weight, she would need to get rid of the sweets and snack foods in her house, because she couldn't seem to eat them "in moderation." She would find herself munching on the high-calorie stuff daily—adding 300 to 500 calories to her regimen. But if she stopped bringing these foods into the house, how would her family react? Should she deprive them of the fun foods she loves so much?

Brittany and I talked about her predicament and discussed the studies that show children learn to prefer the food which is available at home, no matter what it is. Armed with this information and secure in the knowledge that it would be a healthful change for her whole family anyway, she decided to slowly wean herself and her family from these foods.

She didn't announce the change to anyone. In fact, she made it a stealth campaign (particularly knowing that if you try to restrict foods, they all of a sudden become more popular). She didn't completely get rid of the foods at first so no one would notice something was up. She started by offering vegetables and fruit for snacks, and fruit for desserts. She was amazed at how her family simply ate what she offered, especially when she was eating and enjoying the food, too. No one seemed to complain that there weren't cookies for dessert (except her, quietly mumbling to herself!).

One weekend they went on a sailing trip and she was tormented by the thought that she couldn't bring potato chips—they were her tradition and, she thought, important to her family, too. But she also brought tons of fruit for everyone to snack on. Guess what was eaten up first? The fruit! The kids and their friends loved it. Yes, they all started munching on the chips but not until the fruit was gone. Hard lesson: Next time bring more fruit—no one cares about the chips (except Brittany!).

After a while, there were no chips, candies, or cookies in the house on a regular basis—and no one seemed to care. Snacks and desserts were exclusively healthful foods, except on special occasions. After school, the kids would sit down at the kitchen table and munch on carrots and dip, yogurt and granola, or apple slices with peanut butter. No one was the wiser, but Brittany's weight, as well as the general health of the family, reaped the benefits of this stealth campaign.

BOTTOM LINE: Lose 30–50 pounds

Switching from high-calorie sweets and chips to fruit and vegetable snacks could save a minimum of 300 to 500 calories daily. Lose 30 to 50 pounds in a year!

#69. Play Fried-Chicken Charade

No more greasy fingertips when you make this moist and low-calorie version of the All-American standard.

Barbara's family loves fried chicken, mainly because Barbara does. Barbara was raised in a family of Southerners and her love for fried chicken was passed down through the generations. But she decided to stop this particular family tradition with this generation. Barbara had a serious weight problem, and though her children were thin, as she had been when she was young, she wanted to start them off loving healthful foods. She also wanted to lose some weight.

She discovered a delicious way to save tons of saturated fat and calories by oven-"frying" chicken instead.

Barbara's Oven-Fried Chicken

Ingredients:
Skinless chicken breast, drumsticks, or thighs, either whole or cut into strips
1 Egg, beaten
Crunched flaky cereal, such as corn flakes or bran flakes
Salt and pepper to taste
Pinch of rosemary, parsley flakes, or any favorite herb (optional)
Oil spray

1. Place the beaten egg in a bowl large enough to fit the chicken breast. Crunch up flaky cereal, add salt and pepper to taste, and place in a similar-sized bowl.

2. Rinse the chicken and pat dry. Dip the chicken in the egg and coat well. Next dip the egg-coated chicken in the flakes and coat evenly.

3. Coat a cookie sheet with oil spray and bake chicken breasts uncovered

in a 350-degree oven for about 20 or 30 minutes or until the internal temperature of the chicken is 170 degrees and juices are no longer pink.

Variations:

1. Coat the chicken first with milk or yogurt instead of the egg.

2. Coat the chicken first with a mixture of equal amounts of honey and orange juice—and a pinch of ginger and hot pepper, if desired, instead of the egg.

3. Simply buy prepackaged oven-baked-chicken mixes.

Two fried chicken drumsticks contain about 400 calories and 6 saturated fat grams (the artery-clogging kind of fat). Whereas two skinless, baked chicken drumsticks have only 150 calories and 1.2 saturated fat grams. A fried chicken breast contains 364 calories and 5 grams of saturated fat. A baked, skinless breast has 142 calories and 0.8 grams saturated fat.

BOTTOM LINE: Lose 4–8 pounds

Oven- "frying" chicken instead of deep fat frying it saves anywhere from 222 calories for the breast to 250 calories if you're eating two drumsticks. Make the switch once a week, say, every Friday night and lose 4 pounds per year. For every day of the week you make the switch, lose 4 pounds a year. Two times per week, that's 8 pounds a year, etc.

#70. Stop the Portion Distortion

More isn't always better—and that's especially true at mealtimes. Pay attention to how much you place on your family's plates. Chances are, they'll feel full with just a few teaspoons *less* than they're used to!

A lot of people trace the beginnings of their weight problem to the day they got married. The (happy) obligation of spending time together, eating dinner out more often, or making larger meals together all conspire to make eating more calories a grim reality.

The problem is especially acute for women. Gloria, for instance, noticed her portion sizes getting bigger at dinner time. She began serving herself the same amount her much bigger husband was eating. And when her children came along, she did the same for them. Everyone received very large portions.

The problem is that when you get more food, you eat more food—whether you need it at the time or not. We famine-survivors are built that way: to eat food when it's available. But there are no more famines (for most Americans, anyway), so we're storing excess food for nothing. It's just sitting there as body fat.

So how much is enough for you? Go to *Think Yourself Thin*'s "Metabolism Toolbox" on page 461 and figure out your calorie needs. Divide by three and find sample dinner menus that meet your needs. Most women should eat around 600 calories a meal to lose weight. Once you try these portion-controlled meals, it'll feel completely natural to stop eating as soon as you're satisfied (see Tip #87).

BOTTOM LINE: Lose 20 pounds

Save at least 200 calories per dinner by eating the correct portions at dinner time, portions that fit your personal needs, instead of your husband's or kids.' Lose 20 pounds in a year!

#71. Ignore Those Leftovers

Another benefit to serving less is that there's less left over to be wasted–or eaten up by mom.

So many mothers complain they can't keep themselves from finishing what's on everyone else's plates when they're cleaning up after dinner. It's such a waste! Food being thrown away.... But wait a minute, is it better thrown away in the trash or stored as excess fat in your body?

My client Lois found a terrific solution to this problem. She found it impossible to stop eating the leftovers on everyone's plate until she came up with this simple solution: Feed everyone less. Yes, you heard me! Afraid the poor babies might starve? Think again! Studies show very clearly that children will eat until they are satisfied. So you can be assured that if they are still hungry, they'll go back to the serving plate.

This way, you save hundreds of leftover calories and your children become better at self-regulating. If you continue to overfeed them and encourage them to eat what's on their plates, they will begin to lose their natural ability to self-regulate and may develop eating problems.

With this solution, feeding your children and husband a little less than usual—but still very balanced food choices, you're killing two birds with one stone: avoiding extra food on the plates after dinner and fostering a natural way of eating for your children.

BOTTOM LINE: Lose 10 pounds

Save at least 100 calories a night by skipping the leftovers! Lose 10 pounds in a year.

#72. Enjoy the Fresh Air

Research shows we need a certain amount of sunlight and exercise to reduce depression and anxiety. Take time to smell the roses and go play outside!

Connie came to me very depressed. I had worked successfully with her years earlier when she was pregnant with her first baby to help her cope with gestational diabetes. Now she had two little ones at home—one toddler and an infant. She loved them dearly, but she was terribly depressed.

While her husband was holding down a full-time job and going to law school three nights a week, eating became her only interest and pleasure in life, beyond her children. Her weight began climbing and she had been recently diagnosed with high cholesterol and high blood pressure. And because she had a history of gestational diabetes, if she didn't lose weight, a return of her diabetes was a real threat to her.

She said she spent all of her time at home and felt trapped. Her routine had declined to the point where she seemed to be sleeping most of her days away. She would stay up very late at night to eat and spend time with her husband, then wake up late in the morning every day, exhausted. She seemed to only have energy for fixing food for the kids then napping again.

I felt terrible for her. Here was such a vibrant woman, reduced to living a depressed life of eating and sleeping. We talked and came up with a very simple action plan I hoped would start her on her way to a happier way of living—with weight loss naturally to follow.

The first problem I noticed was that Connie rarely went outside into the world and she never did any physical activity. I felt this should be the first thing to change before we attacked anything else. We decided that no matter what, she would get outside every single day. She would bundle herself and her children up and take a long walk with the stroller, see some sights, or visit some friends—on foot.

When I saw Connie for the first time two weeks later, she was like a new woman. I couldn't believe my eyes. She was vibrant, happy, excited—

the old Connie I knew. We made a few other changes, like working on her meal schedule (see Tip #88, Eat by the Clock), but honestly, I believe simply getting outdoors did the trick.

I learned a lot from that experience and have given the same advice to other moms. Patsy came to see me after her first child was born. A former athlete and model, she had turned into a slug, staying indoors. She ate her way into being 30 pounds overweight.

To solve her problem, Patsy bought a baby "jog stroller" so she and her son could get outside daily and walk or jog on a bike path near her home. She took her son for a walk outside and to the park every day, even if she had already gone to the gym. She found there was nothing like getting outside into the fresh air.

Within three months, Connie lost the 20 pounds that were plaguing her, and in 6 months, Patsy lost 30 pounds (it helped that they were both breast-feeding!). I believe spending time outdoors in the fresh air saved both mothers from being depressed and unhappy and from eating their way to oblivion.

BOTTOM LINE: Lose 10–40 pounds

Getting outdoors to walk or move in any way will burn at least 100 calories in 15 minutes. Accumulate 1 hour a day and lose 40 pounds in a year. Accumulate 30 minutes in a day and lose 20. If getting out helps you focus less on eating for entertainment and you save 100 calories a day, you'll lose another 10.

#73. Take up Photography or Film

Is there anything more beautiful than your child sleeping or laughing? Your husband tossing your little girl into the air as she laughs uncontrollably? Capture those moments with a new hobby.

There are moments you'll cherish forever. But you may not remember and won't be able to share them if they're not captured on film. With the advances in technology, anyone can take pictures these days and most people can even take videos.

Problem: Most people's photos are unlabeled, scattered in unmarked shopping bags or shoe boxes and no one can enjoy them. You keep putting off organizing them because it's so easy to say you'll "do it later." Make later *now*. If you don't it may never happen. Memories fade—you could forget half the people or events in the photos by the time you get around to it. Make a project of labeling and organizing your photos so you can display them in ways everyone can have access to and enjoy.

First, spread all the photos on a table. Second, organize them by person or occasion. Throw away bad shots. Pick the best photos for albums. Save the leftovers in a small file box with labels.

Make copies of your favorite photos and send albums as Christmas presents. What could be a better present for any of your loved ones?

Why is this important for a Mom who wants to lose weight? Research shows having creative pursuits helps the mind, spirit, and body. The time you spend with your photos—or doing any other creative act—is time taken away from recreational overeating. You also find fulfillment in life when you are creative. One reason we overeat is because we feel empty, lonely, and unfulfilled.

My hobby of sewing has saved me thousands—if not millions—of calories over the years. Sewing is what I do when everything has quieted down in the evenings. While other people are zoning out in front of the TV, I'm using a needle and thread to make gifts for myself and others. I'm also keeping my body out of the kitchen!

Organizing photographs, of course, is only one suggestion. You could take up gardening, painting, decoupage... you name it. Think about when you were a child. What did you love to do then? Chances are, you haven't changed much. Find your passion and pursue it. Take a class if you need to. I've been taking sewing classes for 20 years, and there's still more to learn!

BOTTOM LINE: Lose 13 pounds

Pursuing a creative hobby saved me hundreds of calories every evening I was engaged in it. If you're able to pursue your hobby just three evenings per week you could save 900 calories a week. Lose 13 pounds in a year.

#74. Find a Quiet Place

What wouldn't you give for just a few moments of peace in your hectic day? Keep stress–and stress-induced eating–at bay with some creative visualization!

Close your eyes. Take a few deep breaths. Imagine you're in a field of lavender in the south of France with no phones, no computer, no people, no work, just you, the lavender, and a lovely ocean breeze.

Perhaps you're lying in the midst of all this on a comfy comforter and a fluffy pillow. With you is your favorite stuffed animal from childhood and a book of fairy tales. Off in the distance, there's even an artist drawing the scene. You can hear tiny birds chirping or dragonflies humming. If France doesn't appeal to you, think of your own favorite scene—on a Caribbean beach or a mountaintop in Virginia. Shouldn't you feel like this every day?

Now, back to real life and a hectic world, where you find yourself multi-tasking nearly every moment of the day. You're on the phone, while you're in the car, while you're calming down your kids, while you're downing the fast food burger. Whew, it's enough to make anyone binge—or at least zone out in front of television every evening from sheer nervous exhaustion.

How can you create a space in your life every day where you can just be calm, just be you? You say you don't have the space? Your special sanctuary can be anywhere. It could be in your own bed—or even your bathtub. It could be a little corner of your bedroom, or in your garden. It could be in a stand of trees at the local park.

Clear your space of clutter, and make it as beautiful as you can. Surround yourself with flowers, or a blanket in your favorite colors. Your space need only be private, calm, quiet and filled with colors, textures things you find delightful. Fill a corner of your room with pillows in your favorite color or photos of calming scenes. If it's easier to play soothing music to get you there, that's okay too. Or read some calming passages from a favorite book.

If you don't have the time, be good to yourself and make the time. It takes only a few minutes to calm down. Take a few deep breaths (see Tip #41) and you'll see just how effective breathing deeply can be for slowing down your heart rate and leaving you more relaxed. The more you attend to these kinds of psychic needs, the less you will turn to food during stressful times.

My special calming place is my bathtub—or my bed. When I'm sitting in bed reading on top of a pile of my favorite pillows, Jack (my significant other) says I'm on my "throne." I sort of like that description! If I need serious calming, the bathtub has always worked for me as well. Throw in some soothing aromatic bubble bath—and I'm in heaven. Soaking in the bubble bath, in fact, saved me from years of nervous eating.

I highly recommend finding a calming place so you can relax completely and reduce your need to snack.

BOTTOM LINE: Lose 20 pounds

Save at least 200 calories of nervous snacking per day. Lose 20 pounds in a year.

#75. Shed Pounds While Killing Time

Moms are always waiting. Think of how fit you could get if you could harness all that time waiting into physical activities.

You wait for the kids to finish soccer practice, you wait for the end of the school day, you wait for the electrician. Think of all the calories you could be burning, muscles you could be building.

My client Alice brings a softball and gloves when she has to wait for her son at soccer practice. She tosses it back and forth with her young daughter. If there's a basketball hoop nearby, she brings a basketball. Sometimes other families join in, and then the fun really begins!

Barbara picks up her daughters from school every day and often from swimming lessons as well. Sometimes she has to wait a while before they show up, so she uses the extra time by walking around the school's track. Another mom brings her bike on the back of her car and rides while she's waiting. Yet another mom wears her running clothes and headphones and jogs.

BOTTOM LINE: Lose 10 pounds

Just adding 15 minutes of physical activity to your day while waiting could burn an extra 100 calories. Result: 10 pounds lost in a year.

#76. Cook with the Kids

Asking your family to help you cook meals prepares them for life and gives them some quality time with you.

Getting your kids to help can be a lot of fun, so you just might find yourself cooking more often for the sheer enjoyment of it. But will this help you lose weight? *Absolutely.* Research shows weight loss maintainers are more likely to eat meals at home instead of going out to restaurants. So anything you can do to increase home cooking is good—asking your children to help or, if they're old enough, giving them the task of fixing a whole dinner for the family (so long as they keep it simple and you okay the menu).

When Lois asked Daniel, 10, what he would like to cook for his first family meal, he chose tacos. Lois was around in case he needed help, but essentially, Daniel did it on his own. He sautéed the extra-lean hamburger with a taco spice mix. Lois helped him put the shells in the oven, while Daniel chopped tomatoes, lettuce, and reduced-fat cheese. Everyone in the family enjoyed this meal, and Lois got many ideas for future meals Daniel could make!

Kids love to make pizza. You can buy a shell already cooked or raw pizza dough that you cook at home. The most fun part is choosing the toppings. Try vegetables sautéed in olive oil and garlic. Some favorites are mushrooms, peppers, onions, spinach, and zucchini. Sprinkle with fresh olives. For meat lovers, look for extra-lean—or even vegetarian—cured meats such as ham and sausage. Let the children pick the vegetables, chop and sauté them, then spread them around the pizza. Try a variety of reduced-fat cheeses: Mozzarella, goat cheese, Provolone. You won't have any picky eaters tonight! And you can be assured that your portion is not only delicious, but nutritious and calorie- and fat-controlled.

The recipes you can teach your children are endless. You're doing yourself and them a favor by teaching them to cook—and saving hundreds of calories every week, to boot!

BOTTOM LINE: Lose 20 pounds

By cooking at home with your family, you're saving at least 200 calories a night by avoiding the greasy spoon. Making your own pizza versus take-out pizza is a huge savings. Lose at least 20 pounds in a year!

#77. Get Creative with Other Moms

When you indulge your creative side, you meet other people with the same interests and this fills your life with more like-minded people and more support.

I'll bet you're a mom who has creativity, get up and go, and an interest in expanding your mind and talents. But you haven't been able to motivate yourself to go it alone.

Next time you see a class you'd like to take, a museum you'd like to visit, or a lecture you'd like to hear, call your friends. Organize creative get-togethers with other moms. Start a bridge club, a (healthful) gourmet club, or a book club. Take furniture painting, pottery, or jewelry-making classes.

There's a fabulous bead shop around the corner from me. One year, I made earrings for all the women on my holiday list. I bought beautiful 14-karat gold hoops and attached delicate pearl, amethyst, or turquoise beads, depending on the personality of the recipient. I organized a "craft day" and several of us got together and made seasonal crafts and gifts all afternoon. We had a blast and got some wonderfully creative and unique presents out of it.

People who do better with their weight tend to be active outside their home, they turn to friends and loved ones in times of trouble, and they have a large support system. And though their families are their priority, they have interests beyond their families.

Finding friends who have the same interests—beyond going out to dinner—fills your life with healthier possibilities. When your creative capacities are engaged, you're less likely to have cravings or eat out of depression or boredom.

BOTTOM LINE: Lose 10 pounds

Save hundreds of calories by developing friendships and interests outside the home. You won't even miss the food! Lose 10 pounds in a year.

#78. Make Mom Exercise Dates

Round up all the neighborhood moms and start your own regular exercise classes. Cheaper than joining a gym!

Have you ever thought about hiring a personal trainer, but just didn't think you could afford it? How about getting several of your friends together and working with a personal trainer—together! If one of you has a large room or basement, you won't even have to go to a gym. Just ask your trainer to recommend some inexpensive equipment you can invest in. Today, trainers are using medicine balls, bands, and free weights—relatively inexpensive but effective tools for getting in shape.

If a personal trainer isn't your thing, start a walking or running club in your neighborhood with like-minded friends. There's nothing like a group for motivation. Get together with your group as often as you can, or even just once a week. Every little bit helps. And watch all of you improve each week. It's amazing how quickly the body rebounds and gets back into shape. A little friendly competition doesn't hurt, either.

Another alternative would be an aerobics class, dance classes, or even tennis classes. Haven't you always wanted to learn to play tennis? How about karate, tai chi, or fencing? When I was in college I took a fencing class—those lunges are great for toning the gluteus maximus. Even if all you do is spend your time running after tennis balls, getting together with your friends is more than half the fun.

BOTTOM LINE: Lose 15 pounds

Being physically active just one more hour a week could burn 300 calories—lose 15 pounds in a year.

#79. Start a Yoga or Meditation Club

Yoga is especially useful during the difficult afternoon period or evening period when anxiety or exhaustion runs high—along with urges to snack on high-calorie treats.

Have you ever wondered if yoga really is as great as everyone says? Or are you someone who tried it and loved it, but just never got around to making it part of your routine? Are you intimidated by going to a class with strangers?

Organize your pals—or family—in a yoga club. You can use an instructional video or take a class together.

While many of the yoga postures look impossible for us normal people, you and your friends will be able to improve and adapt at your own speed. The collective experience will give you comfort and inspiration.

Once you get the hang of some of the basic postures and breathing exercises, you'll find ways to integrate them into your daily life. During stressful moments, you may find yourself springing into a triangle pose instead of gulping down a Snickers bar!

BOTTOM LINE: Lose 25 pounds

Do yoga instead of a Snickers bar every afternoon and save 250 calories. Lose 25 pounds!

#80. You're Getting Sleepy. . . .

Want to stay smart and slim down? Get 8 hours of sleep every night. It's as simple as that!

Studies have found that sleep disorders are correlated with weight problems. The reasons aren't completely clear, but some theories make a lot of sense.

First, when you don't get enough sleep, you're too exhausted to be physically active. I have many clients in this situation. They go to bed late, wake up early, and can't find the energy to exercise. By the end of the day, they're exhausted and can't muster up the strength to do much of anything, let alone be physically active. Night owls also tend to snack more in the evenings, which is another risk factor for weight problems.

Besides weight problems, research shows that lack of sleep could be damaging your health. It raises blood glucose levels and could increase your risk of heart disease and depression. One study found that when people didn't get enough sleep, even their IQ lowered.

If you have problems sleeping, experts say it's important to develop a routine. Go to bed at approximately the same time every evening and get up at approximately the same time every morning.

Find a relaxing bed-time ritual. For me, sewing, relaxing in the tub, or reading a novel all take my mind off matters that may keep my poor little mind whirling and worrying.

In the evenings, if you find yourself naturally drifting off, instead of turning on the boob tube or grabbing a snack to unnaturally keep yourself up later—go with the flow and go to bed! Your mind and body will be happier and healthier for it.

BOTTOM LINE: Lose 30–50 pounds

Going to bed early and saving 300 nighttime snacking calories alone will help you lose 30 pounds in a year. Getting up early with energy enough to be physically active for just 10–20 minutes will burn at least another 100–200 calories, for a total loss of 30–50 pounds in a year.

#81. Surround Yourself with Color

Research by color experts has shown that the right hue can enhance your mood, and as we've seen, mood can have a profound effect on weight loss.

The experts tell us that green is a relaxing and nurturing color. In my experience, this is true. When people sit in my green-walled living room, they feel warm and relaxed. Jack particularly likes the green color on the walls, and when I was considering making a change, he vetoed it. I'm glad he did.

Yellow, the color of sunshine, is uplifting, which is why it predominates in my house. I particularly like a yellow kitchen, as it's associated with happiness and playfulness.

Red is the most stimulating color. It encourages conversation, which is why it's great for a dining room or living room—any room where you want people to feel stimulated and talk. Red probably isn't the greatest choice for a bedroom—it's a little too interesting to promote rest and relaxation. A black and white room is also visually exciting, as are navy with white, and deep brown with white. Combine black and white with primary colors—sparingly—for even more interest. Using contrasts creates drama.

Earth tones, such as antique cream, beige, taupe, honey, terra cotta, and cocoa, on the other hand, are great for relaxing, since they're natural colors and are easy on the eyes. Earth tones create a neutral background that can be complimented with splashier colors here and there but set a calming, elegant tone in the room.

You can also use complimentary colors to create more harmony in a room. Blue and yellow, green and red. When together, complimentary colors balance each other to create a less jarring effect, which is easier on the eyes than with any other color combination.

Sometimes, there's nothing more beautiful or calming than white. In that case, white is the best choice for you. Imagine an all-white room with filmy white curtains all over—white cushions, white everything.

If you find yourself unhappy in any of the rooms in your house, be sure to check out the color and its effect on you. Painting the walls is one of the least expensive but most effective ways to change the mood and tone of a room and a home.

BOTTOM LINE: Lose 5 pounds

Finding colors that are at harmony with your life can give you a sense of calm and togetherness, reducing stress and anxiety. If this helps you avoid stress-eating 50 calories a night, you'll lose 5 pounds in a year.

#82. Call Your Girlfriends

Girl talk and gossip aren't just needless chatter. Chewing the fat rather than chewing on candy will keep you from relying on food in times of stress.

Successful weight loss maintainers call upon their family, friends, and support system when they are troubled. Weight regainers don't. Instead, regainers try to escape from their feelings by eating, sleeping, or wishing their problems away.

A new study has shown that women are more likely to feel their lives are manageable when they call upon their girlfriends in times of need. Somehow, your buddies are often your best bet when it comes to listening and responding to your problems. They may be even more effective than talking with your husband at times, as he's more likely to be too emotionally involved to be helpful.

While I'm not a big fan of cell phones, if you're feeling down and out, go for a little walk and call a friend. This way, you burn a few calories and gain a little serenity and sympathy, which may forestall a trip to the refrigerator later in the evening.

BOTTOM LINE: Lose 9 pounds

If you prevent yourself from downing a doughnut even just 3 times a week by calling a friend, you'll lose 9 pounds in a year.

#83. Stroll While You Shop

Keep your sneakers in the back of the car, head for the mall, and burn off some calories while you're burning up those charge cards!

All of us gals love to go shopping and sometimes we shop rather than exercise (who, me?! NAH!!!). Well, guess what? Shopping is actually a great opportunity to fit some extra exercise into your busy life! How? Simple. The next time you go to the mall, make a point of walking two or three laps around the mall before entering your favorite stores.

It would also help to park as far from the door as possible, especially during the more pleasant months of the year. You'll not only save time by avoiding the problem of finding a parking space, but you'll get a nice brisk walk in before you get to the store. If you decide to drive downtown to shop, take a short walk around the city park before going to the shopping district.

Think of all the time you spend shopping. If every time you shop you spend even just 15 minutes doing some extra walking, you can do some serious calorie-burning!

BOTTOM LINE: Lose 10 pounds

A few steps a day keeps the bulge at bay. Just 15 more minutes of walking a day will burn at least 100 calories. Lose 10 pounds in a year.

#84. Nose Around

Science has shown that scent can increase your energy and elevate your mood, and may be able to prevent insomnia, alleviate pain, improve learning, boost athletic performance, reduce the side effects of chemotherapy, and curb appetite!

Dr. Alan Hirsch, a neurologist and psychiatrist at the Smell and Taste Treatment Foundation in Chicago, who is generally thought the world's leading expert on the effects of odors on human beings, has seen people lose up to 5 pounds of weight per month simply by sniffing the scents of green apple, bananas, and peppermint on a regular basis. It should come as no surprise that what we smell affects our appetite. After all, the scent of freshly baked bread can certainly make us salivate. And researchers estimate that up to ninety percent of what we think of as taste is actually smell. People who have no sense of smell, for example, can't taste chocolate at all.

I can personally vouch for the effects of peppermint. In the evening, if I'm feeling a little antsy—and at risk for nervous eating, I will have some peppermint herbal tea and it nips my cravings in the bud. A new study shows when runners took a whiff of a peppermint-scented towel during their workout, they felt less fatigued and more energized than did a control group. The same researchers found that peppermint scent reduced people's perception of pain. A new study has shown that floral scents can improve performance on mathematics tests.

Aromatherapy is a form of therapy that uses the scents of essential oils—extremely concentrated oils taken from various flowers—to help people relax and reduce depression and anxiety. Usually the oil is put on a warm surface (not your skin!), or in a special dispenser available at health food stores, that fills the room with scent. You may find that you are partial to floral scents or spicy scents. Whatever your favorite scent, make it available when you need it. When you get the urge to eat and you know you're not hungry, it's a sign that you need to calm down, relax. Try rewarding yourself with your favorite scent.

Caution: Because they are so concentrated, many essential oils can be highly toxic if taken internally. Keep away from pets and children.

▌BOTTOM LINE: Lose 5 pounds

Instead of indulging in nervous eating, save hundreds of calories by indulging in your favorite scent. Even if you only save 50 calories a day, that's 5 pounds in a year.

#85. Prevent Bloat

Some tips for avoiding monthly discomfort.

Have you ever experienced progressive bloating as the day moves into night? Many women complain about it. The good news is that bloating usually goes away on its own and is not an indication of a serious condition. The bad news is that it feels terrible and can affect your mood negatively.

Bloating can result from any number of causes. Many women feel bloating for the 2 weeks before their periods and may even gain a few pounds of water weight. This is caused by the buildup of the hormone progesterone, and it goes away with your period. To fight period bloating, consider doing the following:

1. Drink plenty of water; make sure your urine is clear.
2. Watch out for your sugar and refined carbohydrate intake. Foods high in refined carbohydrates can actually cause bloating.
3. Keep sodium intake low. Sodium is known for its bloating side effect.
4. Eat plenty of fiber. Fiber keeps everything moving through your system quickly and easily. Often, bloat is simply constipation. The latest recommendations from the National Academy of Sciences is that women should eat at least 25 grams of fiber daily.
5. Forget fizzy drinks. They cause bloat.

BOTTOM LINE: Lose 4 pounds

Preventing bloating may not help you lose body fat, but it will help you lose water weight—up to 4 pounds during your period.

#86. Mom's Sporting Afternoons

Throw the ball around before dinner; go to the local pool for a cooling swim after supper on soft summer nights.

When I was growing up, the neighborhood dads could often be seen on the ball fields on Saturday or Sunday afternoons playing with their kids, tossing baseballs, kicking footballs. The moms stayed indoors or stood quietly on the sidelines.

Why don't you and your friends organize Sunday afternoon sporting events with the neighborhood kids? It's a good chance to get the kids outdoors doing fun and stimulating activities. Research shows physical activity reduces dramatically in teenage girls. It would be especially helpful to get this group active in your games. It also gets the neighborhood moms in motion—having fun, burning some calories, and keeping themselves young and active.

You can also organize Olympic days with contests and prizes. You can even put together special competitions and walks to benefit your favorite charity. Not only are you burning calories and having fun, you're also sending a message to your kids that physical activity is a lifelong enjoyable pursuit—not just for the guys!

BOTTOM LINE: Lose 9 pounds

Burn 600 calories in 2 hours' worth of activities on the weekend. Lose 9 pounds in a year.

CHAPTER 11

How to Beat Emotional Eating

Especially appropriate for: *Cravers, Bingers, Self-Saboteurs, People Who Are "Hungry All the Time," Those Who Eat Too Fast or With Too Many Distractions, Those Who Are Out of Touch With Their Feelings, Positive Thinkers, Negative Thinkers*

One of my clients, Ellen, complained that she felt hungry all the time. She couldn't control her eating—or lose the 10 pounds that she needed to lose to get back into her favorite clothes.

Gary had a different story. He craved sweets constantly, especially at the office. His doctor told him that he had to lose 30 pounds and lower his cholesterol.

Kelly, another client, told me that she felt out of control. She was bingeing all the time, and was seeing a psychotherapist. But her wedding was in a few months, and she wanted desperately to lose 20 pounds.

Catherine's story really hit home, mainly because it was so typical. She wanted to lose weight, and often she would. But then she'd find herself sabotaging her efforts.

Ellen, Gary, Kelly, and Catherine are all very different people, but with something in common: Their eating habits were a mess. They ate for reasons that had nothing to do with hunger. They didn't understand—or at least weren't able to put into practice—the most basic rules of feeding their bodies appropriately. My job was to help them unlearn the lousy lessons they had picked up from childhood or from years of dieting.

Losing weight often has less to do with specific food choices than with the underlying emotions. People have a hard time understanding that their feelings, and the unconscious self-talk that we all listen to every day, play a critical role in eating decisions.

I've found that most people who have difficulty controlling their weight have never learned how to listen to their feelings or to their bodies. They don't always recognize when they're stressed, depressed, or frustrated, and they certainly don't recognize when they're using food as a way to cope.

My experience has taught me that most people with an "unhealthy" relationship to food, whether that involves out-of-control cravings or anything else, need first of all to understand the importance of careful meal planning and eating meals at regular times. Once their bodies fall into a natural rhythm, it's much easier for them to *feel* the difference—and to stick with the healthy changes.

Weight-related eating problems may seem complicated, but they're not. With sensitive and nonjudgmental self-exploration, nearly everyone can learn to eat normally and keep their weight under control.

#87. Fight the Beast

Hunger is pretty rational. It tells you when you need to eat and when you've had enough. Cravings, on the other hand, are cruel and capricious. They always demand more, more, more!

Food cravings are your enemy. They're the beasts inside you that can make it almost impossible to lose weight—unless you learn to put them in their place.

What's the difference between hunger and cravings? Hunger means your body is running low on energy. Think of it as the warning light that tells you when to eat. Cravings, on the other, live in your emotions. When you're frustrated, tense, tired, depressed, in love, out of love, or whatever, cravings push you toward food in an attempt to quiet the turbulence within.

People who are successful at losing weight have learned to distinguish true hunger from cravings. In other words, they listen to their stomachs, not their emotions.

THE HUNGER TEST

Because we all eat for emotional reasons as well as for hunger, it's not always easy to tell them apart. The real difference between them becomes apparent after you've finished eating. If hunger was in charge, you should feel pretty good—satisfied, but not stuffed. If cravings had the upper hand, well, reach for the Alka-Seltzer!

When you give in to cravings, you are abusing your body, plain and simple. You are forcing your body to store excess calories as fat. You are also abusing a substance—food—by using it for something other than hunger.

My clients are amazed at how much less food they need in order to feel comfortable. Take Ann. She always ate two cups of pasta, even though she left the table feeling uncomfortably full. I convinced her to cut back to one cup, and guess what? She felt terrific, and not ready for a nap the way she had been in the past.

Using a scale of 0–10,* rate your body's hunger signals before you begin eating and when you finish:

0 = **Ravenous:** Irrational... will eat anything
1 = **Empty:** Too hungry, a bit irrational
2 = **Hungry:** Time to eat
3 = **Hungry-or-Light:** You could eat or you could wait
4 = **Light:** You should wait before eating
5 = **Comfortable:** You are no longer hungry; you're satisfied, comfortable without feeling full
6 = **Slightly Uncomfortable:** Very subtly past comfort level
7 = **Uncomfortable**
8 = **Full:** Your waistband is tightening
9 = **Very Full:** You're having to move your belt a notch
10 = **Overstuffed**

BOTTOM LINE: Lose 30 pounds

If listening to your body signals means you don't clean your plate automatically or eat for emotional reasons or if you regularly eat when your stomach registers a "2," and stop eating when it registers a "5," count on saving at least 300 calories a day.

*Adapted from *Eating Awareness Training*, by Molly Groger (Summit Books, 1983)

#88. Eat by the Clock

Believe it or not, the biggest cause of food cravings and bingeing is undereating. Go too long without food, the body becomes ravenous—and the mind becomes irrational.

Your body normally gets hungry every 3 to 5 hours, depending on the size of your meals. Eating regularly during the day gives you the most control over food cravings and bingeing.

I usually advise people to eat five times a day: breakfast, snack, lunch, snack, dinner. If you prefer just three meals, that can work too, provided the meals are balanced, and your breakfast, lunch, and dinner are roughly equal in calories. For most people, that means switching some calorie intake from dinner to breakfast.

This sort of regular routine maintains your body's normal hunger signals, the highest metabolic rate, and the most efficient burning of calories. And, most important, it gives you more control over your impulses.

Let's take a look at this. Impulse eating, or bingeing, is usually a result of poor planning. In other words, you'll find yourself in the wrong place (near a vending machine or a fast-food restaurant) at the wrong time (when you're starving). If you eat at regular times and never let yourself get too hungry, this is much less likely to occur.

Incidentally—and to repeat—I advise everyone to eat dinner at least 3 hours before going to bed. Try to make this the last time you eat because calories that are consumed late are more likely to wind up as fat than calories consumed earlier. Still, be flexible. It's fine to have a light snack—fruits or vegetables are ideal—after dinner if you're hungry. Just be sure that you're not reaching for food for other reasons—because you're bored, for example, or because you're stressed about work or personal problems.

How does all of this add up to weight loss? Let's take a look:

- If you have a fruit snack at regularly scheduled times, you'll be less likely to raid the vending machine. That could add up to 20 lost pounds a year.
- Planning your meals ahead of time allows you to have nutritious home-made food instead of a burger or fries. That could mean 22–30 lost pounds a year.
- Giving up evening snacks (which you won't need because you're eating healthy meals regularly so you're not hungry in the evenings) could knock off 15 pounds.

BOTTOM LINE: Lose 20–80 pounds

This is a very significant change. I think it's clear that you can lose tremendous amounts of weight just by planning meals carefully and sticking to a regular mealtime schedule. And that's without dieting!

#89. Confront Your Feelings

Facing emotions honestly and with acceptance can stop binges before they start.

Jealousy, humiliation, anger, loneliness, and boredom are uncomfortable feelings. But they're *normal* feelings. I have to stress this because the sooner you accept your feelings, whether or not you try to change them, the sooner you'll feel as though a load has been lifted from your shoulders.

No one wants to admit feeling lonely or afraid. We all want to be loved all the time, always in control of our feelings, thoroughly competent and achieving in all respects.

Sorry. Can't be done. The more we deny the ways we really feel, the more we turn to external sources of comfort, food being one of the big ones.

Larry, one of my clients, told me a story. One day in the office, he had a powerful craving for sweets. Since Larry knows himself pretty well, he guessed that the craving had more to do with his emotions than with his stomach. So he thought for a moment, and realized that the real reason he wanted food was because his boss had been yelling at him.

His emotions didn't change. But by understanding why he felt the way he did, his craving disappeared and he was able to avoid responding in an inappropriate way.

BOTTOM LINE: Lose 26 pounds

Larry easily saved 600 calories by not diving into the ever-present plate of office cookies. Assuming he had this type of insight—and restraint—2 or 3 times a week, the year-end weight loss could be dramatic.

#90. Let Yourself Live

The way we talk to ourselves has a huge impact on the way we eat. Are you a perfectionist who's always self-critical? Watch out!

Let me tell you about some of my clients. Julie can buy a box of chocolates and eat one tiny piece each day. Kris, on the other hand, will eat them all.

Lesson: Kris had better not keep chocolate around the house. I call this environmental control.

Here's another example. Renee asked her husband to keep the ice cream in the basement freezer so she wouldn't see it every time she opened the kitchen freezer. Another type of environmental control.

One more story. José wants to eat healthier, but he can't do it if there's nothing in the house to cook. So he plans ahead and keeps the refrigerator well stocked with delicious food that he can prepare quickly. He's learned that the only way to lose weight is to control his environment.

Everyone has different strengths, different weakness, and different food triggers. But you can see what I have in mind. Once you've identified the things that help you eat smarter, and those that send you tumbling off your diet, you can start rearranging your life to accommodate them.

BOTTOM LINE: Lose 31–46 pounds

If you do nothing more than eat healthful, home-cooked meals instead of high-fat food, you'll save at least 300 calories a night. Keep tempting sweets out of the house, and plan instead to enjoy one sweet once a week: Another 150 daily calories saved. And the list goes on and on.

#91. Dream

A decade or so ago, visualization was dismissed by scientists as little more than feel-good snake oil. Well, they're wrong.

No, imagining yourself thin won't solve your weight problems. But without visions of success, you are doomed. As with all things in life, you have to believe that you can be successful before you'll succeed—and one of the best ways to cement this idea in your head is to see the final results as clearly and positively as you can.

There's nothing exotic about visualization. Suppose, for example, you're hoping to lose 20 pounds. Start by visualizing yourself thinner. Form a complete mental picture. Spend some time with it. Picture the outfit the slimmer you is wearing. Imagine the attention you're getting from the opposite sex. Imagine *all* the details—don't be bashful!

While you're visualizing where you'd like to be a few months or years from now, don't rush the process. The more details you create in your mind—sounds, images, textures, and so on—the more real it will seem. And that's the first step to really believing you can do it!

BOTTOM LINE: Lose 10 pounds

People who visualize weight loss—not just on occasion, but every day—will find it much easier to control temptation. Even if your positive thoughts do nothing more than give you the strength to resist a few snacks, you'll easily save 100 calories a day.

92. Do Some Calorie Shifting

Americans traditionally eat a large dinner—one that we attack with zeal. Is it any wonder we gain so much weight?

I never really understood what it meant to "attack" dinner until I watched Jack, my significant other. He would stop at the Chinese takeout for his favorite Hunan shrimp. He would wolf it down, all 1,000 calories, before you could say, "Let's have dinner!"

Calories that are consumed late in the day aren't burned as efficiently as those consumed earlier on. Jack's a big guy who needs about 2,500 calories daily. But he was getting almost half of them at dinner, and that was before the beer.

I asked Jack to keep a food diary for awhile. When I reviewed it, I realized that he was only getting about 300 calories at breakfast. As a result, he started getting hungry earlier and earlier in the day. He would get a full lunch, usually a burger and fries or a fried seafood platter, at an hour most people are only thinking about snacks.

This had a ripple effect. Because he was eating lunch early, there were a lot of hours to go until dinner. He found himself feeding coins into vending machines at the U.S. Capitol, where he works. But snack or no snack, he was starving by the time he left work. He'd usually grab high-calorie takeout on the way home.

A BETTER BALANCE

It was obvious that Jack needed to rearrange his day's calories, and the only way he was going to do that was to do some planning. I advised him to start the day with 800 calories. He got it from healthy servings of granola, muesli, nuts, fruit, and milk.

We also discussed the importance of snacks to tide him over when his belly started to growl. He began to snack on fruit that he picked up at the farmers' market every Sunday, or from a street vendor on the way to work.

He was still hungry by the time lunch rolled around, but he wasn't ravenous any more. Most days, he was satisfied with a grilled chicken wrap—as long as he followed that up with some fruit in the afternoon. At night, he was able to calmly prepare himself a healthy bean and cheese burrito, or a veggie burger and soup.

Does this make sense? Everyone can enjoy a lighter dinner as long as the calories keep coming during the day. It does take some planning and probably more shopping than you may be used to, but the benefits will convince you. It works!

BOTTOM LINE: Lose 30 pounds

Eating relatively light dinners at night, and shifting more of the calories to breakfast and snacks, can easily save you 300 calories a day.

#93. Get Sexy Lingerie

Actually, a personal pat on the back does the same thing. You've worked hard? Reward yourself, darn it!

Americans are real demons when it comes to work and obligation, but we're not very good about rewarding ourselves for jobs well done. That's a mistake, because rewards make repeat successes more likely. Psychologists call this "classical conditioning."

Let's admit, first of all, that losing weight is hard work. Cutting calories is hard. Saying no to dessert is hard. Getting out of bed on a cold morning to exercise—that's hard! Who the heck is going to keep doing all this without some rewards?

Some mornings, I find it so difficult to drag myself out of bed in order to get my workout . . . there's a little voice inside my head that's saying, "I'm so tired, just 30 more minutes of sleep, mmmphhh . . ."

But most days, I get up anyway. I do it because I know I'll feel better for the rest of the day. And to be honest, I can be pretty smug sometimes about my dedication and commitment. I give myself a mental pat on the back and say, "Good girl!" I do the same thing when I finish my workout and leave the gym. I say something like, "Thank you, God, for getting me to the gym. I feel great. (And I'm glad it's over!)"

Patting yourself on the back and giving yourself compliments may feel silly at first. But rewards are more important than you know. Instead of, "Poor me, I have to exercise," say "Exercise makes me feel great, I'm so glad I did it!" You'll be more likely to repeat the performance.

THE GOOD-JOB CLUB

Personal rewards are okay, but I'd rather be complimented by those around me. When you're struggling to lose weight, get some help from your friends. Insist on it, in fact.

Let's say you're getting in the habit of cooking healthful meals. Don't allow your spouse to take it for granted. Ask him (or her) to tell you how good everything tastes. (A few reminders should get the ball rolling.) Did you finish your first week at the gym? That calls for a night at the theater, or a least a bouquet of flowers.

One of my clients, Carol, is so proud of her efforts to lose weight that she asked her husband to reward her periodically—not with the traditional chocolate, but with beautiful flowers, sexy lingerie, and nights at the theater. It worked. It really kept Carol in the mood to continue losing weight and keeping fit!

BOTTOM LINE: Lose 18 pounds

Reward yourself with something that's not a box of chocolates once a week and you'll save at least 1,200 calories.

#94. Listen to the Eagles

Remember the rock anthem that said "take it easy"? It's excellent advice for life in general and it really pays off when you're trying to lose weight.

Maybe it's a sign of a busy world, but we all seem to eat more quickly than we used to. You wouldn't think that plying a fast fork would contribute to weight gain, but it does.

There are sensors in the stomach that tell your brain when you've had enough to eat. But the sensors don't send "full" signals right away. There's a lag of about 20 minutes. The quicker you eat, the more likely you are to keep delivering food to the stomach long after it's had enough.

So slow down already! Rather than loading the fork as soon as it's emptied, put it down between bites. Chew each bit of food thoroughly. Give yourself time to smell it, taste it, and enjoy it.

If you do this all the time, you'll find that you're eating less than you did before. Better yet, you won't leave the table with that stuffed feeling. You'll feel satisfied, but not overwhelmed.

BOTTOM LINE: Lose 21 pounds

Eating more slowly will help you understand the difference between cravings and real hunger. Once you learn to stop eating when you're full (instead of stuffed), you can easily cut out 100 calories at lunch and dinner.

#95. Late Snack

If you regularly feel hungry in the afternoon and begin to forage, or if you attack your dinner as if you hadn't eaten in days, you are a candidate for a planned afternoon snack.

Please, respond to your body's signals. If you're hungry in the afternoon, even if it's close to dinner, have something to eat. Do it now. Approaching dinner in a ravenous state is asking for a binge. (Since you've got the whole night ahead of you, it could be a real doozy!)

It is especially important to eat an afternoon snack if dinner is late. If you regularly eat dinner at 7 P.M. or later, 5 or 6 hours may pass between lunch and dinner. So, plan an afternoon snack to ease your hunger.

Amy, one of my clients, worked out in the evening, just after work, which meant she was ravenous by dinner time. In fact, she often stopped at a fast-food restaurant on her way home from the gym—and she would consume double or triple the calories that she had managed to burn off.

Something clearly had to change. I advised Amy to eat in the late afternoon, about an hour before her workout. It might be a low-calorie frozen dinner that she brought from home and heated up in the office microwave, or the leftover sandwich she had at lunch. The snack menu didn't matter all that much, as long as it was reasonably healthy. This "mini-dinner" helped tide her over until her regular dinner at 8 or 9 P.M. Because of the snack, she was able to approach her dinner—sometimes nothing more than salad, soup, and fruit or yogurt—with relative calm.

Amy began to lose weight. The reduction in overall calories helped, but she was also successful because we customized her eating schedule.

BOTTOM LINE: Lose 30 pounds

Amy's planned snacks saved her at least 300 calories a night. She had more energy, less guilt, and more control. Way to go, snacks!

#96. Don't Go Home

What I mean is, don't go home right after work when your stress levels—and the urge to eat—are strongest. Make a little detour first.

One of my friends recently packed up and moved in order to live closer to the beach. When Linda's done with work for the day, she often stops at the beach before going home. Watching the sunset, walking along the beach, or just listening to the waves gives her a chance to unwind and relax.

There must be pleasant spots in your area where you can unwind at the end of the day. Parks and river walks are great. So is (perish the thought!) dropping by the gym.

You'll notice that I'm not emphasizing the benefits of exercise. The more you give yourself a chance to unwind at the end of the day, the less likely you'll be to resort to unplanned snacking or other unhealthy habits.

Oh, don't forget to throw some casual clothes in your car. Get comfortable and have a great time!

BOTTOM LINE: Lose 15–30 pounds

A lot of my clients only take one walk a week. If you give yourself this relaxing time every day after work, the exercise alone could help you lose as much as 16 pounds in a year. And let's not forget to factor in the "anxious eating" that people often do at the end of the day. Find something else to do, and you'll save an additional 150 calories each day!

#97. Eat Early

Millions of Americans skip breakfast, and millions of Americans are overweight. It's not a coincidence. Eating early is one of the best ways to take the edge off your hunger for the rest of the day.

Donna, one of my clients, thought she had a perfect way to lose weight: skipping breakfast. The only problem: It didn't work.

When we reviewed her eating habits, the reasons became apparent. Without breakfast, she was ravenous around 10 o'clock in the morning, and would reach out to whatever was handy to satisfy her appetite. Usually that "something" was pretty darn fattening.

She's hardly alone. Studies have shown that people who skip breakfast are much more likely to gain weight than those who fill their tanks first thing in the morning.

Breakfast doesn't have to be a complicated proposition. First, have a breakfast that supplies about a third of your daily caloric needs. If you get 1,500 calories a day, then you want a breakfast with 500 calories.

Don't have much appetite in the morning? Then eat a small breakfast, and follow it up with a healthful, planned midmorning snack. That's what I do when I exercise right after breakfast. Most mornings, though, I don't exercise until a few hours later, so I enjoy a full breakfast. Either way, I am not hungry for lunch until 1 P.M.

BOTTOM LINE: Lose 22–30 pounds

When you eat a healthful breakfast, you'll be much less likely to load up on cheeseburgers, fries, or other high-calorie foods later on. This alone can save you 300–400 calories a day.

#98. Satisfy Your Sweet Tooth

I love chocolate. Candy, cookies, ice cream, you name it. But I can't have sweets every day. Neither can you, if you want to lose weight.

I first discovered the connection between sweets and weight during visits to my grandmother in Sweden when I was 19. She would make me hot chocolate with heavy whipping cream and cocoa. It was a perfect accompaniment to the little tray of homemade cookies she also prepared. I loved it, and I looked forward to it every evening.

Oh, and because it was midsummer, there were tender, sweet, perfectly ripe strawberries everywhere. So we sliced them up and topped them with a hefty splash of whipping cream.

I was young, which partly explains why I didn't even imagine that all of this wonderful food was going to have some unintended consequences. Foolish youth! That was when my weight problem began, and it took a long time before I figured out how to deal with it.

SWEETS THAT WON'T BE DENIED
One of the best lessons I ever learned is that sweet-lovers (and we are many!) have to find ways to enjoy these lovely indulgences without negative consequences. It's not easy, because sweets are high in calories relative to the feelings of fullness they provide. One luscious dessert, for example, may provide the same number of calories as a large meal with all the trimmings.

Here's what I do. When I'm going through a sweet-tooth phase, I'm going to want a treat every day. So I look for something with a reasonable number of calories—say, 120 calories per serving or less. I've found frozen chocolate bars that fit the bill perfectly. Even an ounce of good chocolate is okay.

But what if, on the other hand, I want a really luscious dessert? I plan for it and have it once a week. I'll get a lot of calories in one sitting, but that won't be a problem as long as I'm not doing it all the time.

I do draw the line in some places. A bakery near my house has some really scrumptious cookies. But once I realized that each cookie delivered about 600 calories, I decided that the long-term costs just weren't worth the pleasure. So I avoid them.

BOTTOM LINE: Lose 34 pounds

Here's some good advice. If your current dessert of choice has 500 calories, give it up, at least on a daily basis. Find a substitute that only has 120 calories. That's your "everyday" treat. What about that rich dessert? Have it once a week. You'll save 380 calories 6 days a week. That adds up to serious weight loss!

#99. Sing in the Shower

Actually, yelling is more like it. And believe me, when you crank up that cold water, you'll hear some yelling!

There are bath people and shower people in the world. Some of us (me, for example), are "bi"—I love to relax both ways. I spend so much time submerged in water that I hit upon an intriguing way to lose weight.

When you're finished scrubbing and are ready to exit, crank up the water to as hot a temperature as comfort allows. Luxuriate for a moment, then turn it all the way to cold. (Pause for yelling.) Stay under the cold spray for at least 10 seconds. You'll actually feel your body temperature change.

Why in the world would I suggest such torture? Very simply, it's the most relaxing treat imaginable. Regular baths and showers help you relax. But this alternative hot-and-cold finale will give you an unbelievable surge of energy.

The next time you get the urge to eat, even though you're not really hungry, you can assume that you're anxious about something. Now's the time for your bath or shower. You'll feel more relaxed and in control, and less likely to binge unnecessarily.

When I was working out my "nervous snacking" problem, some weekends I'd be in the tub five times a day! I felt it was better than nonhunger, nervous eating.

BOTTOM LINE: Lose 26–31 pounds

Use a daily shower to get you over snacking urges, and you could potentially save 250–300 calories a day.

#100. Kiss Your Spouse

Stress in personal relationships make divorce lawyers very happy. Insult to injury, it can also make you heavier.

Studies show that happily married couples have just as much conflict as unhappy or divorced couples. The difference is that the happily married couples deal with conflicts more effectively.

I suspect they're also more likely to eat wisely, take in fewer calories, and manage their weight effectively.

I've been talking a lot about how stress, anxiety, depression, and other "negative" emotions lead us to eat more than we should, or even more than we want. Troubled relationships—not only within marriages, but also in the workplace or between friends—create tremendous amounts of stress. That's why it makes so much sense to resolve your conflicts as quickly and amicably as you can instead of escaping through food.

One of my clients, Mary, was having a terrible time at work. She just couldn't get along with her boss. Every day, she came home from work and binged.

Sound familiar? We all do this sometimes. Mary, to her credit, wanted to break the pattern. With professional guidance, she began to understand the underlying cause of her cravings, and she took active steps to resolve the conflicts. She ultimately took a new job—but even before that, she began to lose weight because she faced conflict and began communicating with her boss more effectively.

BOTTOM LINE: Lose 7 pounds

Resolving conflicts instead of "solving" them with food and drink could save you 500 calories each Friday night!

#101. Breathe, Bathe, Relax

If everyone in this country would learn to relax a little more, the pounds would melt away like butter.

Mike is a perfect example. A political pundit and journalist in Washington, D.C., he always faces stressful daily deadlines. One of his coping strategies is to buy a bag of candies, take it back to his desk, and devour it while working at his computer.

He wasn't eating because he was hungry. It wasn't because he had a powerful taste for this or that treat. He did it because he was tense—and if snacking allowed him to procrastinate a little, well, so much the better.

There's no question that food gives us comfort. The next time a craving comes out of nowhere, ask yourself how you're feeling. Stressed? Bored? Discouraged? All three? I guarantee you this: Start practicing stress management, and you will lose weight.

Back to Mike for a moment. I suggested that he practice deep diaphragmatic breathing, also called belly breathing. It's a type of breathing in which the exertion comes from the diaphragm, not the chest. It's a great stress-reduction technique because you can do it anywhere, even when you're standing in line at the checkout counter.

Mike belly breathed for a few minutes whenever he felt a craving coming on—and the craving would simply disappear. Needless to say, he started to lose weight.

Years ago, I had the habit of eating when I was anxious, and the extra weight I was carrying was evidence of how anxious I really was. Deep breathing didn't work for me. My trick was soaking in the tub. I started doing it whenever I felt the first twinge of anxiety-induced cravings. By gosh, it worked! Ever since then, I've stayed committed to this particular relaxation strategy, but also, depending on the situation, will take walks, do yoga, call a friend, flip through a magazine, or talk with my significant other. My nervous eating is almost entirely a thing of the past.

Everyone has different ways of controlling stress. Communicating with a loved one is an excellent way to work out your tension. One of my clients, Elaine, always calls her sister after stressful days at work. Conversation calms her down and helps her get in control of her eating.

Another option: Consider getting a pet. Dogs, for example, are happy to take leftovers off your hands! More important, they can reduce stress just by standing near you. Research has even shown that petting a dog, cat, or another pet can lower blood pressure and help you live longer.

BOTTOM LINE: Lose 15 pounds

Once you learn to manage stress with relaxation techniques instead of by eating, you'll eat at least 150 calories less a day.

#102. Love Your Pet

Don't have a dog? Then take a bath. Call your mother. Heck, clean out a kitchen drawer. Just do anything that isn't eating.

One of the most vulnerable times of day is when you first arrive home from work. You're exhausted, stressed, and hungry. Putting food in front of you at this precise time is nothing less than pure folly.

What you need to do is unwind. This might involve nothing more than changing into comfortable clothes. On really bad days, you may want to take a long bubble bath. And your dog does need to go out, right? So get moving. Blow off some of your stress. Do anything that doesn't involve the sight, smell, or taste of food. The more you relax your body and emotions, the less vulnerable you'll be to "anxious eating."

Incidentally, you might not know that people experiencing stress tend to be attracted to the fattiest foods around. You might want to plan for this by keeping plenty of healthy snack foods in the house—plenty of cut-up fresh fruit, for example, or baby carrots.

But the more you learn to unwind, the less you'll turn to food in any event. In fact, people who actively find ways to lower their stress often find that their cravings decrease at the same time.

BOTTOM LINE: Lose 22 pounds

Welcome-home relaxation techniques that divert you from chips, cheese, or other snacks could wind up saving you 300 calories—and that's every work night!

#103. Light a Candle

Don't worry. I'm not suggesting something mystical. But I would like you to turn off the television, the radio, and maybe the overhead light. Get in the mood for eating.

Most of us eat on the run or while we're doing something else at the same time. This kind of automatic eating contributes a lot to weight problems.

Here's why. Your body knows when you've had enough to eat. It tells you so with "satiety signals." But we're all so busy these days, we've stopped paying attention. So we keep eating even when we don't need to eat any more. The bigger portions we're served today make this even more likely.

Eliminate all distractions while eating. Stop working. Get your mind off everything but the food. If it helps, turn off the lights and light a candle. And turn off that TV, for goodness' sakes!

Feeling calm? Good. Now you can focus on the food that's in front of you. Breathe in the aroma. Enjoy the taste and texture, and most of all, appreciate the peaceful space you've just created.

This process of improving awareness may feel unnatural at first, but it quickly becomes natural. You'll also find that you're much more tuned into your body's signals, including the ones that say, "You've had enough."

BOTTOM LINE: Lose 21 pounds

This type of mindful eating almost guarantees that you'll eat less than you did before. I wouldn't be surprised if you save 100 calories at every lunch and dinner.

#104. Get Moving Fast

That's exactly what exercise does. It unleashes floods of chemicals in the brain that reduce anxiety and stress—and, as a bonus, help control appetite.

Exercise is an integral part of any weight-loss plan, but not only because it burns calories. Exercise makes you feel better emotionally and psychologically. And when you feel good, you're less likely to use food as a personal security blanket.

That's an important point. Unlike our ancestors, many of us hardly have to lift a finger in order to survive. We're more sedentary than ever before, and our bodies—and emotions—have paid the price. Maybe you get tired more easily than you should. Or you're always feeling stressed and under pressure. Need an emotional "fix"? Have something to eat!

One of my clients, Tom, is always ravenous after work. But he doesn't eat right away. Instead, he exercises. By the time he gets back home, his "hunger" has decreased dramatically.

How can exercise reduce hunger? Actually, it doesn't. What it does do is burn away stress and exhaustion—emotions that many of us have come to translate as "time to eat." By getting in a good workout after work, Tom found himself more relaxed and able to have a reasonable dinner instead of a pig-out.

BOTTOM LINE: Lose 30–50 pounds

Exercise can save you 300 calories of "anxiety snacking" a day. It also burns calories in its own right. Exercise daily for 30 minutes, lose at least 20 pounds a year. Exercise more, lose more weight!

#105. Examine Your Goals

If you're having trouble losing as much weight as you want as quickly as you want, ask yourself if you've set realistic goals—or if you even care about the goals you've set.

Nothing is more demoralizing than setting goals that you fail to reach. This has nothing to do with determination or discipline. You probably set the bar too high.

My advice is this. Set very modest goals at first. Even if they're so small that they seem insignificant, the satisfaction that you'll feel when you reach them will keep you going.

How do you set good goals?

Be realistic, not a perfectionist. Perfectionists can't help but fail. Permit yourself to be imperfect—and even plan imperfections in your program.

Look at behavior, not numbers. No one can "promise" to lose X amount of pounds. What you can control is your behavior. One goal, for example, might be to eat a good breakfast. Another might be to eat more vegetables. Set goals based on what you'll "do," rather than what you'll "be." Once you start doing the things that you've outlined for yourself, the weight loss will naturally fall into place.

Emphasize the positive. Instead of telling yourself what you won't do, tell yourself what you will: "I will prepare a beautiful bowl of raspberries when I get home from work, " or "I will go for a walk three days this week."

Be flexible. Exercising every day may be admirable, but unforeseen circumstances, if nothing else, will be sure to intervene. Better to make goals that are more flexible: "I will exercise five days every week." If it turns out that you exercise every single day, well, you get bonus points!

Set measurable goals. Specificity makes things happen. "I'll eat more vegetables" is a good goal, but how will you know you reach it? No matter what you plan to do, be specific: "I'll add a vegetable to every lunch and dinner this week," or "I'll exercise for twenty minutes" five out of seven mornings.

Make sure you care. If you consistently fail to meet certain goals, it's possible that they're the wrong ones for you. If the program you've started doesn't excite you, find one that suits you better.

BOTTOM LINE: Lose 31 pounds

Goals that are reachable will make it a lot easier to stay with the program. Even if you only reduce your calories intake by 300 a day, you'll lose impressive amounts of weight in a year.

#106. Eat a Brownie Every Friday

Do you have a particular calorie-rich treat that you crave—and devour—every night? No problem. Here's how to turn cravings to your advantage.

One of my clients, Paul, absolutely loves sweets. He thinks about them all the time, and in the best of all possible worlds, he'd enjoy them with abandon. But none of us can do this for very long without gaining weight.

Here's what Paul does instead. Every Friday night, he allows himself to eat a rich, delicious brownie *without guilt*. In fact, he gloats about it. And no wonder. All week, from Monday through Thursday, he thinks about that brownie. Rather than surrendering to sweets during the week, he reminds himself how much he's going to enjoy that very special treat on Friday.

Is he ever tempted to stray? Of course. But he's able to resist because he knows that weight loss is all about prioritizing.

Suppose, for example, that you're going to a birthday party Saturday night. Let yourself think about the delicious cake, ice cream, and other snacks you're going to have. Then, when a sweet craving pops into your mind, remind yourself about the special treat that's still to come. It's easier to defer your desire for sweets and to make sure they're your favorites than to deny them altogether.

BOTTOM LINE: Lose 30 pounds

At 500 calories per brownie, Paul is hardly depriving himself. Yet by prioritizing his snacks, he manages to forego 2,000 weekly calories!

#107. Learn from Mistakes

Always evaluate what works in your diet and what doesn't—and decide what you can do differently the next time.

The more you fail, the more you learn. I know, it's a tired old bromide, but there's a lot of truth to it. People who are successful don't fail less than anyone else. They just learn from their failures, pick up the pieces, and do it better the next time.

Joanna, one of my clients, tended to emphasize the negative. "I ate too much chocolate" or "I couldn't exercise on Tuesday" was how she started most conversations.

But when I looked at her overall work, I realized that she was doing a lot of things right. Most days she ate well, exercised, and so on. When I pointed this out to her, she began to understand that she was really doing a pretty good job. Her "mistake" was that she didn't recognize her successes!

A lot of diets fail because people set goals that they don't have a prayer of achieving, like losing 30 pounds for an upcoming reunion—next month. I mean, come on! Once you realize what's realistic and what's not, you'll be in a much better position to succeed for the long haul.

BOTTOM LINE: Lose 31 pounds

People who take the time to analyze successes and failures are going to do a lot better overall. Remember, even if you only cut out 300 calories a day, you'll lose more than 30 pounds this year!

#108. Say "No" to Something Bad

People often find themselves gaining weight because they serve other peoples' demands at the expense of their own needs. The solution? Say no more often.

Do you work all the time? Find it difficult to turn down requests? Are you one of those people for whom the demands of career, family, or even pets always come first?

Stop! It's time to take care of yourself. De-stress and unwind. Otherwise, food will have an almost irresistible appeal. You can't eat yourself happy—but nearly everyone tries.

Here's a good exercise. Think about the things you do for others. Now, rank them. Which are the ones that irritate you the most? Now, decide which of the items you should say no to. Don't feel guilty. If you're truly irritated by something, there's a good chance that the other person should be doing it instead, without using you as a crutch.

Of course, we're all willing to help in emergencies and cases of genuine need. But that's not the issue. We're talking about dependency here.

Consider Sheila, one of my clients. She learned to say no to her boss's inappropriate demands for extra work with no extra pay. Thanks to her newfound confidence and sense of self-worth, she stopped bingeing at night—and lost 50 pounds the next year. An extreme case, certainly, but not unusual.

BOTTOM LINE: Lose 5–10 pounds

When you take care of yourself, reduce emotional frustration, and refrain from turning to food for reassurance, you'll find yourself losing weight without even trying.

#109. Say "Yes" to Something Good

It's often easier to say no to things that are irritating or time consuming than to say yes to things that are good for you. Isn't it time to do something nice for yourself?

Maybe there's something frivolous that you've wanted to buy, or a little luxury that you think about, but are always putting off. Well, pamper yourself for a change.

True, making time for yourself may take some getting used to, but all healthy adults do it, and all say that it's worth every second. It's essential to feeling your best and living the highest quality of life possible, as well as being able to give your best to others.

What does emotional health have to do with your weight? Everything! Hunger is one reason we eat, but it's not the only one. We also eat when we're tired, discouraged, or sad. When you feel good emotionally, you're much less likely to turn to food for solace.

So what will it be? A leisurely soak in the tub? A long-distance call to a friend you haven't seen for awhile? Window shopping for things you like? Reading a really trashy book? I'm sure you won't have trouble thinking of something!

Oh, just be sure that your "reward" isn't food-related. There are other pleasures in life, believe me.

BOTTOM LINE: Lose 5–10 pounds

Saying no to things you don't like, and yes to things you do, are the flip sides of the same emotional coin. Take care of yourself emotionally and physically. It's good for your soul as well as your weight.

CHAPTER 12

Getting Organized
and Losing Pounds

Especially appropriate for: *Hassled Moms, Busy Bachelors, Overworked College Students, Workaholics and People Who Live at the Office, Chefs, People Who Forget to Eat or Who Eat "Catch as Catch Can," People Who Don't Plan Their Eating*

Does the phrase "catch as catch can" or "on a whim" describe the way you eat? Maybe you have time in your life for everything except regular meals. You might be so busy pleasing others that your own nutritional health always takes a back seat.

I call this pattern disorganized eating. People who are disorganized eaters often feel as though they need a mother or wife to take care of them because they simply aren't able—or willing—to take care of themselves.

Well, stop it! Treat yourself as well as your mother treated you, or as well as you treat others. Aren't you worth it? A little personal mothering will go a long way toward making you feel important and nurtured. You'll notice improvements in your mood and self-confidence. You'll find yourself making healthful changes that you always wanted to make, but somehow never got around to. You'll discover how good it feels to grow as a person, to learn and to get smarter with every passing year.

I have many disorganized eaters among my clients, and they have a remarkable variety of excuses about why they find it difficult to take the time to eat properly. Take a moment and ask yourself if any of the following situations sound familiar.

- You stuff yourself every time you eat out, and you eat out a lot—not only dinner, but also breakfast and lunch—even though you never really plan to.
- You grab food whenever and wherever you see it. At the supermarket, you might be chomping away while you wait at the checkout counter. If you pass a Dunkin' Donuts, you almost feel compelled to stop. Does the expression "out of control" come to mind?
- You are so busy and focused on your work that you often forget to eat. That is, until you come face-to-face with a vending machine or join your colleagues at happy hour—and then, watch out!
- You're a college student who spends every waking hour studying or in class. You can't find the time to eat, and certainly you're never awake for breakfast. So whenever you find yourself in the vicinity of food, you grab it out of desperation.
- You are too busy taking care of your family to take care of yourself. You eat what is left over on your children's plates. You taste food while you're cooking, but you never seem to sit down for an entire meal. Still, you feel as though you're overweight and can't manage to lose a single pound.
- You're a chef or food service worker who is surrounded by food, but there's never time for a leisurely meal. The only time you can eat is at the end of the shift when all the customers are gone. You might be 30, 40, or even 50 pounds overweight. Your family is worried. Your doctor is worried. You're worried.

Did you find yourself in this crowd? The solution is easier than you might think. If you spend the bare minimum of time that's necessary to organize your life, you'll soon discover that you spend even less time eating than you did before. Why? Because you'll be eating healthy, and healthy eating, with a little planning, is the quickest style of eating you could ask for.

We'll talk more about finding order in chaos in just a bit. For now, I'll just say that mealtime management is 50 percent of the solution. Your willingness to try something new is the other 50 percent. Everyone I know who has taken the time to organize his or her eating swears that it saves time, saves money, and increases energy levels. Which means you'll have even more time to spend on the activities and people you enjoy.

A Success Story

Two of my clients, Jane and Paul, are computer professionals who spend long hours at work. When we first started talking, they were convinced that they had no time for cooking. Just about every meal was at a restaurant, except for meals that they picked up at takeout joints. After several years of living this way, Paul was 100 pounds overweight, and Jennifer tipped the scale at 50 pounds over her desired weight.

They longed for a saner existence. They knew that cooking their own meals and eating at home was an important first step—financially, if for no other reason. And when they did begin preparing meals together at home, they were delighted at the improvements they noticed in just about every part of their lives.

They started losing weight. They felt more energetic and alive. Their relationship improved because they had more quality time with each other, and that helped relieve stress and stress-related eating. They began looking forward to their evenings together, and they enjoyed planning what they might fix for dinner. The changes felt "old-fashioned," but good and very rewarding. They were mothering and nurturing each other.

The "secret" of their success was really pretty simple. Time, or the lack of it, wasn't the cause of their disorganized eating. They just needed to develop a little more focus, and also to establish some new habits. As they soon learned, eating at restaurants because of poor time management actually takes as much time, or more, than preparing meals from scratch.

An Easy Action Plan

If you're a disorganized eater, you'll need to put together a few organizational building blocks—things like scheduling regular meal times, going grocery shopping at regular intervals, stocking your office with quick (and healthful) foods, and so on.

Already feeling overwhelmed? Well, consider this. If you do nothing more than make a few of the changes that I suggest below, you're almost guaranteed to achieve the weight loss you're after. Just a few examples:

Get in the habit of batch cooking. On weekends, make large amounts of soup, stews, and main course salads. Put them in containers and store them in the refrigerator and freezer. Guess what? You've just provided yourself with delicious and nutritious alternatives to restaurant and takeout food for the coming week.

People often think that batch cooking is only useful for dinner fare. Not true. You can use similar techniques to stock up on ready-to-go lunches and breakfasts, as well.

Work exercise into your busy life. I know, no one wants to be reminded to exercise. But my clients have found some ingenious, nearly effortless ways to exercise *without* exercising. In other words, they don't necessarily belong to a gym or watch TV while pedaling a stationary bike. They incorporate physical movement—such as walking or climbing stairs—into their lives without bothering to set aside time for "formal" exercise.

Don't try to do everything at once. You'll find dozens of simple, get-organized techniques in the pages to come. Some you'll try on occasion, and some you'll use all the time. Some won't appeal to you, and others you'll love. The goal isn't to incorporate all of these strategies into your life, but only those that feel most natural for you. They're the ones you'll stick with—and the more consistent you are, the more weight you'll lose!

#110. Shop by the Book

Do you shop for groceries on a regular basis? If your answer is "no," I've got some bad news.

Open the refrigerator and take a look inside. Does yours contain only nail polish, beer, or ketchup? An empty fridge is a sure sign of shopping disarray.

Or, does your refrigerator mainly contain half-empty takeout containers, or a few bowls of moldy something-or-other? Another bad sign.

Disorganized eaters tend to be disorganized shoppers. It's that simple. When you don't have the right foods on hand and ready to go, you have no choice but to improvise. Improvised eating usually translates into splurging at restaurants or stopping at fast-food places and convenience stores. The result, of course, is weight gain.

I have two important pieces of advice. Number one, go shopping every week. Not just when the refrigerator is looking a little bare or when you've reached the bottom of the gallon of Rocky Road. Go every single week. It's the only way to ensure that you always have the ingredients on hand to make nutritious meals that are as quick as they are delicious.

The second piece of advice: Set a specific day and time when you'll *always* go to the store. I admit this will sound draconian to some people, but if you aren't in the habit of shopping regularly, it's the best way to get in the habit. In fact, mark the day and time on your calendar. Choose a time that works for you. Maybe early Saturday, before the hordes arrive. Later in the evening is fine, too. Whatever works best for you.

If you still aren't convinced, let me tell you about one of my clients. She was one of the most disorganized eaters ever. Her routine—her *daily* routine—was to pick up takeout food on her way home. The meals had, on average, about 1,000 calories. I convinced her to start cooking more at home. Guess what? She saved at least 400 calories per meal. With just this one change, she lost 30 pounds in less than a year.

BOTTOM LINE: Lose 20–80 pounds

Organized shopping saves time. That's an important consideration in our busy lives. But that's just the beginning.

Good grocery shopping skills are the flip side of good meal management skills: Both save tremendous amounts of calories. Suppose, for example, you plan ahead for a daily fruit snack: By cutting back on the usual junk food, you could lose 20 pounds a year. Eat homemade lunches every day instead of stopping at the burger joint: another 22 to 30 pounds lost. Enjoy healthy dinners at home instead of splurging or doing takeout: subtract another 30 pounds.

All this just from buying groceries on schedule. Wow!

#111. Don't Cook on Weekdays

Strange advice? Well, I mean it. Life is busy, busy, busy, and if you try to do your weekday cooking on top of everything else, you'll find yourself making reservations at every joint in town.

To take stress out of your life (and calories out of your diet), you want to get in the habit of preparing batch meals ahead of time, preferably on weekends, when you're not as rushed and tired as you are during the week.

This concept is so important that I've added an extra section of recipes for batch cooking.

My clients are sometimes confused about the whole concept of batch cooking. The idea is to prepare quick and easy dinners ahead of time so that you always have something in the freezer or refrigerator that's ready to go on a moment's notice.

Let's say I'm going to make veal stew as my main-course "batch" meal, and broccoli salad as my "batch" side dish. I'll keep enough in the refrigerator for Sunday and Tuesday night dinners; the rest goes in the freezer for dinners on Thursday and Saturday nights.

Other nights, I might have lean burgers (95 percent lean, or game such as buffalo or venison), burritos, or pizza—meals that I can whip up in a hurry. Since I do most of the shopping and cooking on weekends, I spend hardly any time on food preparation during the week. That makes life easy!

Let's get to specifics. For the veal stew, I want to buy enough for eight servings. I make sure that I have olive oil, herbes de Provence, and bay leaves. I'll buy four pounds of veal rump, four carrots, two onions, four ripe tomatoes, six small potatoes, and a bottle of good, dry, white wine. I don't want a cheap bottle of wine ruining my veal stew.

For my broccoli salad, I'll need a pound and a half of frozen or fresh broccoli, a box of raisins, unsalted sunflower seeds, bacon-flavored soy bits, one onion, a small container of nonfat plain yogurt, light mayo (which I already have, for my sandwiches), and small amounts of sugar and vinegar (which I already have in my cabinet).

Finally, for my quick meals, I'll need a half pound of ground lean buffalo, whole-wheat hamburger buns for the burgers (or a package of lean hot dogs and hot dog buns), a frozen pizza, and, for the burritos, whole-wheat tortillas, reduced-fat cheese, a can of black beans, and salsa.

Here's what the week's dinner schedule will look like:

Sunday	Veal stew
Monday	Buffalo burgers with broccoli salad
Tuesday	Veal stew
Wednesday	Burritos with broccoli salad
Thursday	Veal stew
Friday	Frozen pizza and broccoli salad
Saturday	Veal stew

BOTTOM LINE: Lose 36 pounds

Let's say you eat out one night during the week, but the other nights you have these delicious and nutritious meals at home. You'll save at least 400 calories per meal!

#112. The Joy of Index Cards

When you go on your weekly shopping trips, you want to minimize aimless roaming down the aisles of temptation. Your goal should be to head directly for the items you plan to buy. Don't rely on memory: It will let you down every time.

I admit it: Index cards excite me, and I share this enthusiasm with my clients. I advise everyone to keep a few 3x5 index cards in their purses or pockets. When you think of things you need to buy, jot them down right away. I also keep a message pad in my kitchen. This way, you won't have to keep reminding yourself of things—items that you'll probably forget about by the time you get to the store.

When your shopping day rolls around, review all your notes and condense them onto one list. List food items in the order in which you'll visit those aisles or sections of the store. If you know you'll encounter the produce section first, for example, you'll want to list all the produce items together, at the beginning of your list.

This makes for a very efficient trip. You can go straight to what you want, rather than zigzagging back and forth. Apart from saving time, you'll also be less likely to indulge in "hunger shopping," which can add calories (and cost) to your weekly diet.

BOTTOM LINE: Lose 20–80 pounds

Grocery lists are absolutely essential when you're shopping on a once-a-week schedule. Take my word for it: Shopping regularly and stocking up will help you lose tremendous amounts of weight, almost without trying!

#113. Coffee Ain't Enough

I can't count the number of people who tell me that they skip breakfast, and the calories that go with it, in order to lose weight. Wake up! It's a lousy idea.

Donna, one of my clients, thought she had the perfect way to lose weight. She cut out breakfast altogether, except for coffee. She thought it made sense because she was eliminating all of those "extra" calories.

She didn't lose weight, of course. Whether she admitted it or not at the time, she was starving by midmorning. When she was stressed, anxious, or merely ravenous, she would grab something to satisfy her stomach. The calories from her near-constant nibbling really added up.

Donna felt guilty for her lack of discipline. But discipline had nothing to do with it. The problem was hunger and the body's demand for calories. The body has to be satisfied one way or another.

A recent study showed that most people who lose weight and keep it off successfully are breakfast eaters. That's true of adults, and it may be even more true of young people. Teenage girls who skip breakfast are more likely to be overweight or obese.

THE BREAKFAST HABIT

I understand that breakfast, for some people, isn't the most appealing meal of the day. All I can say is, too bad! If you want to lose weight, you have to start the day with a healthful breakfast. There are a few ways to do it.

If you wake up a little earlier than usual and give yourself enough time, you can have a full breakfast that provides a third of your daily caloric needs. If you get 1,500 calories a day, 500 of those calories should come at breakfast.

Still rushed in the morning? You might want to divide those 500 breakfast calories into two meals: half at breakfast, and half as a healthful, midmorning snack. I do this myself when I exercise right after breakfast. Most mornings, though, I don't exercise until a few hours later, so I enjoy a full breakfast. Either way, I am not hungry for lunch until 1 P.M.

My favorite breakfast is a big bowl of oatmeal. I cook it with milk and nuts, and add fruit. I recommend this to a lot of my clients, and most find that they enjoy it. What's more, they're often amazed at how fantastic they feel after allowing themselves this old-fashioned luxury. See the *Think Yourself Thin* menu plans on page 469 for some great breakfast ideas.

The bonus is, they're less hungry the entire day—even up until dinner. One of my most skeptical friends, Dan, tried the big breakfast and reluctantly agreed it controlled his appetite throughout the entire day. For some people, this is the only change they need to make to lose weight and keep it off successfully.

BOTTOM LINE: Lose 22–30 pounds

If you eat a healthful breakfast every day, and the calories you take in make it possible for you to avoid "emotional snacks" or simply cheeseburgers and fries, you'll save 300–400 calories a day. Can't beat it!

#114. Eat Breakfast at Work

Breakfast isn't appealing for some people. No sweat. All you have to do is create an office breakfast stash. It's ready whenever you are!

Perhaps you just don't feel like eating when you first get up. My friend Linda is like that—but she doesn't let it stop her from having a nutritious, filling breakfast.

"I'm not a morning person and I could never get interested in eating breakfast until I started bringing it to work," she says. "On Mondays, I bring in a loaf of my favorite grain bread, a large container of cottage cheese, a box of instant oatmeal, and some fresh fruit that lasts, like apples and pears. I leave everything at the office for the week. With a fridge and microwave at the office, it's no sweat for me to make a nice breakfast when I'm finally hungry, usually around 9 A.M."

Almost everything you normally eat at home can also be enjoyed at the office. Most offices have microwaves, so you can even have some turkey bacon or a veggie sausage. How about whole grain toast with peanut butter and a serving of fresh fruit? Or cereal with milk and fresh fruit?

Even if you don't have access to a refrigerator, there are plenty of wholesome breakfast foods that will fit in a desk drawer, such as mini-containers of cereal, raisins, or high-fiber crackers.

BOTTOM LINE: Lose 22–30 pounds
A satisfying office breakfast can stave off cravings for a cheeseburger and fries—and save you 300–400 calories every day.

#115. Cook More Than You Can Eat

A strange suggestion to find in a weight-loss book? Believe it or not, it's among the best approaches for shedding extra pounds because the foods you cook today become nutritious leftovers for later.

In our frenzied super-busy world, time is the most precious commodity. We never have enough of it. That's why it is so tempting to cut corners and pick up something to eat at a drive-up window on the way home.

My advice: Make the most of the time you spend in the kitchen. Make more than you can eat now. Put what's left in the refrigerator or freezer. You'll be surprised how just knowing that something delicious is waiting for you staves off temptation on the way home. It also makes it possible to invite a friend over at the last moment rather than going out together to eat.

Having food that's ready to go is one of the most important steps you can take, and it's one of the most important tips in this book. It can save you hundreds of calories each and every night because you'll be less likely to order high-calorie meals at restaurants. That can add up to plenty of lost pounds in a year's time, or even a month's time.

BOTTOM LINE: Lose 30–42 pounds

A meal at a restaurant or fast-food joint will easily set you back 1,000 calories. A meal cooked at home, including those delicious leftovers, has only about 600 calories. So cook more—and cook large!

#116. Save Time with Frozen Pineapple Juice

Fresh fruits and vegetables are deliciously wholesome, but frozen or ready-cut produce is every bit as good—and it's more convenient.

You already know how nutritious fruits and vegetables are, so I don't have to sell you on that. The most important thing is to eat a variety of fruits and vegetables, preferably with every meal.

Don't fret about always getting your fruits and vegetables fresh. In the summer, I buy as much as I can from the farmers' market. In the winter, I get all my produce at the grocery store—fresh, frozen, or canned. The advantage of frozen and canned fruits and vegetables is that they're usually picked when perfectly ripe, then frozen or canned immediately. "Fresh" grocery store produce, on the other hand, is often picked early to compensate for the long storage times. Frozen is often the most convenient choice because it's been cleaned and chopped into bite sizes.

When buying fresh: Consider cleaning, chopping, and storing fresh produce in plastic containers or baggies as soon as you get home. That way, it's ready for use all week long. As long as you eat it every day, you won't run the risk of turning your refrigerator crisper into a "rotter." And your kids will have healthy snacks they can grab any time.

BOTTOM LINE: Lose up to 20–50 pounds

If you add a salad to your evening meal, and cut back on portion sizes generally, you can lose 30 pounds in a year. Substituting a fruit snack for a vending machine snack every day will save another 20 pounds!

#117. Eat More to Eat Less

The biggest cause of overeating is undereating. No kidding. People often go too long without eating, then pig out when they're ravenously hungry. Call it poor mealtime management.

Your body is designed to get hungry every 3 to 4 hours. It is important to have a regular progression of meals: breakfast, snack, lunch, snack, and dinner.

This sort of regular routine maintains your body's normal hunger signals. It also boosts the metabolism to its highest rates, making it more efficient at burning calories.

Unfortunately, we tend to focus most of our attention on a few big meals, especially dinner. That's a problem because your body needs calories during the day, when you're active and burning them. It doesn't need large amounts of calories at night, when the body's natural rhythm is to slow down.

Research shows that people who eat their largest meal at night tend to be more overweight and have higher cholesterol levels than those who eat smaller amounts of food throughout the day.

Also, eating more often—and including planned snacks in your routine—is a great way to prevent binges. Binges usually are a result of poor planning: You'll inevitably find yourself at a wrong place (a fast-food restaurant, a vending machine) at the wrong time (when you're ravenous).

A BETTER WAY
Here's what I advise nearly all of my clients:

- Eat your usual supper at least three hours before going to bed. Make this your last meal of the day, if you can.
- Allow for exceptions. You want to eat when you're hungry, and if for some reason you're truly hungry after supper—and you're not merely bored, tired, or depressed—go ahead and have a snack. A piece of fresh fruit is best. Or vegetables, which make a great snack at any time.

• Always plan to have a snack in midmorning and midafternoon. Your body needs the calories—listen to it!

If you do nothing else except plan your meals more carefully, *you're going to lose weight*. I guarantee it. In fact, the amount of weight you'll lose over a year, even if this is all you do, will be impressive.

BOTTOM LINE: Lose 20–50 pounds

The great thing about mealtime management is that it doesn't involve dieting. All you're doing is eating delicious food at the right times! Some examples: Regular meals can eliminate the need for high-calorie snacks; planning for a fruit snack instead of raiding the doughnut box can melt away 20 pounds; and planning a healthful lunch instead of grabbing something on the fly can help you lose 22–30 pounds a year.

#118. Hamburgers Without End

You've been good about substituting lean roast beef or chicken sandwiches for hamburgers, but your cravings can no longer be denied. Don't feel guilty—enjoy!

Hamburgers have gotten a bad rap. As long as you make them at home (rather than *bringing* them home), they're low enough in saturated fat and calories to eat all the time. You can even add Thousand Island dressing for a faux Big Mac.

Put this in perspective: A half pound of burger meat at your favorite burger joint will set you back 800 calories. If you buy extra-lean ground meat and make your own, you'll get 200 calories less.

Better yet: Buy a round steak, have the butcher remove the visible fat, and ask him to grind the rest. This meat is 95 percent lean or better—the equivalent of chicken or game meat like venison or buffalo. You're down to 400 calories, half the amount in the take-out.

The calories in lettuce, tomato, pickles, and so on hardly register. As for dressing, I prefer the regular mayonnaise. Even though it has 100 calories (compared to the 50 in low-fat), the meat-substitute trick keeps the whole thing in the safety zone. And regular mayo, although high-calorie, contains many healthy fats.

To make your burger healthier, use whole-grain bread or buns instead of that nutritional disaster known as white bread.

BOTTOM LINE: Lose 6–18 pounds

Making your own burgers weekly with lean meat and healthy fixings means that you can enjoy them all the time—with only a fraction of the calories that you'd get in ready-made. Make the switch often and lose even more.

#119. Eat Your Office Supplies

Most of us spend more time at the office than at home. The ready availability of fast food, vending machine snacks, and morning doughnuts offer bounteous opportunities for expanding our waistlines.

The typical workday and workplace are almost perfectly designed for gaining weight. Morning is too rushed to eat a proper breakfast, so we stop at a convenience store or fast-food restaurant for a quick (and high-fat) meal. We go out to lunch with colleagues, or ask one of them to bring back a burger meal to eat at our desks. We drop quarters in vending machines for afternoon snacks. And on those days when we work late (and we all have them), we can't face the thought of preparing dinner at home, so we end up, again, at a restaurant or fast-food chain.

Here's a better way.

Most offices today have communal kitchens, with a refrigerator, stove, and microwave. Take advantage of this corporate largess by bringing your own supplies—not only quick snacks, such as pretzels and dried fruit, but also complete meals, which you can prepare whenever you're in the mood for something healthier than the usual office or takeout fare.

It's easier than it sounds. By preparing meals ahead of time and storing them in plastic bags or containers in your office refrigerator, you'll always have delicious and nutritious meals and snacks at your fingertips.

Unfortunately, every office has its share of hungry predators—you know, the ones who won't think twice about raiding your healthful stash. **Hint:** Try putting a "poison" sign on your food containers. And if that doesn't keep the rats out, buy a small refrigerator or cabinet and keep it in your office space.

Let's take a look at some of the payoffs:

• You'll save a lot of time when you don't go out to eat.
• Buying groceries is less expensive than eating out. You're paying dearly for that "convenience," you know.

• You'll almost automatically lose weight because you won't be eating calorie-rich burgers or takeout food.

BOTTOM LINE: Lose 11–60 pounds

At the office you can expect to save at least 300 calories when you prepare your own lunch; 150 calories by bringing your own afternoon snack; and more than 400 calories by eating your own delicious dinner instead of grabbing chow at a takeout dive. Dramatic savings—and that's without going on a diet!

#120. The Secret Is Plastics

For a long time, plastic was a dirty word. Today we know how to use plastic to help us eat less.

Portion control is one of the biggest challenges when you're trying to lose weight. When you use plastic containers, portion control is almost guaranteed: What doesn't fit inside a single-serving container is saved for another day!

Another benefit: You can put leftovers in plastic storage containers and take them to work—or keep them in the refrigerator for those busy days when you're on the go. It's a great way to avoid becoming a "vending machine victim." In the long run, the wise use of plastic containers will help you eat less, lose weight, and potentially save hundreds of dollars a month.

Also, this is an exciting time for plastics. New products make it possible to write the date and contents directly on the container. You'll always know what's inside, and how fresh (or ancient!) it is.

My personal favorite use of plastic is the "salad shaker." You keep the veggies in the larger compartment on the bottom, and put the dressing (vinaigrette, of course) in the compartment above. When you're ready to eat, simply release the dressing and shake. No more soggy salad!

BOTTOM LINE: Lose 10–40 pounds

When you use plastic containers to store meals—especially batch meals that you prepare ahead of time—you'll give up all those calories that come from greasy spoon diners. Go, plastics!

#121. Shop Online

All groceries aren't created equal. Doing your shopping online can save impressive amounts of time—and calories.

If you aren't entirely comfortable with the world of the Internet, the idea of buying fruits, vegetables, meats, or seafood online may seem pretty strange. No matter how enticing and colorful the pictures on your monitor are, they aren't the same tomatoes or steaks that you're actually putting in your grocery bag! No question, grocery shopping on your computer isn't the same as pushing the cart yourself.

But please, consider it. It's a very attractive option, especially when you're trying to stay organized. There's no substitute for shopping regularly and keeping the larder well stocked when you're trying to lose weight.

Shopping online is a great way to save valuable time—and, as we've seen, convenience and time savings are at the core of organized, healthful eating. It's true that online grocery deliveries require you to be home at a specified time, but you may be able to schedule the delivery for a time you're going to be home anyway.

Think about it: If you don't physically go to the supermarket, you have more time to enjoy dinner with your family. True, you'll pay for this convenience with a delivery fee—but the fee is almost certainly less than what you pay a babysitter when you take off to run errands.

What to look for:

• Does the online grocer have the exact products you want, in the sizes and formulations you prefer? These companies have thousands of items, but not as many variations as the supermarket down the street.
• How good and prompt is the delivery service? Is the delivery charge reasonable?
• Do they get your order right? For example, are the steaks and produce equal in quality to those you'd pick out yourself?

- Does the company offer the same specials and bonuses as the supermarket you usually go to?
- Is the Web site easy to navigate? More important, are the time savings worth the loss of control over the shopping experience?

Carole Sugarman, a writer for the Washington Post, compared two online grocers in Washington, D.C., HomeRuns.com and Peapod.com. She liked both. You will want to do some comparison shopping at the beginning, too.

BOTTOM LINE: Lose 20–80 pounds

Your main considerations will probably be convenience and time savings. The weight-loss benefit should be the same as with physically going to the grocery store once a week. Not bad!

#122. Slash Corporate Calories

Sad but true: Too many of us work late at the office—
and the fast-food joints have reaped the windfall.

If you often stay late at work, it's a good idea to have a few dinner items stored in the office freezer. A frozen dinner or made-at-home batch meal will be piping hot in minutes. You'll get your work done without sacrificing good nutrition or the comfort of a good meal at the end of the day.

Of course, if you prepared a hot lunch, you can use some of the same ingredients to make a delicious cold sandwich for dinner. There's no law that says you have to have your big, hot meal at night. Actually, the opposite is better for you: When you have your main meal at lunch, your body has more active hours to burn off the calories.

My client Catherine brings frozen dinner meals and vegetables to work at the beginning of the week. She often gets frozen vegetables prepared in a butter sauce: She likes the taste—and because she saves so many calories by not going to restaurants, she can afford the extra indulgence.

BOTTOM LINE: Lose 6–18 pounds

Office-prepared dinners will easily have 400 fewer calories than restaurant meals. If you work late an average of 3 times a week, this change alone will help you lose about 18 pounds. Those who work late every night could potentially lose 30 pounds a year—but I'd probably advise them to look for a new job!

#123. Eat All-American

Forget doughnuts and other office snacks. An all-American lunch will save loads of calories, satisfy your appetite, and keep your energy high.

What's an all-American lunch? Well, you probably can imagine 50 variations, one for each state. What I think of is a great sandwich, maybe slices of roast turkey, grilled chicken, or lean roast beef. Tuna packed in water is also good.

Bring all your supplies to work on Monday. When lunch rolls around, pack your fillings of choice between slices of whole-grain bread. Apply mustard or low-cal mayo, or a tablespoon of regular mayo. Add all the tomato, lettuce, pickle, salsa, olives, relish, salt, or pepper that you desire. (Use plenty of onion if you aren't planning a one-on-one with the boss in the afternoon!) Add salad or soup, and you've got the perfect all-American lunch.

My client David buys a 6-pound turkey breast when it's on sale. He cooks it on Sunday, has it hot for dinner that night, and has enough left over for another dinner and 2 or 3 lunches at the office.

Also, don't forget those batch meals you prepared over the weekend. An individual-size portion in a plastic container, heated in the office microwave, makes a delicious lunch. Shake things up for variety. Have hot batch lunches on Monday, Wednesday, and Friday, and cold sandwiches on Tuesday and Thursday. Or, heck, do the reverse: It's your choice!

BOTTOM LINE: Lose 22–30 pounds

Substituting an all-American lunch for burgers and fries will save you 300–400 calories a day.

#124. Learn to Count

It sounds elementary, but batch cooking and calorie control won't work unless you know how much to buy ahead of time.

Organized shopping ensures that your larder is always full of nutritious, easy-to-prepare foods. But this approach only works if you know how much to buy for the coming week.

If you've planned to eat 3 servings of your favorite fruit every day, for example, you have to get 21 portions (assuming you're the only one eating it). Some of that can be fresh, some canned, some frozen—but you have to be sure you come home with 21 portions.

On my last shopping trip, I bought 2 pounds of frozen blueberries so I could have a half cup each morning with my cereal. I also bought enough orange juice so that my significant other, Jack, and I could each have 6 ounces every morning.

Using the same sort of calculation, I bought 14 peaches, 14 plums, and 14 nectarines (one a day for each of us), along with 2 quarts of blackberries (Jack has them with his cereal, and I enjoy them as an occasional treat). You get the idea.

Don't forget: Get all the ingredients you need to prepare two large batch recipes for the week.

BOTTOM LINE: Lose 20–80 pounds

Knowing exactly how much you need to buy guarantees that you won't run out of key ingredients during the week. Which means you'll be less likely to make a last-minute run to the fast-food take-out line.

#125. Take Breakfast Shortcuts

I don't know about you, but I'm often rushed in the mornings. The only way I'll eat a nutritionally sound breakfast is to have an ample supply of ready-to-go foods.

When you make your weekly trip to the grocery store, be certain that you get enough breakfast essentials. You don't want any excuses for skipping breakfast, or stopping at a fast-food outlet on your way to work.

First, you have to decide what you like to eat. That's pretty simple for me: I love oatmeal! When I make my grocery list, I make sure I'll have enough of everything. I usually buy a large container of old-fashioned rolled oats, a gallon of nonfat milk, a pound of nuts, a box of brown sugar, a stick of light butter, and a quart of blueberries (or raspberries, just for a change). I also get a jar of toasted wheat germ and a quart of my favorite, fresh-squeezed orange juice.

Incidentally, I buy fresh blueberries in season. The rest of the year, frozen is fine.

BOTTOM LINE: Lose 21 pounds

The great thing about my oatmeal breakfast is that I feel full and satisfied all morning—no need for a vending machine snack. Most important, I don't have cravings that send me to a restaurant for lunch. I'm able to enjoy the simple—but delicious—lunches I've planned. My guess is that starting the day with a healthful breakfast saves me at least 200 calories a day!

#126. Defrost the Freezer

You want to make room for delicious frozen meals. My freezer is always full, which means I don't have to rush out for fast food when I'm hungry. My freezer is a fast-food outlet.

Forget all the nasty things you've heard about frozen foods. Today's supermarkets stock hundreds of items that are nutritious as well as low in calories and sodium. Many of today's frozen foods taste pretty darn good, too.

When buying frozen foods, check the number of calories on the nutrition label. I eat meals with 500 calories or less. Jack, on the other hand, needs about 700 calories per meal. He selects dishes accordingly. If a frozen dinner doesn't include vegetables, I'll buy some frozen vegetable or fresh produce to go with the main dish.

The selection of frozen foods is enormous. I love a macaroni and cheese meal every so often, as well as meatloaf and mashed potatoes, french fries, pizza, and sometimes Thai or Indian food. You'll find most of these at any time in my freezer.

BOTTOM LINE: Lose 18–51 pounds

Stocking up on delicious, wholesome frozen dinners can save you 300–500 calories per dinner—even more if you really go wild when you find yourself at a takeout window. Eat healthful frozen meals four nights a week and you'll drop a minimum of 18 pounds. Eat them more often—and reduce your consumption of rich snacks or restaurant food at the same time—and you'll lose a lot more.

#127. Do Some Fine Dining

Want to eat at the best restaurants in town? Go for it! Just don't break the "calorie bank" by doing it every night.

I love going to a fine restaurant and indulging in whatever my heart desires. My particular favorite: Sitting at the "chef's table" with one of the top chefs in the city taking care of my every whim. Of course, I plan an event like this with some care.

First things first. You can go to excellent restaurants regularly and still lose weight. Even though the food might be swimming in butter or cream sauce, you're not eating it all the time. Life is short. Enjoy.

For many of us, however, restaurants are a fallback from bad planning. We eat out when we're too tired at the end of the day to cook, or when there's nothing in the refrigerator. Do this a lot, and you're going to gain weight.

Personally, I've found that my body can cope nicely if I limit my restaurant indulgences to once a week. Others might be able to do it two or even three times without negative repercussions.

I do advise ordering simply most of the time. Save the real splurges for special occasions, or at least "thank God it's Friday" celebrations.

BOTTOM LINE: Lose 20–30 pounds

Go to a restaurant 3 times a week instead of your usual 5, and you'll save about 500 calories each evening. Heck, be radical—only go once a week. You'll save 2,000 calories!

Chapter 13

Easy Solutions for Your Kids

Especially appropriate for: *Moms on the Go, Kids on Wheels, Dads on Kitchen Duty, Young Athletes, and Budding Bookworms*

The goal for parents is to have a child who naturally loves healthful, wholesome foods, such as fruits, vegetables, and other whole foods. Not only will these foods help keep your child slim and trim, but they will reduce his or her vulnerability to illness as well. As we discussed in Chapter 7, educating your kids' palates may not be the easiest thing you've ever done, but with a little persistence and patience, you're sure to have success. Let's review some of the basics.

First, it's important to have a wide variety of healthful foods available in your home, rather than high-calorie sweets and snack foods. If you keep sugary foods around, you'll have to restrict them, which may actually have a negative effect on your son or daughter. It's been demonstrated that if you restrict a food your child knows is kept in the house, he or she can develop a strong attraction to it and overeat it whenever it becomes available. If your child resists eating more healthful fare such as whole grains and vegetables, remember that it can take up to twenty tries to edu-cate his or her palate to a new taste that isn't sweet. Just keep trying! In the long run, your efforts will be rewarded.

Second, remember that your child should be the one to choose when and how much he or she eats. Studies show that when parents try to restrict or control amounts, the child loses the natural ability to regulate his or her own food intake. We know that when children have a wide array of healthful foods to choose from and are given the freedom to eat how much they'd like, they don't overeat unless they see their parents overeating or are encouraged to overeat. They naturally select just the right amount.

Third, you need to find ways to increase your child's physical activity in fun ways. Turns out the television is one of the biggest dangers in your child's life. As hours of TV watching rise, so does the incidence of obesity, unhealthful eating habits, and smoking. Studies show that children who watch 4 or more hours of TV every day are more likely to be overweight, and are more likely to smoke, be violent, and be inactive than are children who watch only 1–2 hours' worth. These problems are especially pro-nounced in children with TVs in their bedrooms. TV also interferes with a family's ability to communicate with one another. It takes away from fam-ily time and physical activity and teaches negative eating habits. This is why the American Academy of Pediatrics recommends "no more than 1–2 hours a day of good-quality TV programming, video, or computer games."

Fourth, if you have an overweight child, try not to worry. Just be as supportive as you can. If left alone, most children grow out of their chubby phase. My brother Andrew went through one when he was a kid, but no one seems to remember it but me! And this is usually the case. It passes by with no horrible memories or problems.

Finally, your entire family may need to make a few small changes in order to help your overweight child—by eating more healthfully and becoming more physically active. Studies show that children are more likely to lose weight and keep it off if the whole family goes through a weight-loss program. That means if you, the parent, have a weight problem, the best course to take is for you to model healthful eating behavior and a physically active life. This takes the pressure off your child and allows him to keep eat-ing what everyone else is eating and continue to feel a part of the family.

Children are traumatized when they are singled out and put on a diet or food restrictions. It's not fair, and downright cruel, in my opinion, to treat a child in this way. And he'll never forget it as long as he lives.

With these five general points in mind, here are some tips on how to junk the junk food in your children's lives.

#128. Wean Your Child from Sugary Cereals

The first step to developing an appreciation for wholesome foods is to get rid of sugary foods in your house.

Depending on how hooked your child is on sugary foods, you may have to gradually wean him off them and onto healthful foods. The best strategy is to make the change quietly so that he doesn't notice a thing. If you make a big deal of it, he'll start understanding that these foods are restricted and he'll want them even more!

Start with discreetly mixing your child's favorite sugary cereal with a little wholesome cereal, say Kashi or Meuslix. Make sure the cereal you choose has a "whole" grain as its first ingredient. That means it contains more whole grain than anything else. Take a box of each, mix in a container, so that you have about ¼ wholesome cereal to ¾ sugary. As the weeks go by, slowly increase the proportion of wholesome cereal until after about 12 weeks, it contains 100% wholesome cereal. Add fresh or dried fruit to keep it sweet. If your child enjoys nuts, throw some in to add crunch.

BOTTOM LINE: Lose 10 pounds

Nonsugary cereals contain about 10–30 fewer calories per ounce. By replacing cereals alone, over the course of a year, you can save at least 10 pounds. More importantly, the nutritional benefits of additional B vitamins, fiber, and beneficial phytochemicals found in whole grains will help protect your child against cancer, diabetes, and heart disease. You're also helping him avoid a lifelong obsession with sugar.

#129. Wean Your Child Off Sodas

The first step in weaning your children from sodas is to stop drinking them yourself. You simply can't say one thing and do another where your children are concerned. They're too smart for that!

In the past two decades, soda consumption among children has almost tripled, while milk consumption has been cut in half. Today, most teenage boys drink an average of three sodas—that's about 21 teaspoons of sugar—a day. Most teenage girls drink two—14 teaspoons of sugar—daily. Interestingly, the most overweight kids drink the most sodas.

Drinking this stuff poses other health risks, too. Studies show that teenagers who drink soda, drink it instead of milk. As a result, only 36 percent of boys and 14 percent of girls consume the recommended level of calcium. This could have a devastating impact on their bone formation, particularly with girls, as the teen years are the most important for building bone and preventing osteoporosis later in life.

If mom and dad are drinking milk regularly, however, your children will naturally pick up the habit. Have nonfat milk every morning in your breakfast cereal. Or have a glass alongside your whole-wheat toast. It's a good idea to have a glass with your other meals as well.

If you don't like plain milk, try chocolate milk or calcium-fortified soy milk. My clients who don't enjoy cow's milk often like soy milk better. Studies show it takes about 12 weeks for adults to adjust to the flavor of a new food. In 24 weeks, they even begin to prefer it! That's much longer than it takes children to change their preferences, so it's more challenging, but worth the effort in order to model good eating habits for your child.

If it's difficult for you to get off soda, slowly change from soda to Perrier with a twist of lime or add some juice, for instance. Even if it takes a year, it will have a positive impact on your family. At minimum, buy smaller-serving-sized cans or bottles of soda. One of the reasons we drink more today is that bottles are bigger. In the 1950s, a bottle of Coke contained 6 ounces. Today, it's not unusual for a soda to be 20 ounces—more than triple the size, sugar, and calories.

If your children are hooked on sodas already, you can slowly wean them off, without their noticing. Make sparkling water fun by adding lemon or lime slices. To make it sweeter, try adding 100 percent grape juice or apple juice. This way, at least they're getting the nutrients in the juice while they're enjoying the bubbles of the sparkling water. But milk remains a better substitute.

BOTTOM LINE: Lose 15 pounds

Switch from just one soda a day to water and your child will save at least 15 pounds in a year. Switch to juice or milk and you're insuring a healthier future for your child.

#130. Fill the Fridge with Fun Finger Foods

Kids especially love finger foods—anything they can eat with their hands. Fruits and vegetables lend themselves perfectly as kid-friendly —and filling and low-calorie—finger foods.

Interestingly, 75 percent of children eat only 1 fruit or vegetable a day, and it's usually in the form of potato chips or French fries. When you get to the most nutritious vegetables, such as greens, only 7 percent of children touch them. This is a concern because over 200 peer-reviewed studies show that eating at least 5–7 servings of fruits or vegetables daily prevents cancer. A diet high in fruits, vegetables, and whole grains also helps keep blood pressure low and helps prevent heart disease and diabetes. And when you eat more vegetables, you become full with fewer calories, so it's easier to lose weight or maintain a healthful weight.

If you want your child to eat more of these foods, your first step is keep your refrigerator full of them. And make them grab-able and transportable. First, clean and chop fruits and veggies into sizes fit for little hands. Put them in colorful containers to keep it fun and interesting for your kids.

Fruits are easy because they're naturally sweet. Here are some ways you can make fruits grab-able for your kids:

- Grapes: Clean and de-stem, place in plastic baggies in the fridge or on the kitchen counter.
- Bananas: Buy ripe and unripe bananas so your child can grab them for several days.
- Apples: Clean them and place in air-tight containers so your child can grab straight from the refrigerator.
- Berries, cherries: Wash, dry in a strainer. Then place in air-tight containers in fridge. (Delicate raspberries should be washed only just before serving.)
- Peaches, plumbs, nectarines: If hard and unripe, keep on kitchen

counter. As soon as they get soft and ripe, place in baggies in the fridge.
- Melon: Cut in quarters and slices and place in containers or large baggies in the fridge.

Vegetables can be more of a challenge because they're not sweet. If you have them cleaned, chopped, and grab-able, they're more likely to be gobbled up. Keep healthful dips, such as hummus, spinach dip, and yogurt, in plastic containers to make veggies more tasty and fun. Vinaigrette dressings are good to have around in case your child would like to make a salad.

- Carrots: Buy baby carrots, wash them, and keep them in baggies in the fridge. Or buy normal carrots, and scrub and cut them until they're finger-sized. Watch them disappear…
- Celery: Wash and cut stalks so that they're just a few bites long. Fill them with peanut butter or reduced-fat cheese spread. Yum!
- Broccoli and cauliflower: Wash and cut them so they're finger-sized flowerettes. You can marinate them in vinaigrette or serve them with dip.
- Sugar snap peas: Simply wash and place in containers in the fridge. Their natural sweetness will make them eminently popular.
- Radishes, peppers, zucchini, squash—are all great raw. Simply wash and slice into finger-size sticks.
- Jicama: This exotic vegetable is a favorite for crudité platters. Simply peel, then slice the apple-like pulp into baby-carrot-sized sticks.
- Cherry tomatoes: These are fun to eat because they're the perfect size to just pop in your mouth whole. Simply wash them and keep them on the kitchen counter so your child can pop them in his mouth any time he walks by.
- Greens: Wash and drain thoroughly. Then place in a plastic container. Your kids will become accustomed to making their own salads with the array of veggies you already have cut up in the fridge. Always keep tasty, healthful low-fat dips around as a garnish. If they're hooked on high-fat dips, slowly wean them off by using 50/50 high-fat/low-fat sour cream or cream cheese until they get used to the lower-fat versions. It's safe to buy full-fat hummus and salad dressings, since they're made with

healthier oils. And, remember, your child will know when he's had enough if you provide an array of foods at meals and snacks—some high in fat and some low, some fruits, some veggies.

BOTTOM LINE: Lose 10 pounds

Make healthful foods grab-able and save at least 100 calories by avoiding calorie-dense snack foods. Save 10 pounds in a year. And gain thousands of health-enhancing phytochemicals, vitamins, and minerals.

#131. Frozen Fruit Fun

When you have a collection of frozen fruit treats in your freezer, your child knows he can pop by any time for a delicious treat. And you'll know he's eating valuable nutrients for a healthy body.

Everyone loves frozen treats, but standard ice cream comes laden with heart-clogging saturated fat, sugar, and calories.

Children have been amazed at how delicious fruit tastes when it is simply frozen. Take grapes for instance. Wash, de-stem, and pop in the freezer and an hour later you have a natural grape popsicle.

Slice a banana, roll in wheat germ mixed with cinnamon. Stick a tooth pick in each slice. Place on a cookie sheet and freeze. You'll think it's ice cream, it's so creamy and delicious.

Freeze kiwi fruit slices for a sweet-tart kiwi popsicle.

Blueberries—or any berries—are delicious frozen. They're full of natural intense sweetness.

You can also freeze juices and make 100 percent juice popsicles.

For fruity frozen ices, puree frozen or fresh berries with ice or fresh watermelon with crushed ice. Any one of your child's favorite fruits will do. Place in a wine or parfait glass with a long spoon or straw.

You can set up a sundae bar your kids will love. Start with a bowl or parfait dish of vanilla yogurt. Then have bowls of rolled oats, nuts, wheat germ, and cut-up fruit or berries.

Smoothies are also popular with children. Just throw the treats you've frozen into a blender along with low-fat milk or yogurt and voilà! A delicious cold smoothie.

BOTTOM LINE: Lose 10 pounds

Save 100 calories with a healthful frozen treat instead of ice cream. Save 10 pounds in a year.

#132. Make Veggie and Fruit Kebabs

What child doesn't like to build things? You can make
eating healthy a fun, creative exercise with these
easy, kid-friendly sweets-on-a-stick.

Everyone loves shish kebabs, but did you ever think of creating a fruit
kebab? Children naturally love fruit because of the sweetness. But studies show they don't eat enough, probably because it isn't as convenient as
the vending machine. Replace that candy bar or vending machine snack
with a fruit kebab in your child's lunch box. Better yet, have him choose
the fruit and design it himself.

Gather all your favorite seasonal fruits, and chop them into bite-sized
pieces. Try pineapple chunks, peach quarters, apple slices, berries, grapes,
banana slices, and melon balls or chunks. Challenge your child to make it
as colorful as he or she can. That will ensure a wider array of vitamins,
minerals, and phytochemicals and flavors.

In the winter, when choices are more limited, there are always
bananas, apples, and grapes. You can also used frozen and canned fruit,
such as strawberries, pineapple, peaches, and pears.

Place a few pieces of each fruit in a separate bowl.

Get a shish kebab stick, ask your child to choose as many colors as possible to make a colorful kebab with at least three colors: yellow for
banana, apple, or pineapple; orange for peaches; purple or green for
grapes.

Now place the kebabs in plastic containers so your child can grab as
many for his lunch box as he'd like or so that he has a healthful treat when
he gets home from school. If he likes, he can dip in yogurt, rolled oats,
wheat germ, and dried fruit for added flavors and textures. Let him be
creative.

For veggie kebabs, grilling, broiling, or roasting enhances the flavor
and brings out sweetness. Simply cut different vegetables into bite-size
pieces. Ask your child to go for color. Use sliced red and yellow peppers,
mushrooms, zucchini, squash, cherry tomatoes, even sweet onions.

Next, dip a barbecue brush in a little olive oil spiced with salt, pepper, and a favorite herb.

Grill or broil the veggies for 15–30 minutes. Flip at least once so that all sides are cooked evenly, until soft on the inside and crunchy on the outside. Grilled veggie kebabs will become one of your child's favorite foods of all time!

BOTTOM LINE: Lose 10 pounds

Adding fruits or vegetables to any meal or snack could save at least 100 calories because you become full on fewer calories. Save 10 pounds in a year. The nutritional payoff is enormous.

#133. Replace Fried with Oven-Fried

Everyone loves fries. I love fries. You probably do, too. And for sure your kids are fries fans. But deep frying potatoes has health hazards, not to mention the calories, calories, calories!

Recent research shows that French fries and potato chips are loaded with carcinogens called "acrylamides." The EPA limits the level of acrylamide in water to 0.12 micrograms per 8 ounces of water. Swedish scientists discovered that McDonald's French fries contain *700 times* that amount. Something about the extremely high temperatures created during deep-fat frying causes the carcinogens to form.

But guess what! I've discovered a way to make fries without all that fat and with half the calories. As a French-fry lover myself, I can honestly say this method is just as delicious as the real thing!

Katherine's Baked Fries

Ingredients:
Several potatoes, preferably a sweeter version such as Yukon Gold
Olive oil (or oil spray)
Salt, pepper
Herbes de Provence (or your favorite herb)

Scrub the potatoes, but leave the skins on so you'll keep most of the nutrients and fiber. Cut in bite-size pieces or larger cubes, depending on your preference. Place in a large bowl and coat with a small amount of oil so the potatoes are shiny, but there's no pool of oil. Just stir and toss in the bowl until all potatoes are coated. Add salt, pepper, and herbs to taste.

Pour evenly onto a cookie sheet and bake at 350 degrees for 30–60 minutes until brown. The potatoes should be crunchy on the outside and soft on the inside, just like the ideal French fry.

You can also cook carrots, onions, zucchini and other vegetables the same way and they turn out absolutely delicious!

BOTTOM LINE: Lose 10 pounds

This is a great way to make "fried" potatoes they'll love as much as deep-fried French fries and you'll save hundreds of calories per serving. Save at least 10 pounds per year, depending on how often you make this substitute.

#134. Cut Back on TV Time with Crafts

Back in the old days when there wasn't TV (don't yawn!), people actually did productive things in the afternoons or after a hard day's work. So get out there and build a birdhouse together!

Earlier generations interacted with family and friends, they played card games, they had creative pursuits such as knitting, painting, music, or even woodworking. These activities made their lives complete. They weren't just working or in school, then zoning out in front of the boob tube. I work with many adults who have developed the TV habit, and believe me, their lives ain't pretty. They're devoid of hobbies or other interests, and often communicate very little with other people. They complain about being lonely and bored, and having low energy.

Studies show that having creative pursuits, as well as communicating more often with friends and family, actually reduces stress and disease, and prolongs life. When your children are young, it's a particularly good time to introduce creative pursuits so that by the time they become adults, they have developed a keen interest in the outside world. Childhood is the perfect time to get people interested in the arts such as piano playing, singing, painting, sculpting, or dance. Children also enjoy crafts such as decoupage, sewing, knitting, and woodworking.

You might even think about starting your kids on bigger projects, which might include building a bird house, a tree house, or a play house (with parental supervision, of course). Besides keeping them occupied and away from the TV, you'll be teaching them valuable life lessons in patience, reasoning, planning ahead, setting small, realistic goals, and finishing what you begin.

You may have to take him to a class or have a few sessions with an expert to learn about some of these activities, if they aren't taught in school. You could also learn together by buying do-it-yourself kits or books and reading the instructions together! There are plenty of books on arts and crafts in the book stores. You could also go to an arts supply store or crafts store to buy materials for smaller projects such as holiday ornaments and wreaths, Easter eggs, and Halloween pumpkin carving kits. Your child should always have a running project going—and make sure each project is always finished, even if he grows tired of it. There are so many ways this will help him succeed as a child, but also later in life. And think of the great gifts he can make for friends and family members, too!

BOTTOM LINE: Lose 30 pounds

Developing a creative pursuit for your child will keep him from eating at least a handful of chips, and saves 300 calories per day. Save 30 pounds in one year!

#135. Play Games!

One of my favorite activities when I was a child was playing board games and card games with my brothers, parents, grandparents, and friends. My grandmother and I played Scrabble. Of course, being an English Literature major in college, she always won.

Even though she usually won any game we played, it was the interaction with my grandmother that I remember most vividly. We would laugh, look up words in the dictionary, discuss the meanings of words. But the bottom line was, this was intimate time with my grandmother I'll never forget.

I also loved playing card games and board games with my brothers and our friends. It sharpened my sense of healthy competition. It gave me the ability to reason, to plot strategy, and to think fast. It taught me the value of rules and fairness. It gave me the chance to talk with my brothers and to spend time with my parents on fun things. And I had the opportunity to express myself in ways I normally wouldn't.

Choosing games your family would like is easy. They can be as simple as playing "Go Fish!" and "Hearts," played with a deck of cards, or as complex as chess. You can choose games with multiple players such as Monopoly™, charades, or Trivial Pursuit™ or with a single pair of competitors, as in checkers.

There are so many choices today. And for the do-it-yourselfer, there are plenty of books describing card games and games you can make up, which can end up being a life-long family tradition.

One caution: Be sure you're not eating while you're playing. You don't want to create a situation where eating becomes behaviorally connected with the evening game. The goal is to teach your family to eat when they're hungry, and to focus on and enjoy eating during meals.

BOTTOM LINE: Lose 20 pounds

Keeping your child away from the TV alone could save 200 calories daily and will even burn more calories, since anything other than TV watching burns calories. Save 20 pounds in one year!

#136. Encourage Recreational Physical Activities

Studies show children need at least one hour a day of being physically active and that until they reach their teens, activity should consist of play and games rather than exercise.

When I was a kid, the first thing I did after coming home from school was to go outdoors to play. We had tons of kids in the neighborhood and played games like "Kick the Can." Sometimes we marked up a driveway in chalk and played "Four Square," passing a big ball back and forth. We played hopscotch, jumped rope, tossed soft balls and Frisbees back and forth. We played "Hide and Seek" and basketball. Sometimes we would just go bicycling or skating.

I even learned to be a fairly good runner when my neighbor, Sean, chased us girls around the neighborhood with what he told us was an "X-ray vision camera" (really just one of his sisters' Girl Scout cameras). That kept us running . . . and hiding . . . and running . . . and hiding—all of which took a lot of energy.

I know that today playing in neighborhoods may not be so easy for some children as it was when I was growing up. You may have to be especially creative to find physical activities your child can be involved in after school. It's especially troublesome that schools are cutting back on gym class and recess. That makes it particularly important that you take an active interest in your child's physical activity.

It's up to older family members and caregivers to encourage children by being role models of physical activity themselves. In fact, your family life can be centered around physical activity, which would be beneficial for every single family member—from Baby to Grandpa!

Most children are very receptive to going on walks, hiking, swimming, bike riding or simply shooting some hoops with Mom or Dad. If they're done as family outings, these activities are more likely to be perceived as positive and valuable to the child and are more likely to carry over as habits in adulthood. So go sightseeing together. Walk around a zoo or a park.

It's important to integrate physical activity regularly into family routines, like making a rule to avoid the elevator for less than three flights, or picking the farthest parking place for the car when visiting the mall. Make a game of making three circuits around the mall every time you go shopping.

Also, encourage participation in school or community sports programs. Soccer, basketball, hockey, ice skating and many other sports are great ways for kids as young as 7 or 8 to get their physical activity. Tap and ballet are other alternatives. And just allowing kids to play outside for a couple of hours every day helps. Children love to run and jump on their own, if left to their own devices. If there's no safe place to play outside, buy an exercise or dance video. Have a group of friends walk together to school for added safety.

Here some other ways to get your children enthused about physical activity:

• Start new family traditions: Every New Year's Day, your family could take a hike up a mountain; every 4th of July, go sightseeing and visit a national memorial in Washington, D.C.; every spring, watch whales off the coast of California or go bird-watching; for Valentine's Day, go skiing! Whenever there's a picnic, always take a ball to toss back and forth, a softball and gloves, or a volley ball or badminton net.
• Go bowling for birthdays.
• Get your family involved in causes like walk-a-thons or bike-a-thons. It's a great way to teach your children how to healthfully get involved in helping others—in causes important for bettering society.

BOTTOM LINE: Lose 20–40 pounds

Being involved in a daily physical activity could easily burn 200 calories daily—let alone benefiting from all the junk food you're not snacking on. So save another 200. Your child can save as much as 20–40 pounds by increasing physically active fun every day.

#137. Create Family TV Guidelines

TV reduces the time children socialize with family and friends. Children who watch less TV are better at verbal and interpersonal skills, get along better with others, and develop richer vocabularies. And they stay thinner.

Here are some ways you might be able to reduce TV time in your home.

- Monitor TV watching. Keep track of the hours your family watches. Negotiate how you can reduce the time to no more than one or two hours a day on average.
- Find fun substitutes. Decide on activities your children can do on their own and activities you can do as a family that are much more fun than television. Choose from the ideas presented in Tips #134, #135, and #136.
- Never place a television in a child's room. You'll have no way of knowing or controlling his viewing habits. And we know that TV in a child's room is correlated with more weight problems.
- Ban TV watching while eating—at breakfast, lunch, dinner, or snack times. No TV while studying, at bedtime, or on school nights.
- Only watch when there are important events—say, the President's State of the Union Address, PBS's Civil War Special, or a special movie like The Wizard of Oz. Never just sit in front of the boob tube and channel-surf to see what's on.
- Watch TV as a family. It's important that you are there to explain things and answer questions. This way you learn what your child's interests are and you can explore new issues together (assuming you're watching educational programming).
- Teach your children the difference between programs and commercials. TV commercials are loaded with references to unhealthful, sugar-ridden, calorie-laden foods. Slick ads with fit sports figures, rock stars, or super models imply that drinking soda or eating fast food will make you

beautiful, strong, cool, and hip—just like them. Teenagers are especially vulnerable to these come-ons. It's important that you explain the world of commerce and sales and that if these extraordinarily slim, healthy-looking people really ate what they were hawking, they wouldn't be in such great shape for long!

BOTTOM LINE: Lose 10–30 pounds

Reducing TV time could save at least 100–300 calories a night. That's a 10–30 pound savings over a year. The physical and emotional benefits are limitless.

#138. Care for a Pet

Who would have thought that, in addition to being snuggly, Fido or Fluffy can keep you and your kids slim and trim?

When I was growing up, we always had pets. We had dogs and cats who became valued members of the family. We learned to take care of them, feed them, protect them from harm, take them for walks, clean up after them. (That duty was performed mainly by my poor brother, Andrew!)

If your child would like a pet, put him in charge of training and caring for the pet. This will keep him busy after school and away from the TV. It also will provide plenty of physical activity, as you need to walk and play with your pet several times a day.

It will also teach him responsibility. A pet is a member of the family and has certain rights. They have the right to be loved and cared for. They have the right to be trained properly so that they know how to behave within the family. They have the right to be fed regularly and nutritiously.

And of course, there's almost nothing so powerful as the unconditional love a pet can give a child for building self-esteem.

Needless to say, some pets require more time and demand more physical activity than others. While a dog can provide some great opportunities to go walking, for example, a turtle won't. (Turtles are bad for other reasons—they carry salmonella).

One caution, however. As many parents will tell you, children will often try to shift the responsibilities of feeding and exercising their pets back to their moms and dads, so make clear from the start what's expected from them and stick to your guns. If the responsibilities can be shared by family members, it will probably work out better for everyone.

BOTTOM LINE: Lose 10–20 pounds

Save at least 100 calories daily and burn another 100 by avoiding boredom eating and caring for your pet. Save 10–20 pounds a year...

139. Turn Little Diners into Little Chefs

Believe it or not, kids love to cook. It makes them feel independent and gives them confidence. And they love feeling like they're contributing something important to the family's enjoyment and healthy lifestyle.

Those clients of mine who are in the worst shape know nothing about cooking. All their meals are take-out, restaurant, or convenience foods. Can you imagine anything more unhealthful? It's sad because it's difficult to teach an adult if he's unfamiliar with even the basics of cooking. Best to start now when interest and time are abundant.

You don't have to turn your kids into 5-star chefs. Just teach them some basics. This will give them an appreciation of fresh, wholesome foods and will increase their preferences for them. This is invaluable practice for adulthood; what they learn now they will never, ever forget.

Along with cooking skills, of course, come rules for proper sanitation. Be sure to teach your children to wash their hands with soap thoroughly after using the bathroom and before touching any food. Also wash between tasks. It's particularly important not to cross-contaminate, that is, once you handle meat, fish, poultry, dairy, or egg products, wash thoroughly before handling anything else. Do the same for utensils and preparation surfaces such as cutting boards and counter tops.

Teach kids about proper temperature control. To prevent foodborne illness, keep cold foods cold (below 40 degrees) and hot foods hot (above 160 degrees). Don't leave potentially hazardous foods like meat, fish, or dairy products at room temperature, since that's the perfect temperature for bacteria to thrive.

Once food is cooked, it should only be on the table for 2 hours, then back in the fridge for safe keeping. Same goes for any leftovers from the restaurant. They must be in the refrigerator within 2 hours of leaving the restaurant. In fact, if you have any food that will be away from a refrigerator for more than 2 hours—an example might be a picnic or Sunday outing—carry along a cooler with ice and a refrigerator thermometer inside. Make sure it's below 40 degrees.

Obviously, when teaching kids to prepare food, choose age-appropriate skills.

Toddlers can simply help you stir things or pull things from the refrigerator for you. Allow them to choose as many colors as they can to go into the salad bowl. Ask them for something soft, something leafy, something crunchy, something sweet.

Older children can be taught, with close supervision, how to chop safely. They can boil water (with supervision) and cook pasta and rice. They can make a soup by choosing and chopping vegetables and putting them into the pot. They can help with stir fries and browning meats.

While you're teaching kids how to prepare a meal, teach them to plan one as well. The ideal meal has something from every food group. A fruit or vegetable; a lean protein such as seafood, poultry, lean beef, legumes, or tofu; a whole-grain starch; and a little healthful fat. (See some suggested Menu Plans on page 469.) Save the desserts for special occasions so your children don't get into the habit of having something sweet after every meal (that's hard to change once they're adults).

Teenagers can be as competent in the kitchen as an adult. Once a week, plan a meal with your teenager. He or she can choose the entire menu so long as it's balanced. Explore new recipes with your teens. They love being responsible for a whole meal and watching the delighted (hopefully) faces of their family members in response to their labors. It makes them feel grown-up and gives them a sense of belonging. Label their specialty: "Jamie's Caesar Salad" or "David's Bean Dip." Give them credit for their efforts. Make sure they're praised.

Teach your teens to make simple meals, too. One of my favorites is an easy bean burrito:

Dump some canned beans in a tortilla (preferably whole wheat), throw on some reduced-fat cheese, some salsa, and stick the whole thing in microwave for 1 to 1½ minutes. As a garnish, add more salsa, some fat-free sour cream, and some mashed avocado. You can also throw sautéed onions and peppers in the tortilla—really, anything goes. Add fish, chicken, or lean beef pieces.

Always have healthful frozen pizzas in the freezer, veggie burgers, lean hamburgers, low-fat hot dogs, and buns with all the fixings. This way if your child is craving a pizza, burgers, or dogs, he can grab the healthful kind. Frozen French fries are a better alternative to the deep-fried kind. There's nothing wrong—and everything right—with having plenty of frozen foods in your fridge for those times when the kids have a hankering for some fast food. You can save them lots of calories (and they can save money!), when they can make their own "happy meal" from your freezer.

Your children may even love to make more elaborate foods such as pizza from scratch or home-made pasta or crab cakes (see recipe). Teens love having pizza parties or taco parties where they choose their own toppings and design their own creations. Cooking for friends gives them more incentive to do a great job.

If you don't have time to cook throughout the week, *Think Yourself Thin* has great recipes for foods you and your children can make on the weekends and eat throughout the week. The vegetarian chili, vegetable soup, veal stew, white beans with garlic and basil, and stir-fried noodles are all pretty simple and kid-friendly. Have them made up and easy to grab.

If you're not a great wiz in the kitchen yourself, not to worry: Take cooking lessons with your kids! Many cities have cooking schools or chefs who teach classes individually or in groups. It's a great activity for you and your son or daughter to do together.

BOTTOM LINE: Lose 10 pounds

Teaching your children to cook will save them thousands of calories throughout their lifetime and may prevent weight problems. Save 10 pounds a year.

#140. Taste-Test New Veggies with Young Children

When mothers introduce a new fruit or vegetable to 4- to 6-month-old infants, it often takes only one feeding to increase the infant's acceptance of the food. And that acceptance is generalized to other, similar foods. So if an infant has experience with one vegetable, he or she will eat other vegetables more readily.

As children get older, it may take more tries to get them to accept a new food. When 2- to 5-year-olds were given varying numbers of opportunities to taste new foods, it took between 5 and 10 exposures to see an increased preference for them. Repeated opportunities to smell and look at new foods also increased acceptance. By the time kids reach their teens, it may take up to 20 tries before they learn to like a new food. But however long it takes, believe it or not, you can actually raise a child who loves vegetables if you're patient, positive, and consistent, and you love the food as well.

This is why finding fun ways to introduce a new or unusual vegetable is such a good idea. For instance, if you want to introduce broccoli for the first time, try it raw with a low-fat dip. The second time, try a little cheese sauce. The third time, try it sautéed in a little olive oil and garlic. How about broccoli on pizza, or in pasta? You get the idea. The more exposures your child has to the broccoli, the closer he'll get to loving it, especially if everyone else around the dinner table is eating and enjoying it as well.

Just ask him to try it. If he reacts negatively, that's okay. Don't react. Just make it clear that you're enjoying it yourself. And keep introducing it positively. Eventually he'll come around and find his favorite way of eating broccoli (or maybe not). But I would never give up.

My friend Julie serves the vegetable or salad first—as an appetizer, rather than alongside her son's favorite, macaroni and cheese. This way, he eats more of the vegetable because he's hungrier.

Julie's also quite cagey and hides vegetables in the pasta sauce, so that her son gets good nutrition and becomes more accustomed to eating vegetables he thinks he "hates." She also adds mashed banana and grated apple into pancake batter to make them more nutritious. As a result, her son David loves fruits and vegetables.

BOTTOM LINE: Lose 10–20 pounds

Developing in your child a love for vegetables will keep him healthy and trim. Eating vegetables at every meal could save 100 calories per meal because you feel full with fewer calories. Save 10–20 pounds.

#141. Grow Your Own Veggies

We all know kids love to play in the dirt. Why not make take advantage of it? No matter where you live—city, country, or suburbs—you can grow any number of veggies, right in your own backyard or even on a city balcony!

Nutrition education studies show that when children grow their own vegetables, they develop a sense of pride in ownership and are more likely to eat and enjoy them. Many schools have gardens for students to grow vegetables. Some neighborhoods have shared community plots.

In Washington, D.C., youngsters from the inner city planted vegetables at a community garden in the heart of downtown. They were proudly lugging the giant cabbages home for mom and dad to help them cook. You just knew those kids would be future cabbage lovers!

Even if all you have is a windowsill, you can plant miniature peppers, cherry tomatoes, herbs such as basil or rosemary, or spring onions.

Ask your child to pick something he'd like to plant in a pot in your windowsill, on your terrace, or in your yard. Whatever you grow, it will become his favorite food for a lifetime. My client Michael's favorite fruit is a blueberry. When I asked him to try and think about why, he remembered the blueberry bushes in his grandmother's backyard when he was a kid, and how he looked forward to picking them every summer.

BOTTOM LINE: Lose 10–20 pounds

Pride of ownership is a powerful thing. When your kids see the "fruits" of their hard work, they'll enjoy those fruits and veggies even more. This will blossom into a lifelong love of fresh produce, saving them a potential 100 calories per meal. Keep this up and they can lose 10–20 pounds in a year.

#142. Visit a Farm, Year-Round

Another way to create a love for fresh, wholesome foods in your child is to teach him how food is grown and produced. Take him behind the scenes, beyond the shelves of the grocery store.

In the spring, go to a strawberry farm and pick strawberries from the strawberry patches. There's nothing like perfectly ripe, fresh-picked sweet strawberries. Also in the spring, you might find a farm growing asparagus, green beans, carrots, or delicate new potatoes.

In the early summer, berries are around in abundance. Later you'll be able to pick peaches, plums, nectarines, figs, tomatoes, peppers, cucumbers. You name it, you can find it.

In the fall, go to an orchard and pick pears and apples; take your kids to watch apple cider being made. At Halloween, instead of picking up your pumpkin in the grocery store, go to a pumpkin patch and ask your child to pick out his favorite pumpkin. When you get home, carve it together and save the pulp for pumpkin soup or pumpkin pie. Also in the fall, you can pick delicious fresh broccoli—a tastier version you've never had before—as well as all kinds of squash.

In the winter, depending on where you live, your pickings may be slimmer. But you could visit a dairy farm and watch how cheese is made.

When children pick their own food or feel they have had a part in creating it, they're going to be more likely to enjoy and prefer it. You're creating a lifetime of positive food memories here.

If you can't go to a farm, the next best thing is a farmers' market. I go to a "producer's only market," which means there are no middle-men. The farmers sell only what they produce and every dollar goes directly to the farmer.

Of course, the next best thing is to take your children grocery shopping. Give the little ones a kid-size cart or a basket, if available. Let them put something in it, even if all they can carry is just one apple. Ask your older children to choose something exotic—perhaps a jicama or a star fruit. Or ask your teen to bring a recipe along and find all the ingredients. Have them plan the fruit they'll want to eat for the week and buy enough for everyone in the family.

BOTTOM LINE: Lose 10 pounds

Teaching your children where food comes from and letting them pick their own gives them a sense of ownership. They'll grow to love healthful, wholesome foods. Save 10 pounds and foster a lifetime of nutritious eating.

#143. Make Meal Time Family Time

Your child needs to rely on a regular schedule for meals and snacks. And it's your role to insist on sticking with that schedule.

If your child runs off without eating much at meal time, don't give in and give them snacks later—unless it's the usual snack time. They may cry and fuss, but if you start giving them food at any old time, it'll be hard to teach them to eat at meal time. Once they learn about meal time, they'll eat what they need and know that they'll be fed again at the next scheduled meal or snack time and will have time to get hungry before then.

Meal times should be pleasant. Allow everyone to eat in their preferred amount of time and be patient if it's longer than usual or expected. Don't allow distractions from the meal—no phone calls, reading, homework, or TV. Keep eye contact with one another. Make casual conversation. This way, family meal times will forever be a fond memory for your child.

Never encourage your children to clean their plates, or react positively or negatively to any eating behavior. Don't get upset if your child refuses to eat something. When they're hungry, they'll eat. And if they approach a food on their own, they'll be more likely to come back to it. Forcing and cajoling gives your child a signal that this is something she can use for manipulation and it backfires. The best you can do is to provide a model. Enjoy the foods you're eating and offer your child the same foods.

Don't short-order cook. If your child learns that you will stop everything to give him foods that are different from everyone else's, you'll soon have a very troublesome picky eater on your hands.

Do not eat anywhere but the kitchen or dining room table. Today, with so many people multi-tasking, you can observe people eating while running down the street, opening fast food bags on buses, eating while driving, eating in front of their computers while working. Studies show if you gobble your food quickly or without paying attention, your body gets confused and wants more food. You never got the psychological satisfaction of eating a meal.

Even snacks should be eaten at the dining table without distraction. Limit grazing and grabbing behavior between meal and snack times.

The habits your children form now will have far-reaching consequences. One of my clients had a terrible habit of eating chocolate-covered peanuts every night in front of the TV. She knew that if she changed this habit she would lose 30 pounds within 6 months to a year and solve her weight problem. But for the life of her, she just couldn't shed the habit. I asked her to think about her childhood so she could remember the roots of her behavior. At our next session, she told me about a very warm childhood memory she had had of her family gathered around the television in her parent's bedroom. Her father was lying back on his bed with a big bag of—you guessed it—chocolate-covered peanuts on his chest, from which everyone was grabbing.

With this memory, this young lady was able to understand why this was such a difficult habit to change. It made her feel warm and cozy, as if her family was with her snacking on chocolate-covered peanuts. So you can see that what you do today with your child can create habits that will serve him well or poorly throughout his life.

BOTTOM LINE: Lose 10 pounds

Save 10 pounds a year by encouraging your kids to eat only at the right times and in the right places.

#144. Make Breakfast a Family Habit

Breakfast is the most important meal of the day. I know you've heard that before, but let me convince you. Studies show that children can't stay alert or concentrate when they don't eat breakfast.

A myriad of studies since the 1970s have shown that nutrition in the morning stimulates children's learning. With regular breakfast, researchers have found improvements in a child's attendance and behavior, even a decrease in visits to the nurse's office at school. With a good traditional breakfast, your child gets more fiber and vitamins and minerals (especially vitamin C, iron and calcium).

When you don't eat breakfast, you're restless and hungry. That means you don't feel as good as you should. It also means you're more likely to grab unhealthful foods that happen to cross your path (and they're constantly crossing our paths in today's world of abundance).

And if you think skipping breakfast is a great weight-loss method, think again. Recent studies show teenage girls who skip breakfast are more likely to be overweight, while their thinner counterparts were more likely to eat breakfast. The National Weight Control Registry, which keeps track of people who have lost an average of 60 pounds and have kept it off for at least 5 years, found a striking number of breakfast eaters among their successful weight-loss maintainers.

If you don't eat breakfast, chances are your child doesn't eat breakfast either. I've seen time and time again in my practice that when parents begin eating breakfast, a non-breakfast-eating child all of a sudden starts taking time for breakfast as well.

Since we know breakfast is essential to good health and maintaining a healthful body weight, if your child is not eating breakfast, find out the reason. Is there too little time in the morning? Does she need to wake up earlier? Go to bed earlier? Breakfast only takes 10 to 20 minutes to eat and you can even prepare something "to go."

Just try to get as much balance as you can. Choose a whole-grain bread or cereal, fruit or vegetable, a protein source such as low-fat milk or cheese, and toss in a handful of healthful fat like nuts. Set the table the night before to make it easier.

Think Yourself Thin has plenty of quick breakfast ideas for you to choose from.

Here are some you can try:

• Peanut butter sandwich on whole grain bread, fruit and yogurt
• Ham and reduced-fat cheese on whole wheat with a carton of milk
• Homemade banana nut bread or bran-raisin muffins
• Leftover pizza (Yes, pizza!)
• Granola bar, yogurt and fruit

BOTTOM LINE: Lose 10 pounds

Eating breakfast saves you from eating junk food calories later in the day. Save 10 pounds a year.

#145. Pack a Healthy Lunchbox

Despite federal nutrition requirements, today's public school lunches are enough to make you gasp in dismay. Pizza, nachos, and greasy burgers are standard fare. Beat the competition with your own creative lunch ideas, and save calories and money at the same time!

You would think that at school your child is being served wholesome foods for lunch, like vegetables, whole grains, and poultry, meat, or fish cooked in healthful ways. Unfortunately, this is not always the case. A quick look at any typical school lunch menu shows pepperoni pizza, chicken nuggets, hot dogs, hamburgers, and nachos offered on a daily basis. Obviously, it's not a good idea to leave your child's nutritional health up to the local school district.

The solution is simple: Pack your child's lunches. If you have young children, they'll love you for it. It gives them a chance to choose a new lunch box—with whatever design or illustration on the outside strikes their fancy. They'll enjoy the surprise every day of discovering what you've packed for them if you made the lunch by yourself. If you've enlisted their help in preparing the lunch, they'll have fun in making their own choices.

Make sure they're carrying a well-balanced meal with ingredients from every food group in their box when they leave home in the morning. A sandwich, yogurt, and fruit is a great combination. Or use combinations of the "grab-able, transportable" foods you prepared to keep around the house. To give your younger child a delightful surprise, use a cookie cutter to make sandwiches of various shapes—turkeys at Thanksgiving, pumpkins around Halloween, etc.

BOTTOM LINE: Lose 10 pounds

If packing a lunch keeps your child from grabbing burgers and fries, he'll save at least 150 calories each school day.

#146. Teach Mindful Eating Habits

Children are born with the ability to eat just the right amount to feed their bodies properly. Studies show a 3-year-old, when provided with an array of food, will eat just what he needs—no more, no less.

But by the time they're 5 years old, children become more responsive to the environment beyond their own bodies. For instance, if at home, your child is regularly rewarded or somehow encouraged to eat more than he needs or wants by important people around him, he will. If he observes his parents or important people around him eating in response to external cues, he will. Thus, he learns to ignore his natural body signals, which are more likely to keep him healthy and trim, and instead pays more attention to external cues.

An external cue to eat could simply be an encouragement to "clean your plate!" Or it could be using food as a positive reinforcement: "If you finish your homework you can have an ice cream cone!" It could be a negative reinforcement: "You were bad so you can't eat dessert!" An external cue could be using food as an emotional support: "Eat this pie, it'll make you feel better!"

Children are also influenced by observing parental eating patterns. Studies show that when parents eat in response to emotions, when they diet or binge, or when they eat simply because of the presence of tasty foods—regardless of whether or not they are hungry, their children also begin eating for reasons other than hunger. These children lose their ability to self-regulate. This can also happen when parents restrict access to certain foods which are in the home environment. This causes the child to excessively desire those foods and overeat them—even after they've eaten lunch and report that they are no longer hungry—when given unlimited access to the restricted foods.

Children can naturally adjust their calorie intake during a single meal and over a 24-hour period, depending on the caloric density of the diet. To maintain your child's natural ability to eat in response to his hunger signals, try some of the practices listed below.

- Provide a wide array of healthful, wholesome foods to your child at regular meal and snack times
- Allow your child to choose what (within your healthful choices) and how much to eat.
- Never bring food into the house that must be restricted from your child.
- Never use food to reinforce, reward, punish, or bribe.
- Never force your child to eat.
- Eat meals and snacks at the dining or kitchen table mindfully.
- Enjoy and savor your meals and snacks as a family in pleasant surroundings without distractions.
- To introduce new foods, just encourage your child to try a bite, which he doesn't even have to swallow. If it is rejected, don't push and go on about the dinner as normal.
- Don't encourage your child to eat more than he wants.
- Above all, try your best to model the behavior you want your child to emulate.

BOTTOM LINE: Lose 10 pounds

Providing healthful, wholesome food from which your child may choose, and allowing your child to choose the amount he eats at designated meal and snack times based on his internal body signals will save hundreds of calories, or at least 100 a day. Save 10 pounds a year.

#147. Use Show and Tell to Teach Hunger Signals

Using show-and-tell dolls and toys, kids can learn how to judge if they're really hungry, or just bored or eating for the fun of it.

If you're a parent with a weight or eating problem and you've already noticed that your child is modeling some of your less desirable behaviors, or even if your child is already overweight, don't fret. You can teach your child how to listen to his natural body signals and self-regulate, even if you find it difficult to do yourself. Again, these are habits which are so much easier to adopt as a child—as I'm sure you're painfully aware. And as you teach your child, you may learn some valuable lessons as well.

Researcher Susan Johnson, in the journal *Pediatrics*, describes a great way of teaching kids about their own body signals: show and tell.

Through skits, the children were taught about hunger (rumbling in the stomach), eating to fullness (stomach extension, satisfactions), and the signals associated with overeating (stomach distension and discomfort). Then the researchers used doll play to teach about hunger and fullness. The dolls had stomachs (which were actually little plastic Baggies) filled with varying amounts of salt to represent 1) a stomach that was empty, 2) a stomach that was a little full, and 3) a stomach that was very full. When the children ate, they were asked to choose the doll stomach that was closest to how their stomachs felt. The children learned how to appropriately adjust their calorie intake after just 6 weeks of lessons. The lessons successfully overcame the effect of the parent's eating style and weight status.

You can do this at home with your own kids: Buy a doll and fill a baggie with varying levels of rice—showing an empty tummy, a partially full tummy, a full tummy, and a distended tummy. Tie the tummy around the doll's waist. Teach your child the differences between the hunger levels. Whenever your child eats a meal or snack, ask him before and after how he feels. Point to the doll tummies to help him compare how he feels with the doll. Is he hungry (empty bag)? A little hungry (just a little in the bag)? satisfied (full, but with a little space left)? or stuffed and uncomfortable (stuffed bag)? Soon he'll learn to know how he feels and will be able to regulate his eating habits based on body signals. Of course, the more you model and reinforce this behavior, the more natural these behaviors will be to your child. (See Tip #87, Fight the Beast.)

BOTTOM LINE: Lose 10 pounds

When your child learns how to choose the amount he eats at designated meal and snack times based on his internal body signals, he'll naturally want to avoid overeating. You'll save hundreds of calories this way, as much as 10 pounds a year.

CHAPTER 14

The Party Goer's Guide to Perfect Weight

Especially appropriate for: *Party Animals, Anyone Who Entertains (or Is Entertained) Frequently for Pleasure or Business, Those Who Go Home for the Holidays*

The social butterflies among us are very fortunate in some ways. They're often out and about, meeting new friends and entertaining old friends at home. Life is full. Life is great!

But then there's the little (or not so little) issue of weight. Festivities can put a dent in even the staunchest weight-loss resolve. Just about every party, after all, revolves around food. At the very least, there are good cheeses and other snacks, invariably accompanied by beer, wine, and other tasty libations. Just *thinking* about all the calories can make you feel heavier.

Everyone can benefit from the tips in this section, but the people I really have in mind are those who entertain (or get entertained) frequently. It's the repeat offenders who need this section most!

But let's keep things in perspective. If you socialize rarely, go ahead and splurge. Overeating on Thanksgiving Day is not going to add pounds.

However, overeating on Thanksgiving *and* the following weekend certainly will. In other words, don't burn any brain cells worrying about the calories on any one special occasion. Do give some thought to your weight if your calendar is booked for days or weeks in advance.

One of my clients, Estelle, put this theory to the test. She had worked hard (successfully) to lose 30 pounds, and she had no intention of putting it back. But, like all of us, she had to learn for herself. She weighed herself after a Thanksgiving splurge. No weight gain. Emboldened by those apparently "free" calories, she splurged again, weighed herself the next day, and lo, no gain! Naturally, she went for the triple crown and splurged and weighed yet again. Uh-oh—she was up 3 pounds. The human body is one mysterious machine.

My feeling is that parties are a time for celebrating life and for bringing families and friends together. No one's perfect, and it seems almost antisocial to obsess over your weight when everyone around you is having such a great time. Still, parties present a lot of opportunities for overindulging. Even if you've managed to master the daily routines of exercising, eating in moderation, and so on, parties and holidays don't come around all that often. Which means we don't have as much practice reconciling social obligations with our desire to maintain the same waist size.

Okay, the social season is upon you. It is important that you take some time to plan ahead. Sometimes this means controlling your environment. Other times it means distracting yourself from the delicious edibles spread out before you.

In the following pages you'll find a lot of pretty useful tips. My goal throughout is to suggest ways to have fun with your family and friends without making huge sacrifices—or gaining huge amounts of weight.

Parties are *not*—I repeat *not*—only about food. They should not even be *mainly* about food. Not convinced? Well, take a minute to make an inventory of the things that matter to you, that really touch your heart around special occasions and holidays. Here are some of the things that my clients have decided are important to them:

• Looking my best and feeling confident.
• The beautiful holiday decorations and music.
• Showing kindness to others and making sacrifices for those less fortunate.

• Observing the religious significance of holidays.
• Attending holiday events, such as theater and concerts.
• Watching the kids get excited and enjoying the season to the fullest.
• Having enough free time to do special things, like going to museums or spending the morning ice skating.
• Volunteering for charitable work.

Even without knowing you personally, I can say with some confidence that your list of priorities is probably pretty similar. Do we think about food when we go to parties or celebrate the holidays? Of course. But there's also so much more.

In my experience, hosts as well as guests have a better time when social occasions aren't completely dominated by food. You won't feel bloated and heavy at the end of the evening. You won't have to worry about saying or doing something embarrassing after all of those tipsy wassails.

And, most important, you won't have to expend time, energy, or guilt thinking about how you look and feel. Now, that's worth celebrating!

#148. "Happy Hour" at Home

You don't have to go to a bar to enjoy cheap drinks, and you certainly don't have to wake up with regrets about all the chips and beer nuts you wolfed down.

Why not have your next happy hour at home? It's a win-win situation. You'll have a better time with your friends when you're not getting blasted with '80s jukebox tunes. And because you'll control the food and drinks, you'll be able to keep calories to a minimum.

Happy hours are never as much fun as you think they'll be. Real conversation competes with overly loud music and the chatter of hundreds of people. There probably aren't enough stools, and you're always worrying about spilling your drink after getting bumped by the guy carrying three full pitchers of beer. Unless you're using the bar as a "meet market," it gets old pretty fast.

So have your own after-work get-togethers. Stock up some ice and drinks. Invite friends and colleagues, and hang out for awhile. You'll all have a good time, and who knows? A little socializing with the boss just might boost your career.

You'll have to supply food, of course. Put together a feast of healthy snacks—rolled-up smoked salmon, for example, or miniature crab cakes (see recipe on page 444) and a platter of fresh fruits and vegetables.

BOTTOM LINE: Lose 33 pounds

Spend a few hours at a bar and you're almost guaranteed to consume 3,000 calories. At home, assuming you have healthy snacks and a glass of wine, count on knocking that number down to 750. Make the switch every Friday night and you'll save 2,250 calories weekly.

#149. Start a Social Club

It's a lot of fun having a party, but it's also a lot of work. So spread the joy around. Make "home happy hours" a weekly gig, at a different house each week.

I've already talked about the impressive amount of calories you'll save by having parties at home instead of in a bar. But having a party, even a small one, can take a lot of preparation. You don't want to be the only one doing it. The solution is to get enough people involved so that no one person does all the work.

The group should be large and varied enough that it doesn't start feeling "inbred." Figure about a dozen regulars, with other friends and acquaintances showing up from time to time. Larger groups are ideal because it takes the pressure off any one person. If a few people can't make it one week, the flow won't be disrupted.

Have some friendly competition. See who can create the best-tasting—or the most unusual—snacks. They have to be healthy, of course.

Even with a largish group, there will come a time when people feel that it's too much work to host a party. That's when you want to shake things up. Turn your weekly gathering into a potluck. All the host is responsible for is the wine and the venue.

BOTTOM LINE: Lose 33 pounds

Compared to the bar scene, a regular get-together with friends will probably save you about 2,250 calories—and that's just in one night. Party on!

#150. The 25 Percent Blowout

At the height of the holiday season, you might find yourself invited to four parties in a week. Go to all of them—and indulge at one.

Here's some rocket science: What happens when you go to four or five parties in a week, and eat yourself silly at each one? You'll make a good social impression, but the impression on the scale at the end of the week will be even more impressive.

It's difficult for serious party goers to keep calories under control. Every sideboard and dining table is loaded with food, and every bottle is filled with caloric libations.

Don't stay home, for goodness' sake. But try this little trick:

Suppose you've been invited to four gatherings. The hostess of Saturday night's party is justly renowned for her fabulous cooking. Allow yourself to indulge like crazy. Have your fill. But that's it for the week. At the other three parties, feel free to taste whatever healthful offerings happen to be available. Otherwise, limit yourself to a glass of spring water. Won't you be hungry? No, because you were wise enough to eat before leaving home.

BOTTOM LINE: Lose 9 pounds

No matter how much you eat at a special event, remind yourself that you saved at least 600 calories at the other end where you practiced self-control. If you do a similar thing throughout the year, you can plan on saving a whopping 31,000 calories!

#151. Only Eat the Best

Don't waste valuable stomach space on foods you don't really care about. At every party this year, only eat the foods you really, really love.

The scene: Platters are getting passed around the table, and you're taking a little from each one just to be polite.

The trap: You have a mound of food in front of you that an army battalion couldn't finish.

Whoa! Rein in those social impulses that push you to please others without taking care of yourself. You don't need the calories. You don't want the calories. So don't take all the food. The truth is, your fellow dinner guests could care less what's on your plate.

Next time, only serve yourself the foods you like best. It might be turkey, stuffing, and a little gravy. Or maybe you crave cranberries and pumpkin pie. Whatever. Take healthful amounts of your favorites, and pass the others, untouched, to the person on your right.

Believe me, no one's going to notice—not even the person who did the cooking. All of those staring, disapproving eyes are in your head.

BOTTOM LINE: Lose 4 pounds

Let's suppose you really pigged out on stuffing and pie. Even if you had double servings of each, that's a lot fewer calories than you'd get by sampling everything. My guess is that you'll save at least 300 calories this way. In a busy social season, that's a lot of calories!

#152. Eat Before You Party

In order to get their fill of holiday cuisine, most people starve themselves for hours before the big event. What's wrong with this picture?

Your body needs normal amounts of food at regularly scheduled times. If you deprive your body at lunch and again at your usual suppertime, it will go into "survival" mode—and believe me, it's not pretty.

If you don't take in your usual amount of calories, the predictable result is that you're going to devour everything in sight at the first opportunity. Once the serving spoon is in your hand, you aren't going to take dainty servings. In fact, you'll easily wind up taking in more calories at one meal than you would have had you eaten your usual lunch and supper.

More bad news: Most parties occur in the late afternoon or evening. The calories you consume won't have the opportunity to be worked off. They'll be plenty busy, however. "Late" calories quickly convert to fat and make a beeline for your waistline.

Don't let this happen. Eat at your normal times before going out. Get your thrills from nonfood entertainment: good conversation, old friends, and gossip, gossip, gossip!

BOTTOM LINE: Lose 7 pounds

Keeping regular mealtimes helps ensure that you'll stay within your usual caloric parameters. If you show some restraint, you'll save at least 500 additional calories this way—and that's for just one night.

#153. The 30-Second Rule

The minute you arrive at a party, pour a glass of sparkling water.

What kind of wacky advice is this?" you ask. Wait, there's some science behind it.

Water takes up space in the stomach, especially when it has bubbles. Studies have shown that people who drink bubbly water or diet soda before eating usually eat a little less, especially if they wait about 30 minutes before filling their plates.

The water serves a social function, as well. Holding the glass gives you time to relax. This is important because the urge to dive into food declines dramatically with the passage of time. You'll be more in control of your choices. You won't attack food or drink the way you would if you went to the buffet the minute you arrived, all tense from the day's frustrations.

Yes, frustrations. When people go to parties at the end of the day, they generally grab a glass of wine and a handful of cheese puffs even before they see who's in the room. "Outta my way, it's been a terrible day!"

So start out with sparkling water or diet soda. Have a second glass, and then a third. Only then start looking at the food.

BOTTOM LINE: Lose 7 pounds

The typical party goer might have 2 beers (300 calories) and a plateful of snacks (another 300 calories) in the first few minutes. With my plan, you'll have water (0 calories) and probably half as many snacks (say, 150 calories). See the difference?

#154. Score the Best Real Estate

As every realtor will tell you, location is everything. It works at parties, too.

People congregate in the vicinity of food. They just as naturally fill their plates, whether they're hungry or not. Standing alone? A little bored? Take more food!

Hint: Don't go straight to the food table when you walk in the door. And don't stay there after you've filled your plate. The idea is to position yourself as far away from the food as you possibly can. It's a mind game, in a way: "Out of sight, out of mind" really does work. If you're not standing right next to the food, you won't be thinking about it as much, or eating it as much.

There's a convenience factor, as well. It's easy to nosh mindlessly when the food is right there at your fingertips. If you have to walk all the way across the room, you might find something better to do—maybe even talk to the person next to you!

I always tell my friends to find the most attractive member of the opposite sex and start a conversation. It doesn't have to be scintillating. Even a mild flirtation will get your mind totally off the food. And you and your friends can compare notes later!

BOTTOM LINE: Lose 4 pounds

I suspect that you can save yourself about 300 calories just by positioning yourself away from the food table. Even if you only use this trick once a week, the year-end savings will be impressive.

#155. Savor Each Bite*

Particularly at parties, we tend to gulp food without thinking about it very much. You might be getting full—but who notices?

Party eating tends to be unconscious eating. I want you to do the opposite and practice "mindful" eating.

Here's how it works.

Before eating anything, take the food to a table and sit down. Take three or four deep breaths and relax. Focus your full attention on the food you're eating. That goes for each bite.

If you want to talk with someone, put your food down while you talk. When you want to eat, put your full attention on the eating. Enjoy and savor every bite. Don't waste a single calorie by not paying attention to what you are eating.

Notice the point at which you feel comfortable, but not full. That's when it's time to stop eating.

I know this is hard to do in a social setting, but it works. If you're really dedicated, you'll find yourself eating less because you don't have the privacy to enjoy it as much as you know you should. That's a good place to be.

BOTTOM LINE: Lose 21 pounds

If mindful eating keeps you away from a plateful of appetizers, you can easily cut out 200 calories. Do this all the time—at home as well as at parties—and the overall calorie savings, and subsequent weight loss, will be impressive.

*Adapted from *Eating Awareness Training*, by Molly Groger (Summit Books, 1983).

#156. Imagine Every Move

The mind is a powerful thing. Before you walk out the door, imagine in detail all the healthful things you'll do at the party. Guess what? You'll probably do them.

So many times we succumb to situations because they "just happened." You didn't mean to eat 16 chocolate-covered pecans, but they were right there. You didn't want the extra helping of praline ice cream, but the host put it in your hand.

Hey, you're not as helpless as you think. You just didn't plan.

Before going to parties or other social events, spend some time thinking about what you want to do. Form a picture in your mind in which you're avoiding the "wrong" things: ignoring the ice cream, walking right past the buffet table, keeping your fingers out of the M&Ms bowl.

Also, imagine yourself doing the "right" things: having a fruit or vegetable snack before you leave home; grazing from the crudité platter; or simply having so much fun that food (in your mind) doesn't seem important.

Ready? Visualize success! Get a strong picture in your mind of what you want to do. You'll find that your behavior will closely follow.

BOTTOM LINE: Lose 6 pounds

My clients have told me that when they follow this technique consistently, they tend to consume about 400 calories less than they normally would. They also have a better time generally because they know they won't have to deal later on with the guilt of overeating!

#157. Give Away Leftovers

It's not the holiday meal that puts the weight on. It's eating the high-fat leftovers for a week afterward. Get rid of them.

I usually advise people to cook big batches of food so that they'll have delicious leftovers later. But that doesn't apply to holiday meals, which are notoriously high in fat and calories. Splurging is great, but you want to get back to normal eating as soon as possible.

There are two ways to handle this. The first is to cook only enough food for the one meal. That's not easy to do because you're never sure how much people are going to eat or which dishes will be most popular.

The second option is to give away the heaviest treats. Your guests will be thrilled if you neatly wrap half a pumpkin pie and insist that they take it home. Even side dishes—the stuffing with giblet gravy, for example—will get snapped up if you offer them a new home.

You'll probably still have some leftovers—a pound or two of turkey, several sides of vegetables, and the ever-present cranberry sauce. That's good. These are among the leanest dishes on the table, and you can use the leftovers to prepare nutritious, low-fat meals during the following week.

BOTTOM LINE: Lose 7 pounds

If you keep only the low-calorie leftovers, they can easily replace two higher-calorie meals in the coming week. That's probably a savings of 500 calories right there.

#158. Prioritize

Isn't your overall priority to look and feel your best? Keep it in mind during the holidays or when you're out and about with friends.

The people who are most successful (however you define "success") are the ones who keep their minds focused. The more you think about what really matters to you, the more likely you are to achieve your goals.

So put that party buffet out of mind for a moment. Let's focus on some of the things that you really want.

Do you like looking good? Of course you do. So do something to remind you of this priority. For example, buy a copy of *Shape* magazine or *Sports Illustrated*—the fit people may inspire you to look your best. Another trick is always to wear your best-fitting clothes: Unlike loose clothes, they'll remind you that you don't have the option of expanding.

Let's see, what else? Buy an exercise video, and keep it where you'll see it, on the nightstand or the dining room table. You might even pin up some photos of your next tropical vacation. They'll remind you of how you want to look when you're on the beach at Waikiki.

If you keep your priorities in mind during the fun times, you'll feel—and look—better all the time!

BOTTOM LINE: Lose 16 pounds

Using helpful reminders to keep your priorities front and center could easily save you 150 calories a day. Multiply that by 365, and you'll see where positive thinking will take you!

#159. Think Exercise

Keeping up your exercise routine even during the social season—especially during the holidays—will provide a great psychological edge.

It's so easy to excuse yourself from exercise during the party season. You just don't have time, you tell yourself. You've been good all year. Besides, it's cold outside—or not, whatever.

Excuses, excuses. We all have them, and we all tend to gain weight just when our justifications for lethargy are starting to sound believable.

Now for the hard truth. Curtailing calories is only half of the weight-loss equation. Burning calories is the other half. Give up one, and the other isn't going to be effective.

So much for the lecture. Now, let's talk about ways to get your mind back where it should be—on regular exercise. It's all a psyche game. Tell yourself, for example, "Sure, I'm going to have fun during the busy days ahead, and one reason I'm going to have so much fun is that I'm going to stick with my exercise routine. I'll have more energy, and the stress of the season won't get me down."

BOTTOM LINE: Lose 6–14 pounds

There are so many reasons to exercise: more energy, a more positive attitude, and maintaining your desired weight. Even if your exercise routine is minimal—say, walking 1 mile 3 times a week—you can count on losing 6 pounds a year. More exercise, more weight loss!

#160. Serve...Pause...Serve

Do you love your friends? Then treat them as well as you'd like others to treat you—by keeping food out of sight, at least some of the time.

The next time you're hosting a party, do everyone a favor. (You're not the only one watching calories.) Rather than putting out a dozen food platters all at once, pace them. For example, bring out a big platter of shrimp. Wait until it's empty, then bring out the smoked salmon. When that's gone, bring out something else.

Everyone will eat a little less when food isn't just waiting there for the grabbing. The idea isn't for people to go hungry, but to eat at a more natural speed and rhythm and avoid mindless noshing.

This won't work for large recipes that need to be available the whole time, such as fondues or hearty stews. In this case, at least confine them to one eating area—the dining room, for example. You don't want to have food stations all over the place.

Give people, including yourself, an opportunity to get away from the constant sight and smell of food. As I've said before, food that's out of sight is out of mind. Believe me, it works!

BOTTOM LINE: Lose 7–14 pounds

Just changing the way you serve food at parties could potentially save each guest about 500–1,000 calories. Do this once a week. It's not a huge change, but even small calorie savings really add up over time.

#161. Bring Out the Produce

It's not illegal to have fruit and vegetable party snacks between Thanksgiving and New Year's—really!

We're accustomed to seeing baby wieners, buffalo wings, and the like at parties. That's fine. A little junk food tastes mighty good on occasion.

Just don't make it the only food. For your next party, stock up on fresh fruits and vegetables. A lot of your guests will appreciate this more than you know. People don't always admit that they're trying to eat healthier, to feel better overall, and to maintain their desired shapes and weights— but you can be sure you're not the only one who will appreciate the chance to snack on something more wholesome than a sparerib.

Because rich food is so readily available in this country, it's easy to get the idea that fruit and veggie platters are inherently less appetizing. I'd be the first to admit that a huge platter filled with carrot and celery sticks doesn't exactly set the pulse racing, but why be so limited in the first place?

Pineapple, mango, and other tropical fruits are drenched in natural sugars, and they look beautiful when sliced and layered on a plate. Cut radishes into playful shapes. Add olives for color and a hint of salt. How about a few artichokes with a low-fat dipping sauce. Delicious!

BOTTOM LINE: Lose 10–21 pounds

Put fruits and vegetables on your serving table, and eat them in place of high-fat party food. You'll save at least 100–200 calories weekly.

#162. Be a Lousy Host

I really don't mean that. But all too often, we think that being a good host means insisting that people refresh their glasses or take another serving of whatever.

You certainly don't want your guests going without a drink or an extra serving because they're too polite, or too shy, to ask.

But here's another point of view. Sure, they might be hesitant to take seconds, but they'll get around to it eventually. On the other hand, it's very hard for a guest to refuse a host who is foisting food or alcohol on them. The last thing they need is interference.

Go ahead and offer food or drink. Repeat the offer if you wish. After that, consider the matter closed.

I remember when one of my dinner guests refused an appetizer that I had slaved over. I was offended at first, but then I stopped and thought to myself, "Wait a minute. He's here to enjoy himself, not to please me by eating—and raving over—every bite."

Another personal story. When I was much younger, I had two dates with a man who kept pushing food on me. Once, over my objections, he even ordered extra desserts for us to share. He didn't get a third chance.

BOTTOM LINE: Lose 7–15 pounds

If you don't allow yourself to be pushed into taking more than you want, and you don't push others, you can count on cutting out 500–1,000 calories a week.

#163. Lighten Up

Overate? Get over it, and move on.

Nobody's perfect. There *will* be times when you eat in ways that you'll later regret. That's no big deal—but some people are so self-critical! They let their discipline drop over drinks or at a party, then hate themselves the rest of the week.

I've noticed that people who are unusually hard on themselves sometimes use their failings, unconsciously, as an emotional ploy to junk the whole effort. I imagine that their internal tape goes something like this: "I was such a pig at that party last night. I never could control myself, so why bother trying? The heck with the whole thing."

If your plan crashes, and you really do want to forget the whole thing, please be honest with yourself. You may not be ready for the challenge right now. Don't hate yourself.

I think you'll realize, though, that you don't want a small mistake to derail your efforts. That would be like getting so frustrated over a flat tire that you deliberately slash the other three.

Look back at what happened. Learn from it. Use that knowledge to do better next time. Okay? Now, get on with your life.

BOTTOM LINE: Lose 21 pounds

None of my clients gets a 100 for consistency. We all goof now and then. Still, if you manage to eliminate 200 calories on most days (allowing for some slips), you'll still lose about 21 pounds in a year.

#164. The Chocolate Cardiac Challenge

We all need to let loose and splurge on something
now and then. Do it—and use it to your advantage.

Suppose you have this urge for a super-duper dessert. Maybe the infamous Chocolate Cardiac Challenge at your favorite restaurant. You think about it all day. Maybe you even dream about it.

Have the dessert, by all means. But (you knew there had to be a "but") plan for it. Because the dessert is so rich, it doesn't make sense to have it in addition to your regular dinner. So have it instead. Make a real production of it. While your friends are enjoying their entrees, you can be oohing and ahhing over your succulent treat. All eyes will be on your plate, I guarantee you.

Use the same approach for all the wonderful things you enjoy. Don't give them up—substitute. Crave ice cream? Give up a second serving of sour-cream chicken. Have a taste for a chocolate shake? Don't have your usual cola in the afternoon.

Traditional diets are full of "don'ts." They take a lot of the fun out of life, and no one sticks with them very long. My feeling is you should eat what you want. If you keep your overall diet balanced and cut some calories here and there, you're going to lose weight.

BOTTOM LINE: Lose 15 pounds

If you had a full dinner plus the dessert, you'd get a whopping 1,750 calories. Give up the dinner, and your Saturday nights only cost you 750 calories. Not bad for a splurge!

#165. Start a Trend

Social occasions don't have to revolve around food. You won't lose all your friends if you do something else for a change.

We tend to invite friends over for dinner without really thinking about it. It's just what people do, and having a dinner party is, in some ways, the path of least resistance. It doesn't require any creativity beyond remembering what you served the last time so that you don't do it again. (That's considered as bad as wearing the same dress twice around the same people—horrors!)

Next time, get together and do something that doesn't revolve around food. If your friends aren't from the area, bone up on the history of your neighborhood and go on a walking tour. Mix it up by visiting interesting shops as well as historic spots.

Or plan a day trip together. Go to an interesting town. Visit a historic site or a music festival. Heck, rent a canoe and get some exercise! The possibilities are endless. Ideally, pick a place that's no more than 2 hours away, so you don't get car cramps.

BOTTOM LINE: Lose 6–7 pounds

You probably splurge when you're preparing a dinner for guests. By changing to a nonfood event, and eating a normal nonsplurge meal, you are probably saving 400–500 calories. Even if you only do this one night a week, you're going to see the payoff—and you'll have a lot of fun at the same time!

CHAPTER 15

The Calorie Map
for Frequent Travelers

Especially appropriate for: *Frequent Business Travelers, Family or Personal Vacations, Visits to Family or Friends Who Keep Pushing Food Your Way, Happy-Hour Addicts*

Whether you're away from home on business or for pleasure, you know that traveling offers many opportunities for indulgences that can add up to extra pounds. Frequent business travelers face the greatest challenge to maintaining a proper weight, but even the once-a-year family vacation can lead to unhealthy habits that continue even when you return to your regular routine.

Everyone should be able to enjoy their travels fully while still maintaining a healthful weight. Indeed, you'll enjoy your travels even more when you know that you won't have to lose any "travel pounds" when you're back home.

I've often noticed that people tend to admire business travelers. They envy the fullness of their lives, the fact that they're constantly meeting new people, experiencing different cultures, and seeing unique sights.

333

Travel seems exciting and exotic for those who are stuck in cubicles in boring offices.

But there's a downside. If you travel on business a lot, you know all about the harried schedules, the stress of constantly coping with new situations over which you have little control, and being wined and dined by business associates whom you don't know all that well.

Consider Jennifer, one of my clients. She travels to the far corners of the earth for her job with the World Bank. With each assignment, she never knows what conditions she'll find. She doesn't know if she will have access to a gym, or even if it's safe to walk outside. In some countries, eating fresh fruits and vegetables is not safe. She eats a lot in restaurants, which means a lot of unnecessary (and unwanted) calories. Yes, her work is fascinating, even exciting, but it also poses challenges that those of us stuck at home don't have to contend with.

Most of you probably are not frequent travelers like Jennifer, but you do have that family vacation coming up. Occasional travelers face all the same issues as business travelers. Too much restaurant food. Not enough exercise. An utter lack of fresh fruits and vegetables.

Vacations are made for indulging, of course. Nothing wrong with that. But what often happens is that the *routine* of travel continues once you get back home. You might be a little out of shape, so getting back to regular exercise is easy to put off. You've gained a few pounds that stubbornly refuse to budge. You've gotten in the habit of high-calorie eating, and getting back to a healthful routine seems like more work than it's worth.

Steve is one client who has made a concerted effort to avoid these pitfalls. Steve is an inveterate traveler. He makes it a point to trek his family of four to a different destination each year. Sometimes they travel by car. Other trips may require flying to a distant destination, where they stay put for the duration of the vacation.

Either way, Steve knows that he has to maintain the healthy practices he follows at home in order to control his weight. If he doesn't, he'll face the unhappy reality of drifting for two or three weeks in an unhealthy direction, and then fighting to shake off those bad habits once he's back home. Put another way, he can probably count on losing at least two months in his ongoing battle of the bulge. Steve wants to have fun on his vacations, to relax and enjoy them—but he's learned that an essential part of being relaxed is knowing that he's taking proper care of himself and thus avoiding a future showdown.

Even though I planned this chapter with frequent travelers in mind, the suggestions really apply to everyone. Whether you travel every month or just a few times a year, you'll find dozens of easy-to-incorporate techniques that will prevent your time on the road from taking a bite out of your diet plans.

The goal of traveling is to take a vacation from stress and boredom, *not* from the hard-won healthy practices that you've begun to employ. So with that in mind—*Bon voyage!*

#166. Shift Your Appetite Clock

A few days before you travel to a new time zone, shift your meal times backward or forward, as required. You'll be less likely to slip in an "extra" meal.

There are several advantages to getting used to new time zones days before you actually board the plane. Research has shown that people who change their usual routines, including meal times, to accommodate the "new" time zone will have less jet lag and more energy.

A more important benefit, of course, is that this advance preparation keeps you from eating an extra meal on the airplane, or from eating in the middle of the night at your destination. You won't be as hungry for that second breakfast or second dinner if you're already on your new schedule.

It also helps to sleep properly before, and during, your travels. If you're on an extra-long flight, you might consider taking an over-the-counter sleep aid. The idea is to shift your body clock to the new time zone as quickly as possible.

BOTTOM LINE: Lose 9 pounds

If you avoid an extra meal, either en route or after arriving at your destination, you'll save about 700 calories. You'll save even more if you manage to stick to your usual meals and snacks during the trip. Consider this: If you spend 2 days traveling and 5 days at your destination, skipping those "extra" meals could save you 4,900 calories overall. That's 1½ pounds lost (or not gained!) per week-long trip. If you travel six times a year, that's significant savings.

#167. Win with First Class

Enjoy the extra space and comfort. You're paying for it, after all. But try to refrain from the "bonus" foods and drinks that practically get forced on business-class customers.

A first-class or business-class transatlantic trip costs thousands. Everyone is tempted to get the most for their money—but there's no way you can stuff down $5,000 worth of food. Even if you could, do you really want the extra calories?

The food in business class is more extravagant than coach, and there's also more of it. Once it's in front of you, it's hard to resist. I recommend calling the airline in advance and requesting fresh fruit and a low-calorie entree. While you're putting in your order, let them know you only want to be offered water or diet soda, not a calorie-rich cocktail.

Also helpful: Bring along your laptop, or that novel you've been planning to read. The busier you are, the less likely you'll be to use food for entertainment.

BOTTOM LINE: Lose 7 pounds

Suppose you're flying business class from Los Angeles to New York. If you can bring yourself to give up that mini-bottle of wine or champagne, you'll save 150 calories. Forsaking the before-dinner drink will save another 150 calories; giving up one of those gourmet, "even smelling me is fattening" cookies will save at least 500 calories, and resisting the nuts will save 160 calories.

See what you get for restraint? A total savings of 960 calories—and that's just one way! Do it for each of your twelve round-trip flights and save 23,000 calories.

#168. Have a Flying Picnic

Everyone used to complain about airline food. Now they complain about getting no food. Here's the solution to both.

Why go hungry just because you're flying coach? Those little bags of snacks don't cut it. My advice: Bring along a picnic lunch or dinner. It's lower in calories. It tastes better. And it's a heck of a lot of fun.

What makes a good plane picnic? How about a deliciously seasoned chicken breast? I like cold salads—maybe some leftover white beans and shrimp. In addition to the main course, pack a ready-to-go vegetable: raw broccoli florets, for example, or, if you're feeling fancy, some chilled asparagus spears. For dessert, open a container packed with chunks of your favorite fruits. (As you've probably gathered by now, I *love* plastic containers.)

Oh, and don't forget to pack a quart bottle of your favorite spring water. In addition to quenching your thirst, you'll be able to pass up those calorie-rich beers or drinks.

BOTTOM LINE: Lose 3 pounds

Most plane picnics will total around 600 calories. That's at least 200 calories less than you'd get by eating the usual airline food, or the meals that are served in airports. Factor in the water you brought (and the alcoholic drinks you turned down), and you can count on saving 500 calories on each flight.

Put this in perspective: If you fly once a month round-trip, multiply this number by 24. That's a lot of saved calories!

#169. Terminal Snacks

With the added security at airports, we're all spending extra time in the terminals—usually in the vicinity of pretzel and bakery stands.

Eating, unfortunately, is one of the most popular ways of passing the time. The meals and snacks available at airport terminals are getting better all the time, but they're hardly getting healthier. Some might call them, um, terminal.

Consider those cinnamon buns served at most airports: 640 calories each. Those large croissants and gourmet cookies: often about 700 calories. A quick snack while you're waiting for the plane can blow your "calorie load" for the entire day.

One of the best ways to resist airport enticements is to eat before you leave home. Or at least look for food stands that offer a variety of salads or lean sandwiches. Don't go anywhere near those food carts with ready-wrapped sandwiches: They slather them with mayonnaise or other high-fat ingredients, and you have no control over what you get.

Oh, did I already mention that you don't want to get within smelling distance of those cinnamon buns? When you're hungry, the aroma will lasso you in despite your best intentions. Believe me, I know!

BOTTOM LINE: Lose 7 pounds

If you manage to circumvent the gauntlet of food carts, there's a good chance you'll save 1,000 calories each day you spend in airports. You'll do even better if you bring your own meals and snacks, rather than depending on the food served in flight. Travel once a month, multiply by 24!

#170. Steal a Gym

You rush to get to the airport, only to find that your flight has been delayed and you have a two-hour wait. Lucky you.

Yes, lucky you. The delay means that you can get in some extra exercise—assuming, that is, that you had the foresight to pack exercise clothes and shoes in your carry-on bag. I, on the other hand, travel in relaxed "exercise clothes" to make it easier.

I know, exercise isn't the first thing you have in mind when you're traveling. But it's a great way to reduce jet lag—and skim off some of those inevitable "travel calories."

If you belong to one of the airline clubs, there's a good chance they have an arrangement with a hotel gym near the airport. Or, if you're staying at a hotel near the airport and the flight delay is long enough, you can catch a shuttle back for a quick workout.

A third, slightly sneaky option is to hop a shuttle for any airport area hotel, whether or not you're staying there. I have yet to find one that actually checks that the people using the gym are registered guests. At worst, they may charge you a small, one-day fee.It's really no different, in principle, than using McDonald's restaurants along the interstate as "comfort stops."

BOTTOM LINE: Lose 9 pounds

Most people, left alone in the vicinity of an airport snack stand, will consume at least 1,000 calories. By exercising instead, you can count on burning about 270 calories. Not a bad way to use the time. Doing this once a month equals big savings.

#171. Luggage Calisthenics

Rich food and extra meals are only part of the reason that people return from trips heavier than when they left. Exercise—or the utter lack of it—also plays a role.

It's easy to extol the virtues of motel health clubs, but let's be honest: Most of us will never take advantage of them. That's okay because there's an even easier way to burn surplus calories between flights—by logging a mile or two in the terminal itself.

No kidding. Airport concourses are nearly as long as the runways themselves, and you'll expend about the same number of calories (9 a minute) walking as briskly as you would using a treadmill. The only challenge is to find a place to do some brisk walking without appearing as though you shoplifted a magazine and are hiding it under your coat.

Rent a baggage cart for your carry-on luggage. Load it up, then wheel the cart briskly from one end of the baggage area to the other. Or, if the weather is nice, zip back and forth on the sidewalk in front of the terminal.

BOTTOM LINE: Lose 9 pounds

Concourse exercise helps in two ways. You'll be passing up bars and snack stands, where you would have consumed a minimum of 1,000 calories. And the exercise itself will torch about 270 calories. Do this 24 times a year (figuring one round-trip excursion a month), and the weight loss will really add up.

#172. Pretend You're Still Home

The response to this advice generally goes something like this: "Why the heck would I do that?" Calm down and let me explain.

It's very easy to get off schedule when you're traveling. That goes for exercise as well as meals. The problems are even more pronounced at meetings and conventions, where you have very little control over the timing of events.

What usually happens is that people get so off schedule that they become ravenous between meals. That's a bad condition to be in when you're finally confronted with decent food. No matter how much (or how little) you usually eat, see what happens when you starve yourself for a few hours, then sit down behind a full plate. It isn't pretty!

The other problem, of course, is that busy meeting schedules allow little time for exercise, and you probably forgot to bring your workout clothes in any event.

Here's a better way. If you have any flexibility at all, try not to schedule meetings at your regular meal times. Don't be shy about skipping nonessential meetings, especially those that start around 11 A.M. and continue until 2 P.M. Most conventions have tapes of sessions. Go to lunch at your usual time, and review the tape later.

If at all possible, do your exercises first thing in the morning. It's the only sure way to get them behind you. Morning is probably the only time in the day when you'll have a little bit of freedom, so take advantage of it. Besides, exercising early means that you'll have more energy throughout the day.

Ideally, you'll be in a position actually to plan the itinerary. Be kind to your fellow attendees. Discuss the need to schedule meetings that don't conflict with regular meal times, and don't start them so early that people find it difficult or impossible to get in a quick workout. Better yet, follow the lead of some leading corporations: Start off each day's schedule with a group yoga or stretching session. Attendance is optional, of course, but you'll be there to set a good example!

BOTTOM LINE: Lose 14 pounds

Sticking with a regular meal schedule will pay big dividends. You won't starve, because you'll be eating at the proper times. Plan on saving 200 calories at lunch and 200 calories at dinner. Moreover, you won't be as likely to quell your hunger pains with fatty snacks, which will save you another 190 calories. That adds up to 590 calories every day. Good job! Say you travel one week out of every month. That leaves 33,000 calories.

#173. Harass the Hotel

I'm only joking. Most hotels are happy to arrange special meals even before guests set foot in the lobby. But you have to ask them to do it.

Even if you're serious about losing weight, coming face-to-face with good food can send good intentions out the window. That's why I advise people to remove the threat of temptation days or weeks before they travel.

Many hotels and restaurants have begun to post their menus on the Web. Before you leave home, find out what the different hotel restaurants typically serve. What hours are they open? What's on the room service menu? Do they scale back the menu after certain hours?

Suppose you aren't thrilled with what you find. Take a few minutes to browse the Web (or, if you're into primitive technology, pick up the telephone) to see what else is available in the neighborhood. Maybe there's a seafood or vegetarian restaurant nearby, or a farmers' market downtown. Tourist bureaus are great sources of information.

In the age of the Internet, it's easy to "visit" a city before you leave home. With a little bit of planning, you can ensure that your diet doesn't take a hit simply because there aren't healthier options available.

BOTTOM LINE: Lose 14 pounds

There's no reason to settle for second best. When you consider the fat-laden food you might get stuck with, planning ahead can save you at least 200 calories at every meal. If you travel 12 weeks a year, that's a savings of 50,400 calories!

#174. Be a "Shopping Tourist"

Snacking at home is easy. You probably have fresh fruit on the counter or healthy snacks in your desk drawer. When you travel, on the other hand, you won't have the same options. Or maybe you will.

We've been talking about the importance of planning travel meals, but it's just as important to plan travel snacks. You want to have an assortment of fruits or vegetables ready to go when you're attacked by those midafternoon hunger pangs. Otherwise, you'll have no choice but to dive into cheese-covered nachos.

When you're doing your pretrip homework, make sure that hotel room service delivers fruits and vegetables. In addition, get to know the neighborhood. Rather than checking out all the expensive fashion stores, find the delis and supermarkets. Fill a bag or two with healthful snacks, and you're ready to go for the entire week.

Oh, back to room service for a moment: If you're arriving in the evening, call ahead and make sure that a fruit or vegetable platter will be waiting in your room when you arrive. A quick snack on arrival will make it easier to eat moderately if you go out to dinner later on.

BOTTOM LINE: Lose 5 pounds

If you're on the road for a week each month, and you substitute a fruit or vegetable tray for those high-calorie snacks you might have been having, you'll easily save 200 calories a day.

#175. The Briefcase Surprise

Business meetings are notorious for the super-caloric snacks that are offered to innocent attendees. My advice: Set a different agenda.

Got extra room in your purse or briefcase? Good. It's a great place to stash healthy snacks, which you can pull out when your blood sugar drops during those interminable meetings.

During your trip, keep an eye out for fresh food at all times. If you spot a fruit bowl, grab an apple or orange. Help yourself to other fresh fruits every morning at breakfast. Don't leave a restaurant without pocketing leftover raw vegetables or even breadsticks. Wrap things that need wrapping in a napkin or tinfoil, and keep them in your room. When it's time to go to a meeting, take a few of these "surprise" packages with you.

Apart from having an alternative to fatty snacks, you'll be able to keep your appetite in check all day—and you'll be much less likely to approach meals with ravenous hunger.

This is especially important in the afternoon, when so many conventions and business meetings have a "coffee break" that's also a run on the calorie bank. Have a healthful snack before entering the room. If your stomach isn't growling when the meeting begins, you'll be less tempted by those cookies and pastries that are as rich as Bill Gates.

BOTTOM LINE: Lose 5 pounds

When you substitute a fruit or vegetable snack for that high-calorie snack you might have been having, you'll easily save 200 calories a day. Do that on your week-long trips each month and it adds up!

#176. The "First Lady" Technique

Many a healthful diet has gotten derailed during a multicourse banquet. Guess what? You don't have to eat everything. Nobody's going to scold you. Mom didn't cook it just for you.

A client of mine, Tom, once was seated next to Hillary Rodham Clinton, the former First Lady and current senator, at a formal dinner. He couldn't help but notice that Mrs. Clinton didn't touch her dinner.

Tom admitted that he was a little envious. He had tried for years to manage his own weight, and leaving a full plate untouched struck him as a courageous act. But another thought also crossed his mind. Even though Mrs. Clinton totally ignored her food, no one noticed (except for Tom, who was sitting right next to her). Her restraint, he assumed, was probably a necessary defense mechanism for someone who attends multiple events on the same day.

Take a hint from Mrs. Clinton. Nobody really cares if you eat only part of your meal, or none of it, for that matter. The server gets paid for bringing a plate to you and for picking it up later. You won't get a dirty look for leaving food on your plate.

BOTTOM LINE: Lose 4–6 pounds

Consider this: If you travel frequently, there are probably a lot of occasions when you eat just to be polite. Turning down a meal that you don't really want anyway will save at least 700 calories. Do this once a month and save 8,400 calories. Do it weekly and save 36,000 calories.

#177. Join the Snack Committee

Yes, there really is such a thing. Who do you think arranges for all those doughnuts and pastries at office meetings? This is your chance to make a difference.

Modern capitalism would collapse overnight if it weren't for committees. Nearly every decision, from choosing convention speakers to recommending "Friday fun" days at the office, comes out of committees.

So why not join (or convene) a "healthy snack" committee?

Eating healthful snacks will help you lose weight, have more energy during afternoon slumps, and generally work more efficiently. By volunteering to run this operation, you'll also avoid being assigned to tasks that will undoubtedly be dreadfully boring. Plus, your colleagues will be grateful to find some delicious, healthy choices for a change.

Believe me, you'll feel appreciated when your colleagues first catch sight of the attractively nutritious offerings. There's nothing more refreshing than a panoply of fresh pineapple served with sliced kiwi, strawberries, blueberries, pears, grapes, and bananas. Little cups of raw nuts are a good choice. So are dried fruit chips, servings of dry granola.

Bonus: Your colleagues will leave the meeting feeling great instead of miserably stuffed and in a sugar-induced coma for the rest of the day.

BOTTOM LINE: Lose 9-17 pounds

Healthful snacks make an incredible difference. Swapping a serving of fruit for the usual supercookie each week will save you at least 500 calories. Actually, you'll probably save 1,000 calories because no one stops at one cookie.

#178. The Happy-Hour Trap

Business travelers often conclude their meetings at a local bar for happy hour. You can turn these events into your greatest weight-loss opportunity—by avoiding them.

Event organizers think they're doing attendees a favor by capping days of meetings and presentations with a happy hour. It's not a terrible way to dispel pent-up emotion and tension—except, of course, for those who happen to be watching their weight. As I see it, the whole purpose of the happy hour is to blow off steam by eating and drinking—or, more accurately, by drinking and eating.

Happy hour can dump more calories into your diet than lunch and dinner combined. (Plus, many people go out to dinner *after* happy hour). An hour or two of eating and drinking can easily add up to 3,000 calories. Plus, think about all the aspirin that gets consumed the next morning. Yikes!

There's nothing wrong with enjoying happy hour on occasion, but you'll lose a lot of weight if you skip out. (You can always arrange to meet your friends at a restaurant later.) While they're at the bar scarfing beer nuts, you can be enjoying a hot shower and a TV game show or two.

BOTTOM LINE: Lose 31 pounds

Suppose you avoid three out-of-town happy hours a month. You'll lose about 31 pounds in a year. If you're in a hard-drinking crowd that goes out more often, you'll lose even more.

#179. Better than Beer Nuts

Bars don't stay in business by selling health food. If you're lucky, you'll get a cheeseburger to accompany the beer nuts. There has to be a better way.

Everyone snacks when they drink—and the more you snack, the more you drink. Why do you think bars provide free salty snacks, anyway?

Hanging out with friends at bars can be a lot of fun, but you have to find ways to reduce the calorie load. For example, put aside part of a sandwich from lunch, then eat it just before you go to the bar. Less appetite means less snacking, and less snacking means fewer calories.

Or how about drinking a tall glass of sparkling water or diet soda the minute you sit down at the bar? Studies show that sparkling water or diet soda will satisfy your initial thirst, which will make it easier to sip your drinks slowly, rather than pouring them down. They also take up room in the stomach, leaving less room for high-calorie snacks.

What if you're eating at the bar? Instead of a greasy burger, order half a pound of shrimp. Or get a vegetable plate. Traditional bars aren't likely to offer fresh fruits and vegetables, but bars attached to restaurants sometimes do.

BOTTOM LINE: Lose 31 pounds

It's easy to consume 3,000 calories at happy hours. If you drink some water, go easy on the booze, and swap the traditional bar snacks for shrimp, vegetables, or other healthful foods, you might consume about 900 calories, a savings of 2,100 calories weekly. That's worth a toast!

#180. Work Out, then Eat Out

Want to control your appetite at dinner? Spend half an hour in the hotel gym.

People tend to eat more when they travel, and the foods they eat tend to be higher in calories than what they enjoy back home. Exercise makes all the difference.

The main advantage of exercise, of course, is that it burns calories: about 300 in 30 minutes. It's also a great stress reliever. When you're more relaxed, you'll be less likely to succumb to emotional eating and drinking.

If you exercise at the end of the day—and before slipping out to a bar—you might be content to sip a glass of water (maybe flavored with lime) or a diet soda instead of high-calorie alcoholic drinks. Your mind will be focused on health, so you'll be more likely to order a healthful snack. When dinner finally rolls around, you'll order sensibly because you already have some food in your stomach.

BOTTOM LINE: Lose 35 pounds

I've said before that happy hours are a real trap when you're trying to lose weight. But if you exercise first, and follow it up with a healthy bar snack, you might find yourself saving as much as 3,000 calories—and that's not counting the fact that you'll probably have lighter fare at dinner because you'll already have eaten something. Conservatively, that little bout of exercise might wind up saving you 2,500 calories weekly.

#181. Make Faces

I know it sounds weird, but let me explain. Facial exercises will help you unwind at the end of a stressful day. That means fewer calories later on. Really.

Everyone eats more when they're stressed. Not convinced? Well, ask yourself how many times you open the refrigerator after a hard day at work. Compare it to the refrigerator raiding that occurs when you're calm. See what I mean?

Most stress-sensitive muscles are located in the head and forehead. So give them a workout. Start with your forehead. Make it wrinkle. At the same time, stretch your neck and roll your head in a circle. Now, relax.

Next, wrinkle up the muscles in your face. You can't do this exercise and look pretty. In fact, you'll look like a prune. That's good!

Next, squint your eyes. Relax them. Purse your lips. Relax them. Press your tongue to the roof of your mouth. Relax it. Hunch your shoulders. Relax them.

Now, don't you feel a lot better?

BOTTOM LINE: Lose 6 pounds

Stretching your facial muscles doesn't burn calories. But it works wonders for the emotions. By unwinding before you go to the bar or out to dinner, you'll find yourself eating in response to hunger, not tension. I've found that people who get control of their emotions often wind up consuming 400 fewer calories (that's 2 glasses of wine to "relax" and 2 slices of bread eaten nervously) during the evening than they would otherwise. Do it weekly. That adds up to a lot of pounds in a year!

#182. Lose the Minibar Key

Hotel minibars are stocked by people who could care less about your weight. Those little drinks and snacks are very hard to resist. Darn, must have lost the key...

Hunger strikes at all hours. Even if you're not hungry, boredom can drive you toward extra calories—and few things are more boring than being stuck in a sterile hotel room for a few hours or days. There's only one sure way to guarantee that you won't succumb to the lures of the minibar: "lose" the key.

Okay, it's a little gimmicky, but it works. "Accidentally" leave the key at the check-in desk ("Excuse me, I found this on the floor, and thought I'd better give it to you"). Don't be embarrassed—no one will suspect what you're up to!

Other options: Drop the key behind the couch cushions. Kick it under the minibar where you can't reach it. Slip it inside the pages of the Gideon *Bible*. Just get it out of sight. (But remember where you put it so you can put it back in its proper place before you check out.)

BOTTOM LINE: Lose 8 pounds

Minibars can be real killers. Even if you limit yourself to one drink and one snack, you'll tuck in an extra 300 calories. Oh, you usually have 2 drinks or 2 snacks? That's 450 calories. Spend 5 days on the road monthly, and the minibar alone will account for more than 2,200 calories. The only solution: Lose that key!

#183. Get Elastic

They're so lightweight and take up so little room that you can throw them in your luggage without throwing something else out. And they turn your hotel room into an instant gym.

I'm talking about exercise bands and tubes. Made from elastic and available in any exercise store, they take the place of dumbbells and other weights. They're all the rage today, and for good reason.

Exercise bands can be just as effective as traditional gym equipment. In fact, gyms often include them in the workout areas. The tubes can be used for arm stretches, and the bands work well for leg stretches (just follow the directions).

This type of strength training can't be beat when you're trying to lose weight. It burns a tremendous amount of calories, for starters. And as muscles get larger, they naturally burn additional calories, even when you're sitting still!

I've found that people who travel frequently often get hooked on exercise bands and tubes. The equipment makes it easy to keep up with your exercise routine no matter where you're staying. Working out in your room is quicker and more convenient than going to a gym. And we all know that regular exercise helps reduce appetite. You'll have less stress and tension. And you'll get stronger at the same time.

BOTTOM LINE: Lose 6 pounds

At a very conservative estimate, working out with elastic will save you 250 calories a day. Not bad! Do it every day of your monthly week-long trip and burn 21,000 calories in your hotel room!

#184. Bring Your Exercise Instructor

I'm not suggesting that you bring that gym hunk (or doll, for you guys) with you to Cancun. The idea is to pack your favorite exercise tape in your luggage—and quit looking so disappointed!

Seriously, folks, you don't want to disrupt your regular exercise routine while you're on the road. That's a shortcut to feeling bloated and lethargic.

My suggestion is this: Bring an audio or videotape that contains your favorite aerobics routines. Take some time every day to play the tape and get in a bit of a workout.

Hint: Call ahead to see if you can get a room with a VCR.

One of my clients, Georgia, actually lost weight on her last vacation to Mexico. Every day at noon, she put on an exercise video and had her workout on her hotel balcony in Cancun! This was a first for her—and it was the only vacation she could remember during which she actually got in better shape.

Needless to say, this is a lesson she won't forget. She plans to pack that tape, or another one like it, on all her future vacations.

BOTTOM LINE: Lose 10 pounds

Exercising regularly, no exceptions, is the only way to keep the momentum going. It's so easy to get out of the exercise habit—and once the pattern is broken, it's easy to give in to lethargic ways. The immediate benefit, of course, is that you can easily burn 400 calories a day by following the taped routines. Do it each day during your week-long monthly trip and burn 22,600 calories!

#185. Portable Yogis

Travel, even when the final destination is exotic or restful, tends to be stressful—and stress invariable leads to eating. We could all use a personal stress-reduction manager from time to time. Well, this is your chance.

Exercise tapes aren't the only way to curtail travel calories. Another approach is to bring along some stress-reducing yoga tapes. I can't say it often enough: Much of what passes for hunger is really nervous eating. We eat when we're bored, tired, or anxious. Control stress, control appetite. It's that simple!

Call ahead to make sure the hotel has VCRs in the rooms—or a tape player, if that's your preference. You probably already have a set time during the day when you practice yoga. During your travels, maintain the same schedule if you can. Yoga is great for centering your life and controlling out-of-control emotions. Keep it up!

Hint: Check out Om Yoga in a Box, available through the Om Yoga Center, 212-229-0267, www.omyoga.com. For $29.95, you'll get 68 flash cards, a yoga belt, tea candle, sandalwood incense and holder, and two CDs with yoga instructions and music. The flash cards have photos, stick figure diagrams, and detailed descriptions of positions. Compact for packing in your luggage.

BOTTOM LINE: Lose 7 pounds

A yoga or relaxation tape will help keep your mind and emotions centered, no matter how stressful the trip is. If listening to, or watching, a tape keeps you from having that 300-calorie snack each night during your monthly week-long trips, it has more than justified the luggage space it took up.

#186. Heat Up the Day

Hotels usually have steam rooms and saunas. You're paying for the luxury, so use it. Relax and enjoy. You might even lose a few pounds.

It's the end of an event-filled day in a distant city. You're tense, tired, and probably lonely. Hotels anticipate these feelings, and they surround you with "comfort"—in the form of minibars, telephones with the room-service number prominently displayed, and televisions to suck you into sedentary nights.

My advice: Confront your feelings directly. Rather than using escape mechanisms—and food, let's face it, is one of the great escapes—do everything you can to shift your feelings into a healthier mode.

When you're tense or tired, the sauna or steam room can work wonders. Take off your clothes. Get into the water or steam, and let the moist heat envelop your body. Close your eyes. You'll probably feel the tension escaping. Ommm....

Steam rooms and saunas are great any time, but they're particularly appealing on trips when you're a long way from home. The more you relax, the less you'll eat. And because saunas are located in the exercise areas of hotels, you may find yourself tempted to get in a quick workout, as well.

BOTTOM LINE: Lose 7 pounds

At the very least, steam rooms and saunas will help keep nervous eating to a minimum. Besides, the less time you spend alone in your room, the less likely you'll be to raid the minibar or order up an "extra" snack. Saves 2,100 calories each month if you travel 7 days.

#187. Call Home

It's the end of a busy day. Your routine is a mess, and you're lonely. What could be better than calling home?

I understand the impulse to turn to food as a way of coping with negative emotions. We all do it. Food gives us comfort. It makes us feel special and pampered. It distracts us from feelings that aren't very comfortable.

The problem, of course, is that all of this emotional eating can make us fat. If you travel a lot, you really have to be careful not to fall into this trap.

When you find yourself feeling down, discouraged or tired, don't open the minibar. Pick up the phone. Place a call to a loved one. Talk to someone you haven't talked to in months. Even a short call will make you feel better and more connected—and when you're feeling good inside, "extra" food will naturally lose some of its appeal.

BOTTOM LINE: Lose 7 pounds

It's hard to believe that picking up the telephone will help you lose weight, but trust me, it works. Look at it this way. If you feel better after a long, warm telephone call, you'll be less likely to snack for comfort. Giving up that snack can save you 300 calories a night. If you travel often, you could potentially save 25,000 calories or more in a single year. Way to go, Ma Bell!

#188. Travel With Your hobby

A quiz: How can writing, sketching, needlepoint, or photography help you lose weight?

Boredom is among the main reasons that people gain weight when they travel. You're away from home. Time hangs heavy. You've already read *People* magazine or the same trashy novel three times. In the search for amusement, you search for food. And in America, you never have to search very long.

An easy and enjoyable way to fill the time is to bring your favorite hobby with you. By definition, hobbies are things that you enjoy doing. The hours will flash by when you're totally absorbed—and all the time that you spend engrossed with something pleasurable is time that you're not spending eating. Put another way, you'll forget all about the minibar. You'll be less likely to beg room service to empty the refrigerator and cart it up to your room. You'll stay in better shape because you won't be gaining weight.

Obviously, you won't want to bring all your equipment if you're an artist or photographer. But you can still pack the basics without consuming too much luggage space.

If you don't have a hobby, discover one. Think of activities you enjoyed as a child, even a language you'd like to learn. Research shows people who are absorbed in creative pastimes are healthier and happier.

BOTTOM LINE: Lose 7 pounds

Pursuing a hobby or favorite pastime when you're on the road almost guarantees that you'll have fewer snacks. My guess is that you can count on saving at least 300 calories a day and that's 25,000 calories a year for frequent travelers.

#189. Plan Your Dream House

My clients often blink when I mention this tip. "What do you mean, plan a house?" is the usual response. Wait, I'll explain.

"Comfort food" takes on new meanings when you're on the road. Forget it—food can be a false friend. Your goal should be to find comfort in healthier ways.

Before your next trip, jot down a "to do" list. Include some of the things that you've been wanting to do, but never got around to. Focus on fun things, like planning your dream house in the woods, writing a poem, learning to bowl, or whatever. Yes, I know there are more serious things in life, like painting the hen house. Forget it. You're supposed to be having fun, darn it!

Okay, so here you are in your hotel. Take out the list. Pick an item or two, and let your imagination run amok. Daydream, in other words.

My client Monroe fills the time in hotels by planning his next fun vacation. He packs some guidebooks, travel literature, and maps in his luggage—all related to his next travel conquest—and he digs in. Before he knows it, he's mentally transported to Bali, or the Galapagos Islands, or Majorca. He plans his trips in great detail, and guess what? He forgets all about room service!

BOTTOM LINE: Lose 7 pounds

Creative to-do lists can keep your mind occupied for hours—hours in which you're not carting 300-calorie snacks back to your room or hunting down a greasy spoon just because you're bored out of your mind.

#190. Take a Bubble Bath

Hotel bathrooms have all the comforts of home—
except they never feel very comfortable. No wonder
it's hard to relax.

The next time you're packing luggage for a vacation or business trip,
make a mental note to pack bubble bath, lotion, and candles. Believe me,
you'll be glad you did.

Business travel is inherently stressful, not to mention boring. It can be
a challenge to fill the time in ways that don't add inches to your waist.

In a pinch, a hot shower will help you relax. But it can't begin to compare with a lazy, dreamy soak in the bathtub, especially when you've had
the foresight to bring along your bubble bath, a candle or two, and maybe
some fancy lotion as an after-bath luxury.

No kids storming in. No telephone calls to break the spell. Work is
banished from your mind until tomorrow. You'll rarely have this sort of
opportunity at home, so make the most of it on your trip.

BOTTOM LINE: Lose 4–7 pounds

If relaxing in a bubble bath keeps you from having that 300-calorie
snack that you used to depend on to relax, you can count on saving
at least 25,000 calories in a year.

Okay, you may feel that this special experience needs to be celebrated with a glass of champagne. You'll still save 150 calories.
How many of life's pleasures can do that?

#191. Think Active Thoughts

Before your next trip, think about it a little differently. Visualize the active fun that you're going to have. Don't imagine huge meals.

Does this sound like a parlor game? It's not. It's a psychological technique called cognitive restructuring. It means changing the way you think about things, and it can be very effective when you're trying to change your habits and lose weight.

Before your trip, don't let your mind get wrapped up in culinary anticipation. For example, don't allow yourself to visualize French fries every day on the boardwalk. Block out images of juicy steaks, or margaritas in the pool. Instead, think about active things, such as long walks on the beach or hiking a rugged trail.

The purpose of this is to get into an active frame of mind. One of my clients, Cheryl, regularly vacations in Greece. Usually she comes back with 10 extra pounds. But before the last trip, she visualized an active vacation. Guess what? She and her husband walked everywhere. They ate fresh seafood every day. It was the best vacation they'd ever had—and Cheryl brought back not a single extra pound.

BOTTOM LINE: Lose 4 pounds

Being active on vacations means you'll burn calories rather than consuming them. And you'll be eating lighter meals to support all of those activities. You will probably shave at least 500 calories a day off what you'd normally have on 4 weeks' worth of vacation. The amazing power of mind control!

#192. Park the Car

For suburbanites, especially, it's hard to imagine doing anything without hopping in the car. Well, start imagining! For your next vacation, ditch the car in favor of foot and pedal power.

Driving everywhere is an automatic reflex, but most vacation destinations offer countless possibilities for walking, pedaling, or rowing. Indeed, this is a good time to install a bike holder on your automobile—and make the bike an integral part of your vacation plans.

Before embarking on your next trip, use the Internet to scout for walking and bicycle paths, hiking trails, or canoe and kayak rental shops. Another possibility is to take walking tours, either self-guided or as part of a group. You'll be surprised at the variety of tours that you'll find—everything from ghost and architecture tours to bird-walking and history.

Most tourist Web sites will include all the information that you need. When you reach your destination, talk to motel clerks, hotel concierges, or the hosts at bed-and-breakfasts. B&B hosts are usually very knowledgeable about such things. And find the local tourist office or chamber of commerce. The information is everywhere—you just have to look for it.

BOTTOM LINE: Lose 2 pounds

Once you have an active vacation and experience the fun, you'll want to do the same kinds of things at home. The truth is that even modest increases in daily activity—walking to the store, for example—can shave 250 calories a day. On vacation, that means 2 pounds lost, instead of gained!

#193. Be a Culture Vulture

Vacations don't have to be an "escape" from the entertainment and cultural pursuits that you enjoy at home. In fact, you'll have even more fun on the road because you'll discover what the "natives" have to offer.

What is it that interests you most at home? Live theater? Movies? Art shows and exhibits? Concerts? Modern dance? The pop music scene? Ethnic neighborhood festivals? Museums? All of the above? That's what vacations are made for—explore them all!

You can do much of your preparation before you leave on your trip just by checking Web sites for your destination. Many hotels and motels have displays of tourist brochures in the lobby. You can also check with the local tourist office.

Hint: Local newspapers often have a "weekend" or "calendar" section that lists all the goings-on. Or check out the free weekly alternative papers, which are available in most metropolitan areas. These often offer the most comprehensive coverage of the local scene.

Once you narrow your list of possible activities, your only challenge will be choosing among them!

BOTTOM LINE: Lose 3 pounds

An active, fun-filled schedule is a great way to avoid "boredom" eating, so give yourself points for saving 300 calories. Plus, you'll be on the go all day, which will burn plenty of additional calories, say 400. You'll lose 3 pounds instead of gaining it!

#194. Dance!

Want to make friends in new cities? Entertain yourself without spending hours in restaurants or bars? Get a heck of a workout without "exercising"? Dancing is the way to go.

No one thinks of dancing as exercise, but truth be told, an hour or two on the dance floor will burn more calories than a lot of traditional exercises. And it's a lot more fun.

What's your rhythm of choice? Ballroom? Vintage rock 'n roll? Latin? Folk dancing? Cajun and zydeco? Country? Caeli? Whatever type of dancing you like to do at home, there certainly are people at your vacation destination who like it too.

David, a friend of mine, is an avid contra dancer. He always checks the Internet to learn about the dancing scene in cities on his itinerary. In fact, he tries to schedule his business trips around the dances. It's a great way to make instant friendships in a new city.

Before your trip, do some research on the Web or talk to local instructors or dance devotees. Whatever your favorite form of dance, there are probably national organizations that can steer you toward groups or even dance-based bars in different cities.

BOTTOM LINE: Lose 3–6 pounds

A night on the dance floor can burn 500–1,200 calories, depending on the type of dancing you're doing. Add in 300 calories for that evening snack that you're too busy to eat, and you can see how you'll drop a lot of weight in a hurry. Do it every night for 2 weeks, wow, what a difference!

#195. Look for Home Grown

The freshest, tastiest fruits and vegetables are found at local farmers' markets. While you're sight-seeing, take advantage of these wonderful snacks.

You simply cannot beat locally grown produce for taste, beauty, aroma, and nutrition. If you're traveling by car, stop at roadside stands. Stretch your legs and stock up! I really like pick-your-own farms and orchards. Long drives go a lot faster when you have a basket of berries or a bag of fruit on the seat beside you. Plus, picking the produce gives you a chance to stretch your muscles and burn a few calories at the same time.

Nearly every city has at least one farmers' market: Check the "weekend" or "calendar" section in the local newspaper. Hotel clerks and tourist officials usually know what's happening locally. Or, before your trip, check out the Internet: The U.S. Department of Agriculture posts national listings for farmers' markets. The Web address is www.ams.usda.gov/farmersmarkets. Also check out www.farmland.org, which also lists farmers' markets.

Farmers' markets offer more than just great produce. Half the fun is walking around, looking at all the people, and getting a better feel for the city you're visiting. Think of it as a walking tour, with all the fresh food you can eat!

BOTTOM LINE: Lose 3 pounds

Grocery store produce isn't always as fresh or appetizing as it could be. The produce at farmers' markets, on the other hand, is irresistible! So on your 2-week vacation, why not substitute fresh fruit or vegetable snacks for those supersize muffins, bagels, or other 500-calorie snacks.

#196. The Amazing Cooler

When you're on a car trip, you're almost a slave to fast-food chains and convenience stores. Fight back! Keep a well-stocked cooler in the car at all times.

It's crazy not to travel with a cooler. You can pack it with snacks, sandwich fixings, and plenty of cool drinks. The food you bring from home or pick up at grocery stores will be a lot more appealing than the greasy stuff that passes for food on the interstates.

Apart from ice, here are some things to consider for your cooler:

• Bottles of spring water, preferably in container sizes that will fit into your car's beverage holders.
• Sandwich fixings, such as bread, mustard, mayo, pickles, lunch meats, and so on.
• Plenty of fresh fruit and vegetables. Use plastic containers for fruit chunks or vegetable pieces.
• Greens, radishes, peppers, and other salad fixings. Don't forget a "lite" or vinaigrette dressing.
• Utensils, a can opener, plastic containers, paper plates, and seasonings.

Every time you stop at a roadside park and have a picnic, you'll be so thankful that you brought along this gear!

BOTTOM LINE: Lose 5 pounds

On a typical road trip, you might stop for fast food at lunch and at convenience stores for morning and afternoon snacks. Without even factoring in dinner, you can plan on saving 600 calories every day for 4 weeks' worth of vacation.

#197. Rest-Stop Workouts

Highway fatigue can be deadly. That's reason enough to take frequent breaks. And since you've stopped the car anyway, why not hike around and burn a few calories?

Before you leave on your trip, make sure that everyone has comfortable hiking shoes, sun protection (hats and sunscreen), and bug spray. Good, thick socks are a must.

Now that you're equipped, break up the trip with some hikes. Even the busiest interstate will have rest stops, many of which are laced with hiking trails. If you're driving on back roads, you'll find plenty of opportunities for quick hikes.

Expect some wonderful opportunities: short treks to waterfalls or scenic views, for example. In cities, you'll often find former railroad paths that have been converted to hiking and biking trails. Or make your own "trail" by following roads lined with interesting buildings.

Ideally, you'll have one hike just before lunch and another in the evening before you stop for dinner and lodging. Hiking will torch an impressive amount of calories, and the exercise will tame your food cravings at the same time. You'll also avoid "driver's lethargy"—the crash in energy that occurs when you've spent too many hours in the car.

BOTTOM LINE: Lose 15 pounds

It's amazing what a quick hike will do for your energy and your weight. A one-mile hike, for example, only takes about 15 minutes and will burn 150 calories. Do it every day of the year, including your vacations.

#198. Drop Food Hints

Almost everyone gains weight when they spend their vacations visiting family or friends. Politeness demands that you eat—and compliment—the food that's put in front of you. But what do you do when their food choices aren't the same as yours? The solution: Give "invisible" hints.

It took years of visiting my grandparents and extended family in Sweden before I refined my strategy for giving polite hints about foods that I could and couldn't eat. I should have done it sooner because I always felt so uncomfortable and bloated upon my return home.

Time for the truth: These days, I usually return to the United States 2 pounds heavier than when I left. Hey, I'm not perfect! But I used to gain 5–10 pounds on those trips, and it's a lot easier to take off 2 pounds than 10.

My experience seems to be universal. When you're visiting family or close friends, they will show you how happy they are to see you by stuffing you as if you'd just escaped from a prison in Siberia. And their feelings are very, very, very fragile. "I'm on a diet" just doesn't cut it. Whether they say anything or not, what they're thinking is, "Well, if you're on a diet, Miss Goody Two-Shoes, you can afford to splurge this one time. And after all the trouble I went to!"

Nothing works 100 percent of the time, but my usual approach is this: I let it "slip" that what I've really been looking forward to are those traditional foods that I never get at home. What I don't mention is that the foods just happen to be healthier than the meatballs in gravy that I usually get.

Try this on for size: "When I come to Sweden, I love to experience seafood as much as possible. It's the best in the world!" Or, before a trip to Maine: "I've been so excited because now I can eat lobster every night!" You get the idea.

Don't be shy about stating your preferences in a positive way when asked. If someone asks what you'd like for breakfast, don't feel guilty and express a preference for that fattening cheese you got before. Say something like, "Oh, in the morning I really enjoy cereal with milk, and maybe a fruit to cut up in the bowl."

It's important to keep it positive. Give your relatives the benefit of the doubt. They really do want to make you happy, even though their efforts seem misguided at times. What they want to know is *how* to make you happy. So give tons of clues and positive reinforcement ("I love your salads more than anything else!") And you'll get what you want, eventually.

BOTTOM LINE: Lose 4 pounds

If you can manage to shave 300 calories off each meal (by the standards in my family, at least, that's a very conservative estimate), you'll have a much better chance of returning home from vacation at the same weight, or nearly so, as you were when you left.

#199. Compliment Lavishly

This is the flip side of the previous suggestion. Use positive reinforcement to let your hosts know subtly which foods you like (and which won't make you resemble a whale).

As I mentioned before, my way of politely steering my hosts toward the foods I prefer is to innocently let slip the fact that I've been looking forward to specific (read: healthier) items.

Every now and then, they actually listen, and I make sure that they feel well rewarded. You can do the same thing. Suppose you're in the middle of a fresh salad, or a vegetable dish that isn't swimming in butter. Single out the dish for some lip-smacking compliments: "Oh, I just love salads, especially the ones with shaved carrots."

If you really want to lay it on thick, add something like, "That was delicious! We can't get anything even close to this in Washington!"

Do this consistently, and pretty soon your friends and relatives will have a fair idea of the kinds of foods you like. Notice, you never uttered turn-off words such as "healthy," "diet," or (worst of all) "low fat." By the time you're gone, your Aunt Thelma will have made a mental note that you're the niece who loves vegetables so much.

BOTTOM LINE: Lose 4 pounds

If you can convince your family to serve a few healthful dishes at every meal, you can potentially save 300 calories. Multiply that by a few meals a day, and you can see the power of stealthy hints!

#200. Stretch!

No one thinks of stretching as a weight-loss tool, but I know from experience that it's hard to beat.

How does stretching help you lose weight? For starters, it gives muscles that have been stuffed in car or airline seats a chance to recover—and muscles that don't hurt are muscles that don't scream at the very idea of exercise. Stretching gives a quick surge of energy, which naturally leads to thoughts of exercise. It's also a great distraction when you're starting to think about snacks.

Here's a great stretch everyone can do:

• Stand with your feet shoulder width apart.
• Keep your heels flat, your toes pointed straight ahead.
• With your knees slightly bent, bend forward at the hips. Keep your arms and neck relaxed.

Hold the stretch for 10–20 seconds. Then return to an upright position, keeping your knees slightly bent.

BOTTOM LINE: Lose 2–3 pounds

If stretching gives you the energy you need to wake up early and exercise for just 15–30 minutes, you will burn about 135–270 calories each morning. If stretching in the evening takes away your appetite for a "little" snack, you'll save 300 calories more. Lose 2–3 pounds on vacation instead of maintaining!

CHAPTER 16

Restaurant Eating Without the Bulge

Especially appropriate for: *Social Butterflies, People Who Take Frequent Vacations, Business Executives, Busy Singles or Couples, Culinary Adventurers*

I love going out to restaurants. Apart from the fact that it gives me a respite from cooking (and doing dishes—ugh!), the whole ambiance is delightful. I enjoy the solicitude of the staff, watching the people, and simply taking a quiet hour or two to relax and enjoy good food.

For me, eating out is a special occasion. For millions of Americans, however, it's a way of life. I know more than a few people who eat out 5, 6, even 7 days a week. That's when restaurant food could start to present some problems.

Let's face it, one reason that the dishes we get in restaurants are so delicious is that they're swimming in richness. Chefs ladle butter on just about everything, and they choose their ingredients and cooking methods for their effects on the palate, not for their health properties or low-calorie contents. An occasional splurge won't do any lasting damage.

Indulging—or, to be frank, overindulging—on a regular basis will add some serious weight if you aren't careful.

If you eat out frequently, I recommend setting some priorities. Suppose, for example, you've booked 3 dinners out this week. You certainly won't lose weight if you eat with abandon each time. What you can do, however, is decide in advance that one of those nights is going to be your "splurge night." Order anything you want. Enjoy every bite. Savor each and every one of those special calories. On the other two nights, order more carefully. Get the seafood (preferably steamed or baked) rather than the 12-ounce steak. Go easy on the cocktails. Fill up on salad or non-creamy soup rather than extra appetizers or bread. You'll still enjoy the experience of dining out, but you won't take in more calories than your diet can handle.

Obviously, you can't control what goes on in restaurant kitchens. Dishes that you think are healthy might turn out to be real calorie bombs. The only way to maintain a measure of control is to order dishes with clearly identifiable ingredients, such as sandwiches, salads, grilled meats, fish, seafood, sushi, and so on. You know that everything you order is going to be higher in fat and calories than anything comparable that you'd make at home, but at least there won't be too many caloric surprises hiding in there.

Some diet plans forbid, or at least discourage, eating at restaurants. I can't agree. Eating out with friends is a wonderful experience. Being waited on is a joy. Professionally prepared food offers taste sensations that are hard to match. Despite all of the health benefits of homemade food, I would never advise someone to give up the pleasure of restaurants altogether.

What I do advise is eating (and ordering) smart. By all means, enjoy your meals away from home—but take a few simple steps to keep the calories under control.

Some restaurants today have Web sites that list calorie information. Or ask your waiter or manager if the information is available. The Center for Science in the Public Interest, a consumer group in Washington, D.C., has written a book, *Restaurant Confidential* (Workman Publishing, 2002) that you may find helpful. You can order it at their Web site: www.cspi.cc.

#201. Watch Out for Calorie Creep

Lunch is probably the best time to eat out. Prices are lower, portions are smaller, and you have hours ahead of you in which to burn off the excess calories.

If you have to choose between eating out at lunch and going out for dinner, definitely choose the lunch. You'll get fewer calories overall, and many lunch offerings—sandwiches, salads, and soups, for example—tend to be lighter than the usual dinner fare.

That said, lunch can easily turn into a caloric disaster. The main risk is from what I call "calorie creep." No matter how healthful the entree, all of the add-ons that come with it—croutons, creamy dressings, gobs of mayonnaise, French fries, or soft drinks—can change the whole equation. In fact, it's not uncommon for the calories in these little extras to exceed the calories in the main course.

Keep your orders simple. Get the sandwich, the soup, or the salad—but don't get all the extras. Drink water instead of soda. Pass on the appetizers. Ask the waiter to put the salad dressing on the side.

BOTTOM LINE: Lose 7–37 pounds

The typical burger-and-fries lunch has a whopping 1,100 to 1,600 calories. You'll do much better with a lean sandwich and a salad on the side—or a salad as the main course. My guess is that this will save you about 500 calories every time you eat lunch out if you make this switch. Do it once a week for a 26,000 calorie savings... or do it every work day.

#202. Drown Yourself

The human body is awash in water. Eliminate the water, and we'd all weigh about as much as Labrador retrievers.

Which is another way of saying that drinking water is integral to our health and well-being. It's also among the most powerful ways to control appetite and limit your daily intake of calories—that is, if the water is bubbly or incorporated into the food. A plain glass of water doesn't seem to do the trick.

Studies have clearly shown that eating high-water-content foods, like fruit, vegetables, soup, and bubbly water or diet soda with a meal can dramatically reduce the amount of calories you take in. When water is incorporated into the food, it empties from your stomach more slowly than a plain glass of water, making you feel more full with fewer calories. The water also increases the volume or weight of your food, which signals you that you're full, even though you're eating fewer calories. In addition, drinking sparkling water means that you're not drinking regular sodas or other high-calorie beverages such as alcohol.

Speaking of alcohol, how many times have you sat down at the table and quickly downed a cocktail or a glass of wine? You may appreciate the alcohol, but undoubtedly you were also taking care of your thirst. Studies demonstrate that drinking sparkling water or diet soda the minute you sit down, and keeping it flowing, or ordering a salad or soup, will help you eat 100 calories fewer at the main meal, and will make it easier to drink less alcohol, or none at all.

BOTTOM LINE: Lose 4–21 pounds

A glass of wine has 100 calories. If drinking water allows you to drink two fewer glass of wine over dinner, you'll save 200 calories right there. Drink water instead of a cocktail, and you'll save 150 calories. Add soup or a vegetable or fruit to lunch or dinner and save 100–200 calories. It adds up fast!

203. Eat Simple Breakfasts

If you order "traditional" breakfasts at restaurants, you'll get so much fat and calories that you'll blow your diet for the entire day.

Bacon and eggs. A sky-high stack of pancakes. Belgian waffles drenched in butter and syrup. Is your mouth watering? Mine too! I would love to start the day with an over-the-top American breakfast, but I know too well what the consequences will be.

Of all the calories in all the meals in your day, breakfast calories are probably the easiest to control. Every restaurant, from the humblest greasy spoon to the most expensive hotel dining room, offers an abundance of healthy choices.

Whole-grain hot or cold cereals, for example, are loaded with fiber. Apart from improving digestion and protecting the circulatory system, fiber is Nature's appetite suppressant. Eat a high-fiber cereal, and you'll naturally eat less later on.

Other healthful breakfast offerings include bagels, fresh fruits, and whole-grain toast. Add a glass of orange juice or skim milk, and you'll get all of the calories that you need for energy, without the excess calories that you're trying to avoid.

BOTTOM LINE: Lose 6–30 pounds

A hearty breakfast of cold cereal, 2 percent milk, fruit, and juice only provides about 500 calories—about 400 calories fewer than the Belgian waffle. Make this one change 5 mornings a week, and you'll lose about 30 pounds a year. Good morning!

#204. Fish for Health

After all of this talk about the dietary dangers of meals out, I think it's worth mentioning one standard entree, seafood, that always pays off.

A few decades ago, seafood was something of a rarity on American menus. Even when fish was offered, it invariably was fried or battered beyond recognition.

Thank goodness things have changed. Today, you'll find seafood of all types—salmon, tuna, mussels, shrimp, swordfish, you name it—on just about every menu. Please, order it!

Seafood starts out so lean and low in calories that even when the dish is drenched in butter, as it probably will be, the result won't bust your buttons. You'll certainly get fewer calories than you would if you ordered a meat dish. Plus, seafood contains important fats called omega-3s, which have been shown to lower cholesterol and reduce the risk for heart disease and other diseases.

If you're really being conscientious, order seafood that's grilled, broiled, or poached. It will have a lot fewer calories—and less saturated fat—than its fried counterparts.

BOTTOM LINE: Lose 22 pounds

A comparison: A 16-ounce cut of prime rib has 1,300 calories. The baked potato and sour cream that come with it add 330 calories. Oh, and the Caesar salad packs 310 calories. If you order grilled or broiled seafood and a side of vegetables instead, you'll save about 1,500 calories—and that's just in one Saturday night!

#205. Read the Fine Print

So many people have shifted toward healthier meals that restaurants have tried to make things easy by highlighting menu selections that are lower in calories.

Take advantage of them. It's an excellent way to keep an eye on your calories without having to do the math yourself.

Many restaurants work with major health organizations, such as the American Heart Association, to create meals that are much lower in fat, calories, and sodium than the usual offerings. You might see a little heart symbol on the menu, or the words "light" or "healthy."

In some cases, dishes with these symbols must meet certain dietary requirements; other times, they're more subjective. Don't abandon your common sense. A broiled chicken dish with the "light" symbol is probably a good choice, but the rules go out the window if the chef drenches it with a cheese sauce. It's difficult to enforce the accuracy of what the restaurant advertises.

If you're serious about watching your weight, don't be embarrassed about asking the waiter to explain what, exactly, is in a dish. It's your food. You're paying for it. You have a right to know what's in it.

BOTTOM LINE: Lose 4–10 pounds

You can assume that "light" entrees—grilled chicken with a salad, for example—will have at least 250 fewer calories than many traditional meat dishes. If you eat out frequently, making this one change could help you lose 10 pounds in a year.

#206. Words Count

Unless you graduated from cooking school, a lot of menu terms are probably a little mysterious. (Just what is "fricassee," anyway?) Get to know the main ones if you're serious about losing weight.

People who count calories tend to spend a lot of time thinking about ingredients. They know that beef is fattier than fish. That butter packs more of a health wallop than olive oil. That chicken breast is probably a better choice than a pork chop. I can't argue with this approach, but it only tells part of the story.

Cooking techniques have just as much (or, in some cases, more) influence on the final calorie content of a dish than the ingredients themselves. Menus don't always provide clues about how dishes are prepared, but usually they do. When you see the words "fried," "sautéed," or "stir-fried," you can be sure that the dish is high in fat and calories. "Crispy" is another danger sign.

Now, here are some "good" words: "grilled," "poached," and "steamed." What makes these cooking methods better? They require little or no added fat, which means you'll get a lot fewer calories.

BOTTOM LINE: Lose 8–40 pounds

Steamed lobster, rice pilaf, and a vegetable will have about 550 fewer calories than a *fried* seafood combo. Multiply this savings by one meal a week, and you'll lose at least 8 pounds; multiply it by 5 weekly meals, and you could lose as much as 40 pounds in a year!

#207. Naked Salad

Time for a science class: A single gram of fat contains 9 calories. Fill a tablespoon with fat, and you wind up getting about 120 calories. Oh, did I mention that salad dressings are little more than disguised fat?

Salads are among the healthiest foods you can eat—but oh, the dressings! A creamy blue cheese or Thousand Island dressing almost overflows with saturated fat and calories. Even vinaigrettes are about two-thirds oil (the other third is vinegar), so the calories can add up.

I often get a sinking feeling when my clients describe the "healthy" salads they eat every day—drenched, in many cases, with these or other high-fat dressings. Think about the last salad you ordered in a restaurant. I'll bet that there was a little pool of dressing floating around at the bottom of the bowl. That's because restaurants normally add way too much dressing in order to get the desired taste.

Keep ordering salads, by all means. But ask for the dressing on the side. Dip your fork in the dressing. Take a bite of salad. Dip your fork again, and on and on, or use just 1–2 tablespoonsful directly on your salad. Believe me, if you do nothing else but limit the amount of dressing on your salad, you'll lose weight without even trying.

BOTTOM LINE: Lose 2–16 pounds

Let's put this dressing issue in perspective. Suppose you order a chicken Caesar salad. If you get the dressing on the side and only use about two tablespoons, you'll get at least 150 fewer calories than if you'd ordered the salad "dressed." Make the switch once a week and lose 2 pounds; every day takes off 16.

#208. Eat Plenty of Filet

I admit, "plenty" is a relative term. I'm not suggesting that you order a grilled steak every night. But choosing filet mignon over other, fattier cuts will save you a heck of a lot of calories.

The diet police would have you believe that all beef is inherently evil, but that's simply not true. There's a remarkable variation in the amount of fat in different cuts of beef. Some cuts, it's true, contain more fat than you even want to imagine. But others are nearly as lean as chicken or pork.

The next time you eat out, pay attention to the different cuts on the menu. The ones with the most fat and calories are prime rib, New York strip, and porterhouse. Sirloin, on the other hand, is respectably lean. Filet mignon, the prize jewel at restaurants, is also lean.

This doesn't mean, of course, that every filet you see on menus is low in fat. It really depends on how the meat is served. Sauces will add tremendous amounts of calories to even the leanest cut. If you can, order your meat sans sauce.

BOTTOM LINE: Lose 7–70 pounds

If you order a filet mignon instead of a 12-ounce prime rib, you will save 480 calories. For those real carnivores who eat out a lot and order meat at lunch as well as dinner, those "saved" calories could help you lose 70 pounds in a year!

#209. The Power of Doggie Bags

Restaurants are well aware of the gargantuan American appetite. Most meals that you get away from home will contain enough food—and calories—for two meals. So take some home.

Have you noticed that restaurants no longer use normal-size plates? The darned things are the size of platters. Given the sheer volume of the amount of food served in restaurants today, anything smaller just doesn't work.

There's no evidence, of course, that today's humans require platter-sized portions. It's just that restaurants have gotten in the habit of serving two or three times the normal portion sizes.

Don't even try to eat it all. It's an accepted practice for diners to ask for a "doggie bag" for the leftovers. Take the extras home. Eat them for lunch the next day. Heck, you might even have enough for dinner. While you're at it, mentally thank the restaurant for its largess: You've just been served 2 (or 3) meals for the price of one!

BOTTOM LINE: Lose 6–49 pounds

Suppose that your chicken fajita has 840 calories. Eat half, and your meal will supply a respectably low 420 calories. The same principle works for that delicious shrimp in garlic sauce. Eating half and saving the rest will save you 475 calories at that one meal. Do this every time you eat out, and you'll give up a tremendous number of calories in a year. And think of all the time you'll save by not having to cook the next day. Thanks, restaurants!

#210. Break the Rules

There isn't a law that says you have to order an entree every time you eat out. Don't take my word for it— look it up!

I'm being a little silly here, but most of the people I know are under the impression that eating out requires ordering selections from the appetizer, entree, and dessert sections of the menu.

Okay, if you're ordering from a fixed-price menu, your liberties may be abridged somewhat. But most of the time, you really do have freedom of choice. The next time you go out to eat, ask yourself this: "Am I really so hungry that I need to order every course? For that matter, do I really want the entree?"

Listen to your appetite. Maybe your hunger will be amply satisfied if you only get a dinner salad. Or soup and bread. Or even an appetizer alone—today's appetizers are often fairly large. Don't feel coerced into ordering more than you want. You're the customer, which means that you're calling the shots. Let anarchy reign!

BOTTOM LINE: Lose 4–20 pounds

When I eat out, I might get a side order of steamed shrimp, accompanied by a salad on the side. This order will supply about 250 fewer calories than the entree with all the fixings. Even if you only eat out once a week, that could add up to 4 lost pounds a year!

#211. Have a "Premeal"

Do you ever find yourself dreaming about a special dinner—one that's so fancy that you'd gladly starve yourself before going? Look out! Your dream is about to turn into a nightmare.

I understand the temptation to eat less during the day to make room for a big meal out. It sounds reasonable, in a way. After all, if you're going to be taking in a lot of calories at night, why not cut back the calories you consume during the day?

Alas, it doesn't work. If you don't get enough calories during the day, your appetite will expand to impressive proportions. By the time you finally get to the restaurant, you'll probably order more appetizers, more drinks, and a bigger entree. Even the breadsticks won't be safe. The calories at dinner will more than offset the calories you "saved" at home.

Another problem is that you get the lion's share of your daily calories at night—and calories consumed late are more likely to be stored as fat than burned as energy. (Tossing and turning in bed doesn't count as exercise.)

My advice: Eat normally during the day. Maybe even have a snack before going out to dinner.

BOTTOM LINE: Lose 15–75 pounds

Arriving at a restaurant in a ravenous state almost guarantees you'll order an appetizer. That fried calamari packs about 1,000 calories. Eat normally during the day and skip the appetizer, and you'll automatically lose an impressive amount of weight over time.

#212. Irritate the Waiter

Just joking. You never want to annoy the person who's serving you dinner. But I do suggest shaking up the usual order of things by not ordering an entree right away.

Think about all of your restaurant experiences for a moment. How many times have you been almost full by the time the entree arrived? Even if you didn't fill up on free bread and butter, the combination of appetizers and a salad may have been enough to take the edge off your appetite, or even quell it entirely.

For those who order their entrees in the usual order, there's always the doggie bag option if food is left over. But you can avoid this situation altogether by finishing the salad or soup *before* ordering the entree. You may find that by the time you're finished with the preliminary courses, you really don't need anything else. Or that a smaller entree will work just fine.

Sure, everyone else at the table will be following the script, but dare to be different. The waiter may resist, but insist. After all, there's very little extra work involved, and, after all, you're the customer. Tip appropriately.

BOTTOM LINE: Lose 6–42 pounds

Look at it this way: If starting with a salad or appetizer takes the edge off your appetite, you might wind up ordering a modest chicken dish instead of the calorically dangerous lasagna. Count on saving at least 400 calories for the evening.

#213. Start with Salad

I avoid buffets. They simply offer too many opportunities for overindulging. But once you're standing in line, about all you can do is damage control.

Start with a salad. Carry it back to the table. Eat it slowly, and eat it all. (You did remember to get your dressing on the side, I hope!) Now, check out your appetite. You're probably still hungry, but since the salad took the edge off, you'll be able to reapproach the buffet in a rational frame of mind.

This might seem like a gimmick, but it's not. Studies have shown that when people are served (or serve themselves) more food, they eat more food. This is probably a holdover instinct from our days as cave dwellers, when food was hard to come by.

Eating the salad first gives you time to determine realistically how hungry you really are. The great thing about buffets is that you can customize your serving sizes and the variety of foods you take to accommodate your actual (not imagined) hunger.

I'm certainly not suggesting that you go hungry. But do yourself a favor and take only the food that you really need, not the amount that's required to fill one, two, or three plates.

BOTTOM LINE: Lose 10–20 pounds

The salad-first approach will easily save you 100 calories in a single meal. If you indulge in buffets often, you can count on losing at least 10 pounds—and probably a lot more—a year!

#214. Do a Hunger Check

Research has shown that when people are in groups they tend to eat more than when they're dining alone.

The reason? They're having such a good time that they're not paying attention to their natural hunger signals. And restaurants, let's face it, want you to have a good time. The more you eat and drink, the larger your bill—and the more likely you'll be to come back another time.

Eating out is supposed to be a festive occasion, of course. I would hardly suggest putting on a dour face and merely poking at the breadsticks. But you do want to focus your attention on how you feel as you eat. Are you eating because you really need the food, or are you just doing it mindlessly as part of the occasion?

Hint: Eat much more slowly than you usually do. We're often so rushed that we stuff ourselves silly long before the brain and stomach have a chance to say "enough." That's why people are more likely to feel uncomfortably full after leaving a restaurant than when they eat at home.

BOTTOM LINE: Lose 3–49 pounds

I've found that people who pay attention to their hunger signals will often quit eating when they've finished about two-thirds of their restaurant meals. This alone could save you 250–500 calories in a single meal.

CHAPTER 17

Mix and Match to Lose
Whatever You Want

In this chapter, I've arranged all of the strategies in *Think Yourself Thin* by pounds you can lose. It's designed so you can mix and match your own tips. The beauty of *Think Yourself Thin* is that it's painless. Start by analyzing your normal eating routine, and look over the strategies outlined in the previous 214 tips. Look for changes that are simple enough for you to live with. Your personality and preferences should dictate what you decide, not some stringent diet police dictating your plan.

Then, start perusing the "Lose 2 to 5 Pounds" category, which follows. Are there a few painless techniques you can try that would be a snap to do? How about "doing a hunger check" or "choosing surf over turf?" Next, peruse the "Lose 6 to 10 Pounds" strategies. Would it be simpler for you to "eat before you party," or "mine-sweep for calorie bombs?"

I tell everyone—those who are very overweight as well as those who simply want to drop a few pounds—that it makes more sense to set modest initial goals, and to achieve those goals by tinkering with, rather than completely overhauling, their diets and lifestyles. Drastic diets can certainly result in impressive weight loss, but they're not healthy, and no one sticks with them very long. I'd rather see people set reasonable goals and achieve them than shoot for the moon and fail completely.

Losing 10 pounds in 2 months is a great first goal. For some people, that's all they'll need to lose in order to feel better—and to fit into some of those clothes that are hanging in the back of the closet! For those who need to lose more, setting an initial 10-pound goal makes the entire process less daunting. I've seen the excitement build as the pounds come off a little bit each week. People start getting giddy as they approach the 10-pound mark—and by the time they reach it, they're almost always eager to keep going.

Nearly everyone can lose a pound a week. Losing a total of 10 pounds in 2 months, for instance, is easier than most people imagine.

Now take a look at the higher weight loss categories, where the strategies may be slightly more challenging. In the "Lose 16 to 20 Pounds" category, are you ready to "buy better dairy," "eat more to eat less," or "turn on your VCR"? Only you can decide what you're ready for.

In all, choose several tips from each category. Find the ones that fit your lifestyle, that you would actually enjoy doing. Mix and match to decide how much you want to lose. Be creative. Make sure the tips fit your personality. And have fun.

Lose 2 to 5 pounds

TIP#	TIP	LBS
#6	Baked not fried	3
#12	Hold the tuna salad	3–6
#14	Choose "surf"	4–18
#17	Add the whipped cream	3–16
#27	Eat more pizza	3–6
#33	Reduce noise pollution	5
#62	Fitness gifts: Easy exercise equipment	4–5
#69	Play fried-chicken charade	4–28
#81	Surround yourself with color	5
#84	Nose around	5
#85	Prevent bloat	4
#108	Say "no" to something bad	5–15
#109	Say "yes" to something good	5–15
#154	Score the best real estate	4
#168	Have a flying picnic	3
#174	Be a "shopping tourist"	5
#175	The briefcase surprise	5
#176	The "first lady" technique	4–6
#190	Take a bubble bath	4–7
#191	Think active thoughts	4
#192	Park the car	2
#193	Be a culture vulture	3
#194	Dance!	3–6
#195	Look for home grown	3
#196	The amazing cooler	5
#198	Drop food hints	4
#199	Compliment lavishly	4
#200	Stretch!	2–3
#202	Drown yourself	4–21
#205	Read the fine print	4–10
#207	Naked salad	2–16
#210	Break the rules	4–20
#214	Do a hunger check	3–49

Lose 6 to 10 pounds

TIP#	TIP	LBS
#1	The sundae solution	9–35
#2	Set your alarm	6–14
#4	Do the bed stretch	7
#8	"Pedal" while you prattle	10–42
#11	Eat more slowly	10
#13	Say "no" to pushers	7
#16	Eat, then shop	9
#20	Minesweep for calorie bombs	10–29
#21	Beware the burger blast	6–16
#25	Cook with spray	10–31
#30	Lose with tailoring	9
#32	Join Martha Stewart	9
#45	Walk somewhere . . . anywhere	6–14
#47	Make exercise dates	9
#58	Shed the car, shed some pounds	10
#60	Serve soup as an appetizer	10–20
#61	Sneak veggies into dinners	10–20
#64	It takes two to tango	7
#66	Dads are people, too	7
#71	Ignore those leftovers	10
#72	Enjoy the fresh air	10–40
#75	Shed pounds while killing time	10
#77	Get creative with other moms	10
#82	Call your girlfriends	9
#83	Stroll while you shop	10
#86	Mom's sporting afternoons	9
#91	Dream	10
#100	Kiss your spouse	7
#118	Hamburgers without end	6–18
#120	The secret is plastics	10–40
#122	Slash corporate calories	6–18
#128	Wean your child off sugary cereals	10
#130	Fill the fridge with fun finger foods	10
#131	Frozen fruit fun	10

Lose 6 to 10 pounds (CON'T)

#132	Make veggie and fruit kebabs	10
#133	Replace fried with oven-fried	10
#137	Create family TV guidelines	10–30
#138	Care for a pet	10–20
#139	Turn little diners into chefs	10
#140	Taste-test new veggies with young children	10–20
#141	Grow your own veggies	10–20
#142	Visit a farm, year-round	10
#143	Make mealtime family time	10
#144	Make breakfast a family habit	10
#145	Pack a healthy lunchbox	10
#146	Teach mindful eating habits	10
#147	Show and tell for hunger signals	10
#150	The 25 percent blowout	9
#152	Eat before you party	7
#153	The 30-second rule	7
#156	Imagine every move	6
#157	Give away leftovers	7
#159	Think exercise	6–14
#160	Serve…pause…serve	7–14
#161	Bring out the produce	10–21
#162	Be a lousy host	7–15
#165	Start a trend	6–7
#166	Shift your appetite clock	9
#167	Win with first class	7
#169	Terminal snacks	7
#170	Steal a gym	9
#171	Luggage calisthenics	9
#177	Join the snack committee	9–17
#181	Make faces	6
#182	Lose the minibar key	8
#183	Get elastic	6
#184	Bring your exercise instructor	10
#185	Portable yogis	7
#186	Heat up the day	7

	Lose 6 to 10 pounds (CON'T)	
#187	Call home	7
#188	Travel with your hobby	7
#189	Plan your dream house	7
#201	Watch out for calorie creep	7–37
#203	Eat simple breakfasts	6–30
#206	Words count	8–40
#208	Eat plenty of filet	7–70
#209	The power of doggie bags	6–49
#212	Irritate the waiter	6–42
#213	Start with salad	10–20

	Lose 11 to 15 pounds	
TIP#	TIP	LBS
#10	Substitute oil for butter	12
#18	Take up yoga	13
#19	Less creamy, more oily	13
#22	Take center stage	12
#39	Say "hi" to your feet	11–22
#40	Win with gadgets	12–52
#54	Stealthy, healthy superbowl party	15
#56	The cookout or tailgate party	15
#59	Recreational day trips/spa weekends	15
#63	Subscribe to fitness or health magazines	15–20
#73	Take up photography or film	13
#78	Make mom exercise dates	15
#96	Don't go home	15–30
#101	Breathe, bathe, relax	15
#119	Eat your office supplies	11–60
#129	Wean your child off sodas	15
#164	The chocolate cardiac challenge	15
#172	Pretend you're still home	14
#173	Harass the hotel	14
#197	Rest-stop workouts	15
#211	Have a "premeal"	15–75

Lose 16 to 20 pounds

TIP#	TIP	LBS
#5	Pour another glass	17–22
#7	Think positive thoughts	20–30
#9	Eat more salads	20
#15	Tighten a muscle	19
#23	The dilution solution	18
#26	The "whole" story	21
#31	Splurge on expensive delicacies	20
#38	Buy better dairy	16
#41	Breathe deeply	17
#42	More snacking, fewer calories	19–26
#43	Turn on your VCR	16–66
#48	A breakfast bar is not enough!	20
#70	Stop the portion distortion	20
#74	Find a quiet place	20
#76	Cook with the kids	20
#88	Eat by the clock	20–80
#93	Get sexy lingerie	18
#110	Shop by the book	20–80
#112	The joy of index cards	20–80
#116	Save time with frozen produce	20–50
#117	Eat more to eat less	20–50
#121	Shop online	20–80
#124	Learn to count	20–80
#125	Take breakfast shortcuts	21
#126	Defrost the freezer	18–51
#127	Do some fine dining	20–30
#135	Play games!	20
#136	Encourage recreational physical activities	20–40
#158	Prioritize	16

Lose 21 to 25 pounds

TIP#	TIP	LBS
#24	Muffin madness	21–52
#35	The amazing sandwich	21
#37	Lead a snake dance	24
#44	Listen when you chew	21
#46	Write it and lose it	23
#50	Send him off with his favorite lunch	22–50
#79	Start a yoga or meditation club	25
#94	Listen to the Eagles	21
#97	Eat early	22–30
#102	Love your pet	22
#103	Light a candle	21
#113	Coffee ain't enough	22–30
#114	Eat breakfast at work	22–30
#123	Eat all-American	22–30
#155	Savor each bite	21
#163	Lighten up	21
#204	Fish for health	22

Lose 26 to 30 pounds

TIP#	TIP	LBS
#29	Steal a TV	27
#36	Hit the ground running	28–42
#49	Send him to work with terrific snacks	30
#51	Healthy, light dinners	30
#52	Fill your home with healthy snacks and desserts	30
#53	Negotiate ground rules for eating	30
#55	Teach him to cook	30
#58	Shed the car, shed some pounds	30
#67	Change family rewards	30
#68	Do the healthy snack switch	30–50
#80	You're getting sleepy…	30–50
#87	Fight the beast	30
#89	Confront your feelings	26
#92	Do some calorie shifting	30
#95	Late snack	30
#99	Sing in the shower	26–31
#104	Get moving fast	30–54
#106	Eat a brownie every Friday	30
#115	Cook more than you can eat	30–42
#134	Cut back on TV time with crafts	30

Lose 31 to 35 pounds

TIP#	TIP	LBS
#90	Let yourself live	31-46
#98	Satisfy your sweet tooth	34
#105	Examine your goals	31
#107	Learn from mistakes	31
#148	"Happy hour" at home	33
#149	Start a social club	33
#151	Only eat the best	31
#178	The happy-hour trap	31
#179	Better than beer nuts	31
#180	Work out, then eat out	35

Lose 36-plus pounds

TIP#	TIP	LBS
#3	Walk the dog	46–88
#28	Shop at the farmers' market	36
#34	March for a cause	60
#57	Stretch out with yoga	50
#65	Teach him "plate geography"	40
#111	Don't cook on weekdays	36

PART III

Fast and Delicious
Batch Recipes
from the Best Chefs

In today's fast-paced world, many people end up grabbing whatever food is available. And in our society, that isn't good. It probably means whatever you're grabbing is higher in calories and other unsavory ingredients than you would prefer or even suspect.

Maybe you get take-out or don't think much about your food choices because you want to save time. In our superfrenzied society, time is the most precious commodity. We never seem to have enough of it. That's why it is so tempting to cut corners and pick up something to eat at a drive-up window on the way home.

Of course, there's an easier and more pleasant way to live. My advice is to make the most of the time you spend in the kitchen. To take stress out of your life (and high calories out of your diet!), get in the habit of

preparing these delicious and simple batch meals ahead of time, preferably on weekends, when you're not as rushed and tired as you are during
the week.

This concept is so important that I've included this section of recipes
of batch cooking in *Think Yourself Thin.*

My clients are sometimes confused about the whole concept of "batch
cooking." The idea is to prepare quick and easy dinners ahead of time so
that you always have something in the freezer or refrigerator that's ready
to go on a moment's notice.

Let's say I'm going to make "Veal Stew with Carrots La Boutarde" and
"Chile Non Carne" as my main-course "batch" meals for the week. I'll
make "Vegetable Soup" as my batch side dish. Once I make the batches,
I'll divide them into serving sizes and keep them in air-tight containers in
the refrigerator. It's important that I have enough servings for the whole
family's dinners for the week—and even some lunches.

In the end, it doesn't take more time than ordering take-out. It actually saves time (and money)—especially when you consider the time
wasted feeling starved during the day, and stuffed and miserable every
evening, and all the negative economic, weight, and health consequences
that go along with that.

This is one of the reasons I'm such an advocate of gourmet batch
cooking. You get to save time, but eat wonderfully, and much better than
you can get in most restaurants, in my humble opinion. You simply prepare two or three "batches" on the weekend, store them in serving-size
containers, and use them throughout the week. Just imagine the frenzy of
your office mates or the anticipation of your family when they smell the
wonderful aromas emanating from the microwave as you heat up...let's
say...White Beans with Garlic and Basil? Savory Pot Roast? Baked Shells
with Ricotta and Eggplant? How about Crab Cakes for dinner? They're
all home-made, and all you need is a few minutes to reheat your meal!

Studies show you (and your family) are more likely to eat whatever is
in your environment. I have found that to be true for myself and my
clients. If you surround yourself with delicious, healthy, wholesome foods,
that's what you and your family will end up eating. It's simple physics. We
naturally take the path of least resistance. So why not make things easy on
yourself? Stack things up in your favor by planning a few batch meals to

make on the weekend so you and your family will have wonderful food at your fingertips all week long. Einstein said genius was 1 percent inspiration and 99 percent perspiration. I've always liked to say losing weight is 99 percent planning and maybe 1 percent inspiration!

Having food that's ready to go is one of the most important steps you can make toward successful weight loss, and it's one of the most important tips in *Think Yourself Thin*. Gourmet batch cooking can save you hundreds of calories each and every night because you'll be less likely to order high-calorie take-out when you've got delicious and tempting meals in your fridge, ready to go. That can add up to plenty of lost pounds. As I mentioned earlier, a take-out meal will easily set you back 1,000 calories, usually more. A meal cooked at home, including those delicious leftovers, has the perfect amount of calories for you, depending on your needs, maybe about 600 to 700 calories. That amounts to a savings of 300 to 400 calories per dinner and a potential loss of 30 to 40 pounds in a year!

No matter how many pounds you're looking to lose, or what tips you choose to get you there, batch cooking is an integral part of *Think Yourself Thin*. Make these recipes on the weekend, and you have great dinners ready to go on Tuesday, Thursday, and Saturday nights. Just knowing that you have delicious meals ready to go in minutes will keep you away from high-calorie, disorganized eating. Plus, batch cooking saves you time and money and nurtures your spirit all at once.

I recommend the following main-course, hearty stew and soup recipes because they're delicious and satisfying. You won't go hungry. They're perfect for the chilly seasons, when most people's tastebuds sway toward the hearty. And the Main Dish Salads are perfect calorie reducers for warmer months. Try a few of them; try them all! The flavors will bring you culinary ecstasy!

MAIN DISH STEWS

The French Culinary Institute's Veal Stew with Carrots, La Boutarde

This veal stew is the perfect meal for a brisk fall or winter day. The aromas will fill your home with warmth and comfort. This is also a very simple recipe. The preparation is fast, but I add an hour to the cooking time because I double the vegetables and the herbes de Provence. I also use wine only (no water). The beauty of this recipe is that the measurements are not precise. You can cook to your own taste.

The veal rump can be found at a butcher's or a specialty market, if you can't find it at your grocery store. A substitute would be veal shoulder, which is typically used for stews, but is not as lean as the rump. If you're on a budget, beef round is an excellent—and very lean—substitute.

4 servings

Ingredients

1 tablespoon olive oil

2 pounds veal rump, well trimmed and cut into 2-inch cubes and seasoned with salt and freshly ground white pepper

2 medium carrots, cut into ½-inch slices

1 medium onion, chopped

1½ cups dry white wine

1 cup water

2 medium very ripe tomatoes, peeled, cored, seeded, and chopped

2 teaspoons herbes de Provence*

1 bay leaf

3 small all-purpose potatoes, peeled and quartered

Directions

Warm the oil in a large sauté pan over medium-high heat. When hot, add no more than half the veal and sear for 3 minutes, or until the veal has evenly browned on all sides. Do not crowd the pan or scorch the meat. Using a slotted spoon, transfer the veal to a Dutch oven. Continue searing the veal until all of the meat has been browned. Season with salt and pepper.

In the same pan over medium heat, sauté the carrots and onions for 3 minutes, or until the onions are translucent. Reduce the heat and stir in the wine. Using a wooden spoon, stir vigorously to lift the browned bits from the bottom of the pan.

Pour into the Dutch oven. Add the water, tomatoes, herbes de Provence, and bay leaf.

Place the Dutch oven over medium heat and bring the stew to a boil. Reduce the heat to medium-low, cover, and simmer for one hour.

Add the potatoes and simmer for 35 minutes, or until the potatoes are tender.

Taste and adjust the seasoning. Remove and discard the bay leaf.

Chef's Note: Herbes de Provence is a mixture of dried herbs that often includes basil, lavender, rosemary, sage, thyme, and others. Look for it in the spice section of your supermarket.

Per Serving

calories	437	total fat	12g
saturated fat	4g	total carbohydrate	22g
dietary fiber	4g	protein	60g

"Veal Stew with Carrots, La Boutarde" originally appeared in *The French Culinary Institute's Salute to Healthy Cooking*, by Alain Sailhac, Jacques Pépin, André Soltner, Jacques Torres, and the Faculty of the French Culinary Institute.

©1998 The French Culinary Institute.

Graham Kerr's Turkey Pot Pie

This is a lighter take on the traditional American comfort food. The dish is basically a flavorful turkey stew in a creamy sauce topped with savory cheese biscuits. It's delicious with all of its flavors and textures, the strong, crunchy turnips balanced by the sweet parsnips. This saves beautifully in the refrigerator for lunches at the office or midweek dinners.

4 servings

Ingredients
1 teaspoon nonaromatic olive oil
½ sweet onion, cut in ¼-inch pieces and diced (1 cup)
2 turnips, peeled and cut in ½-inch pieces
2 small parsnips, peeled and cut in ½-inch pieces (½ cup)
1½ cups homemade turkey or low-sodium chicken stock
¼ teaspoon salt
⅛ teaspoon pepper
1 pound broccoli
2½ cups cooked turkey

Sauce:
¾ pound parsnips, peeled, roughly chopped, and steamed until tender
1 cup evaporated skim milk
¼ teaspoon salt

Cheese Biscuits (adapted from *Eating Well: Secrets of Low-Fat Cooking*)**:**
1 cup all-purpose flour
1 cup cake flour
1 tablespoon sugar
1½ teaspoons baking powder
½ teaspoon baking soda
¼ teaspoon salt
1½ teaspoons cold, hard, butter-flavored margarine, cut into small pieces
¾ cup buttermilk
1 tablespoon nonaromatic olive oil
¼ cup grated low-fat sharp cheddar cheese
1 tablespoon low-fat milk to brush on top

Directions

Heat the oil in a chef's pan or skillet on medium high, sauté the onions, turnips, and parsnips on medium heat 3 minutes. Pour in the stock and season with salt and pepper. Bring to a boil, reduce the heat, cover and simmer until the vegetables are tender, 6 minutes. Whiz the steamed parsnips in a blender with the salt and a little of the evaporated milk until smooth and velvety, another 30 seconds.

Biscuits:
Preheat the oven to 425 degrees. Coat a baking sheet with oil spray. Whisk together the flours, sugar, baking powder, soda, and salt in a bowl or combine in a processor.

Scatter the pieces of margarine over the top and cut in with 2 knives or pulse 2–3 times in a processor. Make a well in the center of the dry ingredients and pour in the buttermilk and oil. Stir with a fork until just blended or pulse 2–3 times in a processor.

Knead the dough very lightly on a floured board. Pat or roll out about ½ inch thick and cut into 4 large (3½-inch) biscuits. Place on the prepared baking sheet, brush with milk, dust with cheese, and bake 15 minutes or until golden.

While the biscuits are baking, lay the broccoli on the simmering vegetables and cook 6 minutes or until tender but still bright green. Stir in the turkey and parsnip sauce and heat through.

Biscuits by the nature of their chemistry are high in calories and fat. To reduce the risk, make a whole recipe, cut the tops off 4 to use in the recipe, and save the bottoms and extra biscuit to toast for breakfast.

To serve: Spoon the turkey mixture into 4 hot soup plates and lay the biscuit halves on top.

Per Serving

calories	438	total fat	9g	dietary fiber	5g
saturated fat	2g	total carbohydrate	51g	protein	38g

Graham Kerr is an internationally known culinary consultant, television personality, award-winning author, and colorful motivational speaker. His focus is on serving people who want to make healthy, creative lifestyle changes, and he believes that the only lasting changes are the ones that we enjoy.

Jacques Pépin's "Poule Au Pot"

Poule Au Pot is a rich, aromatic, easy-to-prepare main-course meal in one pot. The dish, according to Pépin, originated in the sixteenth century under the rule of Henry IV. But Pépin lightens the stew by removing the fat from the chicken stock. The French make the most flavorful stocks, and cloves is one of their secret ingredients. Combined with thyme, rosemary, and bay leaves, this creates a surprisingly fresh and savory flavor. Store in your refrigerator and pack in plastic containers for meals at the office.

4–6 servings

Ingredients

1 chicken (about 3½ pounds)
4 quarts water
1 teaspoon dried thyme leaves
1 teaspoon dried rosemary
3 bay leaves
12 cloves
2 teaspoon salt
1 teaspoon black peppercorns

Garnishes:
16 slices from a baguette (2 ounce total), toasted in the oven
½ cup grated Gruyère cheese
cornichons
hot mustard

Vegetables:
2 large leeks (about 12 ounces total), cleaned
4 medium onions (10 ounces total), peeled
4 carrots (about 1 pound), peeled
1 small butternut squash (1 pound), peeled, seeded, and quartered
1 small savoy cabbage (about 1 pound), quartered
4 large mushrooms (about 4 ounces)

Directions

Place the chicken, breast side down, with the neck and heart in a narrow stainless steel stockpot. Add the water, and bring it to a boil over high heat. Reduce the heat, and boil gently for 10 minutes. Skim the cooking liquid to remove the fat and impurities that come to the surface.

Add the thyme, rosemary, bay leaves, cloves, salt, and peppercorns to the stock. Cover, and continue boiling gently for another 25 minutes. Remove the chicken from the pot; save the stock. When the chicken is cool enough to handle, pull off and discard the skin. Pull the meat from the bones, keeping it in the largest possible pieces. Set the meat aside, covered, in about ½ cup of the stock. Place the bones back in the remaining stock, and boil gently for another hour.

Strain the stock twice through a strainer lined with paper towels. Rinse out the pot and return the stock to the pot. (You should have 8 to 9 cups. If necessary, adjust with water.)*

* This procedure should remove much of the fat. But if you have time, you could chill the stock until the remaining fat solidifies on top. Once it hardens, it's easy to remove and discard so that you have a fat-free stock.

For the vegetables:

Add the leeks, onions, carrots, squash, and cabbage to the stock, and bring to a boil, covered, for 15 minutes. Add the mushrooms and cook for another 5 minutes.

Reheat the meat and the surrounding liquid, and arrange the meat in the center of a large platter. Remove the vegetables with a slotted spoon and arrange them around the chicken. Ladle some of the stock into 4 to 6 small bowls, and serve it with the baguette slices and cheese. Pass around the cornichons and hot mustard at the table.

Per Serving

calories	402	total fat	9.4g
saturated fat	3.5g	total carbohydrate	40g
dietary fiber	8g	protein	42g

Jacques Pépin is a master chef, author, and teacher to a generation of famous chefs—as well as millions of enthusiastic home chefs. One of America's best-known cooking teachers, Pépin has published 19 books and numerous articles and has hosted acclaimed television cooking shows, including a two-hour public television special, *Chez Pépin,* that celebrated his 50 years in the kitchen.

John Ash's Grandmother's Pot Roast

Chef John Ash says his grandmother had a real touch for wholesome, comfort foods like this savory pot roast. The meat is cooked until falling off the bone—stracotto, as it would be called in Italy. Styles may change; dishes like this won't. That's why I decided to include it in *Think Yourself Thin*. It's lean and a great source of protein, iron, and vitamin A. You can keep it in your refrigerator for up to 3 days and slice it for a sandwich or toss it in a salad using Dan Puzo's Red Wine Vinaigrette (page 449).

6–8 servings

Ingredients

3 pounds tri-tip or bottom round of beef
salt and freshly ground black pepper
4 tablespoons olive oil
3 cups sliced onions
1 cup leeks, sliced into rounds
1½ cups celery, sliced on the bias
1½ cups carrots, cut in wedges
¼ cup slivered garlic
¼ teaspoon red pepper flakes
4 cups hearty red wine
3 cups rich beef stock
2 cups seeded and diced tomatoes
2 large bay leaves
1 teaspoon fennel seed
2 teaspoons each minced fresh thyme, sage, and oregano leaves
  (1 teaspoon each dried)

Garnish:
Roasted potatoes and sautéed shiitake or wild mushrooms

Directions

Trim beef of all visible fat and season with salt and pepper. In a large, heavy-bottomed roasting pan, quickly brown the meat on all sides in the olive oil. Remove meat and add the onions, leeks, celery, carrots, and garlic and cook over moderate heat until vegetables just begin to color and onions are translucent.

Return meat to the pan and add pepper flakes, red wine, stock, tomatoes, and herbs. Bring to a simmer, cover, and place in a preheated 375-degree oven for 2 to 2½ hours, or until meat is very tender and almost falling apart.

Strain the liquid from the meat and vegetables. Allow the liquid to sit for a few minutes so that the fat will rise to the surface. Strain off and discard fat. Return the liquid to the pan and, over high heat, reduce by approximately ⅓ to concentrate flavors (if desired, thicken with 2 teaspoons cornstarch dissolved in wine or water). Correct seasoning with salt and pepper.

Return meat and braised vegetables to pan and warm through. Slice meat and arrange in shallow bowls along with some of the braised vegetables. Generously ladle reduced sauce around and garnish with roasted potatoes and mushrooms.

Per Serving

calories	430	total fat	14g
saturated fat	4g	total carbohydrate	16g
dietary fiber	3g	protein	40g

John Ash established his restaurant, John Ash & Company, in Northern California's wine country in 1980. Soon, he was selected by *Food & Wine* magazine as one of America's "hot new chefs." The restaurant has regularly been recognized as one of America's best by leading critics. He has written an award-winning cookbook, *From the Earth to the Table: John Ash's Wine Country Cuisine* (Dutton).

Kaz Sushi Bistro's Asian Vegetable Noodles

This is a perfect basic stir-fry recipe for great batch meals. You can use any number of vegetables or meats. Add one pound of shrimp, chicken breast, or tofu, and you have a complete dinner. Try a variety of fresh vegetables—just about any will do. The aroma of the sesame oil, ginger, garlic, and soy sauce will make you feel like a genuine Asian cook.

4 servings

Ingredients
½ pound vermicelli noodles or rice
1 tablespoon vegetable oil
½ Spanish onion, julienned
½ red bell pepper, julienned
5 dried shiitake mushrooms (or any type of fresh), julienne
½ carrot, shredded
1 bunch scallions, julienned
¼ cup soy sauce
1½ tablespoons sugar
black pepper
4 tablespoons sesame oil
1 teaspoon ginger, grated (optional)
1 teaspoon garlic, minced (optional)

Directions

Soak dried shiitake in warm water until soft (about 1 hour), if not using fresh shiitake mushrooms. Cut all vegetables.

Cook noodles in boiling water for 5 minutes, drain, and toss with 1 tablespoon of the sesame oil, set aside.

Sauté onion, ginger, and garlic in pan with the vegetable oil until soft. Then add carrot, shiitake, red bell pepper, and scallion with soy sauce and sugar.

Add noodles into the pan, toss with the vegetables, and add the remaining 3 tablespoons of the sesame oil and black pepper.

Chef's Note: Sesame oil adds a rich flavor but loses some of the flavor in cooking. This is why vegetable oil is used for the vegetable sauté and sesame oil is saved for the tossing.

Per Serving

calories	440	total fat	18g
saturated fat	2.5g	total carbohydrate	61g
dietary fiber	5g	protein	10g

Kaz Sushi Bistro's chef-owner **Kazuhiro Okochi (Kaz)** was the first to introduce an original new concept—"Free-Style Japanese Cuisine." "My goal," says Kaz, "is to create simple and authentic Japanese cuisine as well as innovative dishes with a Western touch." The Washington, D.C., Bistro has garnered many awards, including Highest Rated Sushi Bar by the *Zagat Survey, 2001.*

Nora Pouillon's Ratatouille

Ratatouille is an authentic Provençal ragout of onions, eggplants, peppers, zucchini, and tomatoes, stewed slowly in olive oil and flavored with garlic and fresh herbs. Cutting up the vegetables is time consuming, so I like to make double the amount and use the leftovers . . . at room temperature the next day with grilled chicken or fish; mixed with eggs and cheese for a quiche; heated and stirred with beaten eggs, spiced with chilies, and served with sliced ham, Proscuitto, or cooked lean sausage reheated and used as sauce for freshly cooked pasta, garnished with feta or goat cheese, with the addition of pitted black olives; as minestrone, heated with vegetable or chicken stock, adding a can of drained cannellini beans and maybe a spoon of pesto on top.

The trick of a good ratatouille is not to overcook the vegetables. They have to be added one after the other, depending on the amount of time they need to cook to be just tender.

6–8 servings

Ingredients

½ cup olive oil
1 large onion, chopped
1 tablespoon garlic, minced
1–2 eggplants (2 pounds) cut into 1-inch cubes
2 peppers, red, green, or yellow, cut into 1-inch squares
2 zucchini (1½ pounds) cut into 1-inch cubes
1½ pounds tomatoes, peeled and cut into 1-inch cubes
salt and freshly ground black pepper
1 tablespoon fresh thyme, minced
½ tablespoon fresh rosemary, minced
2 tablespoons fresh parsley or basil, minced

Directions

Heat olive oil in a large skillet until hot.

Add the onions and stew for 10 minutes until soft. Add the garlic, then the eggplants and peppers. Cover and cook slowly for 20 minutes.

Add the zucchini, cook for 5 minutes, then, last, add the tomatoes and cook for an additional 5 minutes or less.

Season with salt and pepper and the minced herbs.

Per Serving

calories	220	total fat	16g
saturated fat	2g	total carbohydrate	18g
dietary fiber	6g	protein	3g

Nora Pouillon is the chef and owner of two of Washington, D.C.'s most popular restaurants. Featuring organic, multi-ethnic cuisine, the internationally known Restaurant Nora opened in 1979 and has been praised for its delicious, high-quality food and healthy approach to eating. In 1999, Nora became the first certified organic restaurant in the country. Nora received the 4-star rating from *Mobile Travel Guide 2000* and was voted one of the "Top 10 Healthiest Restaurants" by *Health* magazine.

Phyllis Frucht's Chicken Lentil-Curry Stew

This recipe is one of the quickest and easiest batch recipes to make—about 20 minutes to prepare and 20 minutes to cook. Yet it's one of the most aromatic and elegant dinners you'll have. One chef I know gives this savory stew with an Indian flair a "3-D rating" for delightful, delectable, and delicious! Even though the okra is optional, I say "go for it."

The recipe may be prepared a day ahead, and it freezes well, too. To save time, use a large package of your favorite frozen vegetable blend. For a heartier meal, add cooked brown rice. Leaving the bones in the chicken thighs improves the stock and the flavor.

8 servings

Ingredients

1 tablespoon vegetable oil
2 pounds chicken thighs (without skin)
2 garlic cloves, minced
1 medium onion, peeled and minced
1 14.5-ounce can tomatoes, chopped
2 carrots, peeled and cut in ½-inch cubes
1 pound potatoes, peeled and cut in ¾ inch cubes
¾ pounds okra, sliced (optional)
1 pound dry lentils
4 cups water
2 tablespoons curry powder
salt and pepper to taste
2 tablespoons cilantro, chopped (optional)

Directions

Heat the oil in a 5-quart saucepan with a tight-fitting lid. Season the chicken with salt and pepper. Fry until golden brown in the vegetable oil, a few minutes on each side. Remove from the pan. Sauté the garlic and onions in the same pan, scraping up bits from the bottom of the pan, until soft and golden.

Add the vegetables and mix to coat well. Add the lentils, chicken, water, and seasonings, except for the cilantro. Bring to a boil and lower the flame. Cover and simmer for about 20 minutes until the potatoes and lentils are soft.

Sprinkle with cilantro and serve.

Per Serving

calories	370	total fat	8g
saturated fat	2g	total carbohydrate	49g
dietary fiber	15g	protein	29g

Phyllis Frucht is a chef and a teacher specializing in international cuisine from the Orient to India, Europe, the Middle East, and the Caribbean. She gives instruction in Washington, D.C., in elegant hands-on classes that include generous samplings of the foods with matching beverages and wine. Her menus often reflect the fusion of cross-cultural traditions and flavors.

Tallmadge's Chili Non-Carne

I love this simple, quick chili recipe. Of course, there're zillions of ways to make chili, but this recipe is easy to follow and it's meatless. And believe me, you won't miss the meat. This batch is packed with flavor. Use however much garlic or chili powder that appeals to you. I like mine hot and spicy!

I usually double the recipe so I have plenty for the week. This dish makes a great lunch or dinner alongside a green salad. I also serve it at parties as a dip next to fresh tomato salsa, light sour cream, and guacamole. It's perfect rolled up in a tortilla or stuffed in a taco with some cheese.

4 servings

Ingredients
1 tablespoon olive or canola oil
1 large onion, chopped
3 large garlic cloves, minced
3 tablespoons hot chili powder
1 large fresh green pepper, chopped
1 28-ounce can Italian plum tomatoes, chopped, including the liquid
1 1-pound can kidney or black beans, whichever is preferred
½ cup water or bouillon (to hydrate the bulgur)
½ cup bulgur (cracked wheat)
2 seeded jalapeño peppers, chopped, if desired
salt and pepper to taste

Directions

Sauté the onions and garlic in the oil over low heat in a large pot until soft, 15 or more minutes.

Add the chili powder and simmer for a few more minutes. Then add the fresh green pepper and cook until al dente. Meanwhile, soak the bulgur in the boiling water for 15 minutes.

Add all remaining ingredients including the bulgur and simmer slowly over low to medium heat until flavors are well blended and vegetables are cooked to the desired consistency.

Adjust seasonings to your preference. Since many canned items were used, additional salt will probably not be needed.

Per Serving

calories	320	total fat	7g
saturated fat	1g	total carbohydrate	60g
dietary fiber	14g	protein	12g

Xiomara's Arroz con Pollo

This creamy, filling, and luxurious one-pot meal is rich enough to serve to guests, but it's deceivingly light (just don't tell the party; it'll spoil their fun). The pungent garlic and oregano combined with the tart juice and beer will transport you to the smells and sounds of Cuba. And it tastes even better the next day, which makes it a perfect batch recipe.

6–8 servings

Ingredients

8 garlic cloves peeled

1½ tablespoons salt

1 teaspoon black pepper

¼ cup fresh chopped oregano

¼ cup sour orange juice (or a 50/50 mix of sweet, fresh orange juice and fresh lime juice)

4 pounds skinned chicken thighs, and legs (with bones)

½ cup olive oil

2 medium red onions (peeled and finely chopped)

1 large red bell pepper, cored, seeded, and finely chopped

3 cups chicken broth (defatted)

6 strands saffron toasted in a dry skillet over medium heat for about 30 seconds, or until they lose their moisture

½ cup tomato sauce

2 cups short grain rice

2 bottles of beer

1 cup of frozen peas (thawed)

Directions

Mash the garlic into paste with the salt and pepper.

Add the garlic paste to the mixed citrus juice and pour over the chicken. Cover and refrigerate for about an hour.

Heat the oil over medium heat in a wide shallow pan.

Pour the marinade off of the chicken, and set the marinade aside. Blot the chicken before browning the pieces in the hot oil, and then set them aside.

In the same oil, sauté the onions and red pepper until the onions are translucent, about 4 minutes. Add the broth, beer, saffron, oregano, tomato sauce, marinade, and the chicken and simmer for about 5 minutes. This a very moist dish. If needed add more beer or chicken broth.

Add the rice and stir just enough to cover it with liquid. If the rice is not fully covered, add more broth or beer. Simmer uncovered, until all the liquid is absorbed and the rice is cooked, about 30 minutes. Add more broth or beer if needed.

Remove pan from the heat and add peas 5 minutes before serving (the heat from the rice will cook the peas), and mix.

Suggestions from Xiomara:

In my home, after cooking the chicken I debone just before serving. Cooking with the bones adds necessary flavor."

"When cold, this dish may dry out a bit. Just add a cup of chicken broth when reheating."

Per Serving

calories	540	total fat	19g
saturated fat	3g	total carbohydrate	52g
dietary fiber	4g	protein	33g

Xiomara Ardolina, chef-owner of Xiomara's in Pasadena, California, was born in Cuba and came to the United States at the age of 13. She established herself as one of the top restaurateurs in Southern California. In 1991, she opened Xiomara in Pasadena, featuring French cuisine. It was recognized as one of the finest restaurants in the Los Angeles area. In 1996, Xiomara began serving Nuevo Latino cuisine, and she's continued receiving high praise from the critics.

Tallmadge's White Beans with Garlic and Basil

I love these beans. They taste deceptively rich, and they're easy to make. After I've made and stored a batch, I'll ladle a heap into a bowl and microwave for lunch, with a slice of whole-grain bread topped with smoked turkey, lean ham, or light cheese (or all three!) and some crunchy lettuce. Slice a spicy chicken sausage into a bowl, top with the beans, and pop in the microwave. Add a green salad and tart dressing and you've got a winning dinner. I usually double the recipe to have plenty during the week. Without meat, it will last more than a week refrigerated.

4 servings

Ingredients

½ pound dried small white (cannellini) beans, or 24 ounces canned, rinsed beans
1 tablespoon olive oil
1½ onion, chopped
4 garlic cloves (more or less to taste—I double it)
1 quart defatted chicken stock
salt to taste
12 ounces (3 medium) fresh or canned tomatoes, drained, peeled, and chopped
1 large handful of fresh basil
juice from 1 lemon
freshly ground pepper

Directions

If you're using dried white beans

Soak the beans in 1 quart of water overnight or up to 24 hours. Drain and rinse.

Add one quart chicken stock to the beans along with one clove of garlic and ½ onion. Bring to a boil, reduce heat, cover, and simmer 1½ hours or until the beans are almost tender. Add more water or stock to keep moist. Add salt to taste and cook until beans are tender.

Continue with your cooked dried beans or start here if you're

using canned white beans

Heat oil in a large, heavy soup pot or casserole and sauté the remaining onion and garlic over low to medium heat for 10 or 15 minutes or until soft.

Add the tomatoes, and more salt to taste and bring to a simmer. Simmer about 10 minutes then add the beans with their cooking liquid and simmer 15–20 minutes. If you used canned beans, rinse the beans, then use enough stock (approximately 1 cup) to keep the beans moist while cooking.

At the end of the cooking time, add the fresh basil (it will get bitter if overcooked), fresh lemon juice, and freshly ground pepper. Mix together.

Let the beans sit at room temperature overnight to let the flavors blend.

Refrigerate and heat to serve.

Per Serving

calories	290	total fat	4.5g
saturated fat	0.5g	total carbohydrate	45g
dietary fiber	16g	protein	19g

Adapted from *Mediterranean Light*, by Martha Rose Shulman (Bantam Books, 1989).

MAIN DISH SOUPS

Aquavit's Marcus Samuelsson's Corn Soup with Smoked Salmon

If you love corn, this is the soup for you. Though corn is not a typically Swedish food, Chef Samuelsson uses it liberally here, combined with very typical Swedish ingredients: potatoes, salmon, tarragon, and sour cream. This soup uses the salmon bones to give the stock a depth of flavor to support the sweetness of the puréed corn and potatoes, but it can also be made without them. It is a delicious soup served warm or even at room temperature. You'll love it all week.

4 servings

Ingredients
6 ears of corn, shucked
6 fingerling potatoes or small new potatoes
2 tablespoons canola oil
Bones from 2 salmon (get these from your fishmonger), optional
2 shallots, finely chopped
1 garlic clove, finely chopped
1 quart chicken stock
1 cup light sour cream, optional
salt and freshly ground black pepper
2 sprigs fresh tarragon, finely chopped
2 sprigs fresh cilantro, finely chopped
6 ounces smoked salmon, cut into ½-inch cubes

Directions
Preheat the oven to 400 degrees. Put the ears of corn and potatoes on a baking sheet and roast them for 25–30 minutes, until the potatoes are cooked through. Remove from the oven and let cool.

Cut the corn kernels off the cobs and set them aside. Break each corn cob into 2 or 3 pieces and set aside. Peel the potatoes, and set aside.

Put the canola oil in the bottom of a soup pot and turn the heat to medium high. Add the salmon bones, shallots, and garlic and sauté for about 3 minutes, until the shallots start to soften. Add the corn cobs and chicken stock and simmer for 30 minutes.

Strain the stock, and combine it with the corn kernels and potatoes. Purée the soup in a blender, return it to the saucepan, and heat through over medium heat.

When it's hot, turn off the heat, stir in the sour cream, and season to taste with salt and freshly ground black pepper.

Garnish with tarragon and cilantro and top with cubes of smoked salmon.

Per Serving Without Sour Cream

calories	470	total fat	15g
saturated fat	2g	total carbohydrate	77g
dietary fiber	5g	protein	19g

With Sour Cream

calories	550	total fat	20g
saturated fat	6g	total carbohydrate	81g
dietary fiber	5g	protein	23g

Owner **Håkan Swahn's** goal with Aquavit, when he opened it in the heart of Manhattan in 1987, was to serve the finest Swedish cuisine available. And the restaurant has met with resounding success. Swahn and executive chef Marcus Samuelsson are basking in the glow of a 3-star review by *The New York Times,* and Marcus's 1999 James Beard Foundation award for best "Rising Star Chef."

Border Grill's Turkey Albondigas Soup

What could be more hearty and inviting than a soup full of delicate meat balls and plenty of garlic, hot peppers, vegetables, and tomatoes? This dish is a spicy main course perfect on a cold day as it warms the soul. The Border Grill is renowned for serving zesty Latin street foods and this is a perfect example.

6 servings

Ingredients

¼ cup olive oil

8 garlic cloves, peeled

2 bunches cilantro, leaves only

1 tablespoon salt

1½ teaspoons freshly ground black pepper

1 pound ground turkey or chicken, preferably dark meat

1 large egg, beaten

⅔ cup fresh bread crumbs

⅓ cup vegetable oil

1 large leek, trimmed, washed, and thinly julienned

4 medium carrots, peeled and diced

¼ head white cabbage, cored and thinly sliced

1–2 jalapeño chilies, stemmed, seeded, and thinly julienned

3 medium Roma tomatoes, cored, seeded, and diced

2½ quarts chicken stock

3 tablespoons white vinegar

Directions

Combine the olive oil, garlic, cilantro, and 1 teaspoon each of the salt and pepper in a blender. Purée until smooth.

In a large bowl, mix together the turkey or chicken, egg, and cilantro paste. Add the bread crumbs and mix only until combined. Roll into small walnut-sized meatballs in the palms of your hands and place on a tray in the refrigerator.

Heat 2 tablespoons of the vegetable oil in a large stockpot over high heat. Sauté the leeks and carrots with the remaining 2 teaspoons salt and ½ teaspoon pepper for 2–4 minutes. Add the cabbage, jalapenos, and tomatoes and cook, stirring frequently, until the vegetables are limp, about 3 minutes longer. Pour in the chicken stock. Bring to a boil, reduce to a simmer, and cook, uncovered, 15 minutes.

Meanwhile, heat the remaining oil in a medium skillet over medium heat until nearly smoking. Add the chilled meatballs in batches, shaking the pan to prevent sticking, and brown on all sides. Transfer with a slotted spoon to paper towels to drain.

When all the meatballs are browned, transfer to the simmering stock and cook an additional 5–10 minutes. Stir in the vinegar and serve hot.

Per Serving

calories	460	total fat	31g
saturated fat	7g	total carbohydrate	28g
dietary fiber	4g	protein	20g

Mary Sue Milliken and Susan Feniger, chef-owners of The Border Grill and Ciudad in Santa Monica, Los Angeles, and Las Vegas, are the stars of the popular Television Food Network show *Too Hot Tamales.* Though they are multimedia figures of television and radio, have written cookbooks, and own several restaurants, the two never lose sight of the pleasure that cooking brings them.

"Turkey Albondigas Soup" was reprinted from *Mesa Mexicana*, by Mary Sue Milliken and Susan Feniger, published by William Morrow ©1994.

Café des Artistes' Seafood Gazpacho, Sixty-Seventh Street Style

Gazpacho epitomizes the feeling of summer. When I purée my gazpacho, I leave it coarse and chunky. The garnish of fresh dill, scallions, cucumber, and croutons is essential to the soup's success. The added crunch and flavor go a long way to satisfy your senses. Adding shrimp to the gazpacho makes this a main course dish—one you can keep in your refrigerator for up to 3 days.

8–10 servings

Ingredients

2½ pounds red ripe tomatoes, peeled, seeded, and chopped
1 cup coarsely chopped Bermuda onion
½ cup each chopped green pepper and chopped carrot
1 clove of garlic, peeled
5 cups tomato juice
⅓ cup red wine vinegar
salt and freshly ground black pepper to taste
2 tablespoons olive oil
8 ounces tiny shrimp, shells removed, deveined, and lightly cooked
dash of Louisiana-type hot sauce

Garnish:
¼ cup chopped fresh dill
6 medium scallions, white part only, washed and cut into ¼-inch dice
1 large cucumber, peeled, seeded, and cut into ¼-inch dice
1 cup freshly toasted croutons

Directions

Process tomatoes, onion, green pepper, carrot, and garlic in a food processor until the mixture takes on a rough texture.

Stir in tomato juice and vinegar, and season with salt and pepper. Whisk in olive oil. Chill for at least 3 hours.

Add shrimp. Adjust seasoning with hot sauce, and serve sprinkled with dill in chilled bowls, with crocks of scallion, cucumber, and croutons on the side.

Per Serving

calories	120	total fat	4g
saturated fat	0.5g	total carbohydrate	17g
dietary fiber	3g	protein	7g

(This dish is a great source of vitamins A and C.)

Since June 1991, *Thomas Ferlesch* has been the executive chef of the 3-star Café des Artistes, one of the 10 most popular restaurants in New York City, as ranked by the *Zagat Survey 2000.* The Café, owned and operated by Jenifer and George Lang, was named one of the "50 Best Restaurants in the United States" by *Conde Nast Traveler.*

Judy Zeidler's Hearty and Versatile Vegetable Soup

Vegetable soups are fast and simple to make. They can be prepared in advance and stored in the refrigerator for a week or more until ready to serve. Most soups are even better the next day, and the longer they cook the more concentrated they become. Garnish this soup with chopped vegetables, sautéed mushrooms, or grilled onions.

Purée the leftover soup, and it can be used as a sauce for pasta on the second night and a sauce for fish on the third night (see the following recipes).

6 servings

Ingredients

¼ cup olive oil
2 medium leeks, finely diced
2 cloves garlic, minced
4 medium carrots, finely diced
4 stalks celery, finely diced
2 small new potatoes, unpeeled, finely diced
1 large zucchini, finely diced
¼ cup minced fresh parsley
6–8 cups water (or fat-free stock if preferred)
salt and freshly ground black pepper, to taste
2 tablespoons fresh basil, thinly sliced
freshly grated Parmesan cheese (optional)

Directions

In a large heavy pot, heat olive oil over medium heat. Add leeks, garlic, carrots, celery, potatoes, zucchini, and parsley. Sauté 5 to 10 minutes, stirring until tender.

Add water, bring to a boil over high heat, reduce heat and simmer, partially covered, for 30 minutes, stirring occasionally. Season with salt and pepper to taste.

Add basil and simmer until vegetables are soft, about 15 minutes more. Ladle 1 cup of soup into blender and purée; return to soup and mix well.

Ladle into heated soup bowls and sprinkle with grated Parmesan cheese.

Hearty Vegetable Soup with Sautéed Fish

6 servings

Ingredients

Hearty Vegetable Soup (see recipe)
1 pound salmon fillets or white fish
¼ cup Panko Crumbs or bread crumbs
¼ cup olive oil

Directions

Place soup in a food processor and purée. Transfer to a saucepan and set aside.

Dice the fish fillets into 1-inch cubes. Dip in Panko Crumbs and place on paper towels.

Heat olive oil in a nonstick skillet and sauté prepared fish fillets on both sides until lightly brown. Transfer to paper towels until ready serve.

To serve, heat the soup, ladle in heated bowls, and spoon the sautéed fish in the center.

Pasta with Vegetable Sauce

6 servings

Ingredients

2 cups puréed vegetable soup (see recipe)
6 ounces dry spaghetti or tagliatelli
Parmesan cheese

Directions

In a large skillet heat the puréed soup. Bring a large pot of water to a boil and add spaghetti or tagliatelli. Cook until tender.

Drain, add to the sauce, and toss to coat pasta. Serve in heated shallow bowls and sprinkle with Parmesan cheese.

Per Serving: Vegetable Soup

calories	160	total fat	9g
saturated fat	1.5g	total carbohydrate	19g
dietary fiber	4g	protein	3g

Per Serving: With Sautéed Fish

calories	400	total fat	27g
saturated fat	4g	total carbohydrate	22g
dietary fiber	4g	protein	18g

Per Serving: With Fish and Whole Wheat Pasta

calories	495	total fat	27g
saturated fat	4g	total carbohydrate	43g
dietary fiber	7g	protein	21g

Judy Zeidler is the author of the widely acclaimed *The Gourmet Jewish Cook* as well as *Judy Zeidler's International Deli Cookbook*, among others. Her weekly syndicated television show, *Judy's Kitchen,* airs on the Jewish Television Network. Zeidler is a regular contributor to the *Los Angeles Times* and the *Jewish Journal.*

Kjerstin's Simple Hot and Sour Soup

This recipe of my mother's is so irresistible that friends have told me they've finished off the whole batch in one evening. Use it as a first course or a main course.

4 servings

Ingredients

4 diced dry black (shiitake) mushrooms or fresh mushrooms
5 cups chicken broth
1 chicken breast
¼ cup bamboo shoots, slivered
½ cup rice wine vinegar
2 tablespoons soy sauce
1–2 green onions, cut into 2-inch slivers
1 tablespoon finely chopped cilantro
1 teaspoon Tabasco sauce
½ teaspoon pepper
3 tablespoons cornstarch
¼ cup water
1 egg, lightly beaten

Directions

Soak mushrooms in warm water for 30 minutes. Drain, cut off, and discard stems. Thinly slice caps.

Bring broth to simmer, add chicken, and cook 3 minutes. Stir in vinegar, soy sauce, Tabasco, pepper, bamboo shoots, cilantro, green onion, and mushrooms. Return to simmer.

Combine cornstarch and water. Stir into mixture. Simmer until slightly thickened, stirring constantly.

Remove from heat and slowly drizzle in egg, stirring constantly.

Per Serving

calories	160	total fat	7g
saturated fat	2g	total carbohydrate	12g
dietary fiber	less than 1g	protein	11g

Margaret Ferrazzi's Spiced Red Lentil Soup with Mint-Cilantro Raita

This exotic lentil soup is rich in aroma but the hot Indian spices don't overwhelm. A dollop of the cooling yogurt relish will balance the flavors and add a creamy texture. Double your serving size and this vegan soup becomes a substantial main course. It'll keep for a week or more in the fridge.

6–8 servings

Ingredients

2 quarts of chicken broth, defatted
2 cups dry red lentils
3 large carrots
3 celery stalks
1 large brown onion, peeled
3 cloves garlic
2 inch chunk of ginger
¼ cup extra virgin olive oil
juice of ½ lime
salt and freshly ground black pepper to taste

Spice Mix:

1 tablespoon mild curry powder
1 tablespoon paprika
½ tablespoon turmeric
½ tablespoon garam masala
½ teaspoon ground cinnamon
Raita (Yogurt Relish):
1 pint nonfat plain yogurt
½ cup fresh cilantro leaves
½ cup fresh mint leaves
salt to taste

Directions

Drain the yogurt by adding a little salt and putting it into a fine sieve set over a bowl. Place in the refrigerator. It's surprising how much water will be removed this way and it makes the nonfat yogurt nice and thick.

Cut the carrots, celery, and onion in fine dice. Peel and mince the ginger and garlic finely. Combine the powdered spices until well mixed.

Heat the olive oil in a large heavy saucepan. When very hot, add the diced vegetables. Stir briskly for a couple of minutes until they begin to release their juices and aromas. Add the garlic and ginger and stir, turn the heat to low, and cover the pot tightly. Let these vegetables "sweat" for 10 minutes until softened.

Stir in the spice mix and leave for a couple of minutes to let the dry spices cook to bring out the flavor. Add the chicken broth and the lentils and bring to a low boil. Cook uncovered until the lentils are tender (about 20 minutes). Do not overcook or they will become mushy.

Add black pepper and salt to taste. The lime juice completes the seasoning.

Chop the herbs fine and add to the yogurt. Pass the bowl of raita and help yourself.

Per Serving

calories	270	total fat	8g
saturated fat	1g	total carbohydrate	33g
dietary fiber	12g	protein	18g

Margaret Ferrazzi is a culinary consultant, cooking teacher, caterer, and chef to Hollywood celebrities and executives. Her clients have included Steven Spielberg, Ted Danson, Paul Reiser, and Matt Groening. Her love of aromatherapy and passion for fresh, seasonal foods is reflected in this recipe.

Michel Richard's Chicken, Mushroom, and Barley Soup

Nothing could be simpler or more delicate than this dish. The flavors are rich and earthy. The texture creamy. It contains all the elements of a complete meal. It's nutritious and filling, to boot. I'm delighted that Michel Richard provided this recipe for *Think Yourself Thin*. It fits perfectly as something you can cook, store in the refrigerator, and eat for several meals. And it's low in calories.

4 servings

Ingredients

2 tablespoons olive oil
2 small onions, peeled and diced
1 pound mushrooms, ends trimmed and thinly sliced
2 quarts unsalted chicken stock (defatted)
½ cup soy sauce
6 tablespoons pearl barley
4 cloves garlic, peeled and minced
salt and freshly ground black pepper to taste
4 large chicken breasts or thighs, boned, skinned, and sliced into bite-size pieces, at room temperature
1½ cups (about 3 ounces) freshly grated Parmesan cheese (optional)

Directions

Heat the oil in a heavy, medium-size saucepan over medium-low heat. Add the onion, cover, and cook until translucent, for about 10 minutes, stirring occasionally.

Add the mushrooms, increase heat to medium-high, and cook uncovered until lightly browned, for about 5 minutes, stirring occasionally.

Add the chicken stock, soy sauce, barley, and garlic. Simmer gently for 45 minutes to cook barley and then blend flavors.

Season with salt and pepper.

This can be prepared ahead, cooled, covered, and set aside at cool room temperature for up to 4 hours or refrigerated for several days.

To serve, bring the soup to a boil, add chicken, reduce heat, and simmer just until the chicken becomes opaque, for about 2–3 minutes. Ladle into 4 soup plates. Pass Parmesan, if desired.

Per Serving: Without Parmesan

calories	320	total fat	10g
saturated fat	2g	total carbohydrate	26g
dietary fiber	6g	protein	34g

Per Serving: With Parmesan

calories	500	total fat	22g
saturated fat	9g	total carbohydrate	28g
dietary fiber	6g	protein	48g

Michel Richard and his restaurant, Citronelle, in Washington, D.C., have received numerous awards. In 2001, *Zagat Survey* named Citronelle one of the five best restaurants in Washington, D.C., and *Gourmet Magazine* rated Citronelle in the top 20 of all restaurants in the United States. In 1988 Richard was inducted into the James Beard Foundation's "Who's Who in American Food and Wine." Richard is renowned as a genius with ingredients, using surprising combinations of textures and flavors.

Oodles Noodles' Spicy Chicken Noodle Soup

I love to stroll down the street to Oodles Noodles, a local "noodle bar" in downtown Washington, D.C., and order this soup. The flavors explode in your mouth, and the combination of hot chili, lemongrass, Thai spices, and the fresh vegetables, noodles, and chicken makes this a full-course meal that's hard to beat.

If you want to make extra servings to save in your refrigerator, go ahead and cook the noodles and clean and chop the garnishes, but keep them in separate containers apart from the soup. The noodles are so delicate, they'll disintegrate if left in water. And it's nice to have crispy, fresh onions, bean sprouts, and cilantro to add at the last minute for maximum effect.

4 servings

Ingredients

½ pound bag Oriental-style rice noodles (banh pho)
1 pound chicken breast
½ pound mushrooms
4 stalks lemongrass stem
5 slices galangal
4 pieces kaffir lime leaves
7 cups chicken stock (defatted)
4–5 tablespoons fish sauce
4–5 tablespoons fresh lime juice
3–4 tablespoons Thai chili paste (namprik pao)

Garnish:

3 ounces spring onion, chopped
3 ounces cilantro, chopped
½ pound bean sprouts

(Note: The galangal and lime leaves are not edible. They're meant only to float in the bowl to impart their distinctive flavors.)

Directions

Soak the rice noodles in cold water for at least 4 hours. Cut the chicken breast into thin slices. Slice the mushrooms. Set aside. Cut the lemongrass into short lengths.

Add the lemongrass, galangal, and kaffir lime leaves to the chicken stock and bring to boil. Season to taste with fish sauce, lime juice, and chili paste, then bring to another boil. Add chicken and simmer until cooked, in a few minutes.

Boil the noodles in hot water until soft, no more than 10 seconds.

To serve, divide the noodles in 4, place in 4 soup bowls.

Sprinkle on top of the noodles in each bowl one quarter of the bean sprouts, spring onions, and cilantro.

Pour the hot soup over the noodles and garnish. Serve.

Chef's Note: Many of the ingredients, particularly the lemongrass, galangal, kaffir lime leaves, fish sauce, and the oriental noodles (banh pho) can be found in an oriental market.

Per Serving

calories	460	total fat	3.5
saturated fat	1g	total carbohydrate	62g
dietary fiber	6g	protein	43g

Jessie Yan, Vanessa Lim, and William Tu own Spices, Oodles Noodles, and Yanyu restaurants in Washington, D.C., all of which are popular and critically acclaimed. Oodles Noodles, an informal "noodle bar," has received rave reviews for serving fresh, light, innovative ingredients at very reasonable prices.

Goody's Vegetable Soup

I first experienced this soup at a pot luck dinner with a group of colleagues in Les Dames d'Escoffier, a professional group of women in the food and wine business. My fellow Dame Goody Solomon made it and when it was passed around, I was mesmerized by the soup's delicate aroma. When I tasted it, I was surprised that a simple vegetable soup could be so delicious. The tender vegetables imparted a sweet and complex flavor. I couldn't get enough. This was the only dish I got seconds of. Goody says she serves her vegetable soup often—for lunch with good bread, to start dinner, at a pot luck event, as part of the Thanksgiving feast. It's always a winner. I just love it and swear by it as a weight-loss aid. Serve this with every meal and you'll not only be bowled over by its flavor and look forward to every meal, you'll see results.

10–12 servings

Ingredients

4 quarts defatted chicken stock
1 large can of tomatoes, with juice
2 parsnips
1 large potato
5 carrots
¼ head large cabbage
2 stalks celery
1 medium peeled onion
½ teaspoon butter or light margarine, per serving

Bouquet garni:
1 large clove garlic
4 sprigs of fresh parsley
2 sprigs of fresh dill

Directions

Cut all of the vegetables into bite-size pieces.

To make the "bouquet garni," place the garlic, parsley and dill in a cheesecloth and tie with a string.

Put vegetables and bouquet garni in the chicken stock and simmer until potatoes and carrots are soft, about 40 minutes.

When serving, garnish each bowl with 1/2 teaspoon of butter or light margarine.

Per Serving

calories	120	total fat	2g
saturated fat	1g	total carbohydrate	14g
dietary fiber	3g	protein	10g

Goody Soloman is the executive editor of the Food Nutrition Health News Service in Washington, D.C., in which she reports on government policies affecting food, nutrition, and health. Her career has been multi-faceted and included stints as an award-winning syndicated food columnist, a restaurant reviewer, consumer correspondent, magazine writer, television personality, book author, public speaker, and teacher.

The Oceanaire Seafood Room's Carrot Soup with Blue Crab and Cilantro

Rob Klink, executive chef of this fun restaurant in Washington, D.C., ensures that twenty-five to thirty varieties of the best and freshest seafood available are secured daily for the restaurant. Whenever possible, Rob features local produce and seafood on the award-winning restaurant's menu. This is a great batch recipe for just yourself or a real treat to serve for company on a crisp autumn evening!

6 servings

Ingredients

3 tablespoons olive oil
1½ pounds carrots, peeled and cut
1 onion, peeled and diced
1 celery stalk, diced
2 cloves garlic, chopped
2 small potatoes, peeled and diced
4 cups chicken stock
1 cup milk
1 tablespoon cilantro, minced
1 tablespoon cilantro leaves, reserved for garnished
6 ounces jumbo lump crabmeat
Salt and freshly ground pepper, to taste

Directions

Heat the oil in a heavy stock pot and sauté the onions, celery, garlic, and carrots over medium heat for about 5 to 10 minutes or until translucent. Add the potatoes and chicken stock and bring to a boil.

After the stock comes to a boil, turn down heat and simmer for about 20 minutes or until the carrots and potatoes are tender.

Take the soup off the heat and place in a food processor and puree until smooth. Return the puree to a clean pot over medium heat.

Stir in the milk, minced cilantro, and salt and pepper. Cook for about 3 to 5 minutes.

Remove the soup from the heat and immediately place into 6 soup bowls.

Divide the crabmeat and cilantro leaves and place on top of the soup to garnish. Serve immediately.

Per Serving

calories	250	total fat	11g
saturated fat	2g	total carbohydrate	28g
dietary fiber	5g	protein	11g

Native Marylander **Rob Klink** is a seafood expert and executive chef at Washington D.C.'s Oceanaire Seafood Room.

MAIN DISHES FOR GREAT LEFTOVERS

Kjerstin's Crab Cakes

My mother's recipe for crab cakes is very light, but tastes rich. These crab cakes are versatile, too. I've served them for brunch alongside fried eggs and hash browns, and they make a great crabcake sandwich when placed between slices of toast.

You can hold the crabcake mixture in the refrigerator for up to 3 days and make fresh crabcakes in an instant.

4 servings

Ingredients
1 pound crab meat, fresh or canned
¼ cup bread crumbs
1 egg
2 tablespoons reduced-fat mayonnaise
1 tablespoon Old Bay seasoning
½ tablespoon mustard
juice of 1 lemon
dash of Worcestershire sauce
dash of cayenne pepper
a few drops of Louisiana-style hot sauce (or Tabasco)

Directions

Mix the crab meat lightly with the bread crumbs. In a separate bowl, mix the egg, mayonnaise, bay seasoning, mustard, lemon juice, Worcestershire, cayenne pepper, and hot sauce.

Mix it all together and make 8 small patties.

Fry in a pan over low to medium heat with a little oil, butter, or oil spray until lightly brown on each side.

Per Serving

calories	230	total fat	10g
saturated fat	1.5g	carbohydrate	7g
dietary fiber	0g	protein	26g

Patrick O'Connell's Chilled Charcoal Grilled Salmon in a Mustard Crust

This is a delightfully different treatment for a whole salmon. The fish can be grilled ahead over charcoal and beautifully presented as a whole side, or it can be individually portioned and served chilled as a refreshing summery dish. The cooked salmon makes a versatile leftover flaked into a pasta salad, scrambled eggs, or a cocktail spread. Ask your fishmonger to split a whole salmon, removing the head and all of the bones, but leaving the skin, which helps keep the salmon intact on the grill. The salmon can be cooked under the broiler, as well.

9 servings

Ingredients
1 side of salmon, head and bones removed (about 3½ pounds with the skin on)
1 cup dried mustard seeds
1 bunch fresh dill, lightly chopped
1 medium onion, thinly sliced
¼ cup extra virgin olive oil
salt and freshly ground pepper to taste

For grilling:
½ pound hickory wood chips, optional

Directions

Lay the side of salmon flesh side up, salt and pepper liberally, and coat with the mustard seeds, then cover with the chopped dill, followed by thinly sliced raw onions. Finish with a sprinkling of olive oil.

Remove the rack from your charcoal grill and ignite the charcoal. Sprinkle the wood chips on top of the fire, letting the flames subside to glowing embers.

Lay your rack on the top of the flesh side of the fish. Pressing the onions, dill, and seasonings in place with the rack, quickly flip the rack over the fire with the skin side facing up. Lower the lid if your grill has one and cook for 10 minutes. The fish will continue to cook somewhat after it is removed from the fire.

To remove the fish from the fire, use tongs or oven mitts to lift off the grill rack with the fish in place and set on a large metal tray or cookie sheet to cool. Gently remove the skin.

To serve, place a serving tray or platter on top of the fish and holding the rack in place, turn the fish over onto the tray. Pick off and discard any burned bits of onion and dill.

The salmon may be served whole or individually portioned by cutting into vertical strips about 2 inches wide.

Per Serving

calories	480	total fat	31g
saturated fat	5g	total carbohydrate	9g
dietary fiber	3g	protein	40g

Patrick O'Connell, chef and owner of the award-winning Inn at Little Washington, is a self-taught chef who pioneered a refined, regional American cuisine in the Virginia countryside. He has been referred to as "the Pope of American Haute Cuisine." America's first 5-star country house hotel, the Inn has been named "Restaurant of the Year" by the James Beard Foundation. O'Connell himself was named "Best Chef in the Mid-Atlantic region" and was honored with the "Outstanding Chef Award for 2001."

"Chilled Charcoal Grilled Salmon in a Mustard Seed Crust" is from *The Inn at Little Washington, A Consuming Passion,* published by Random House, 1996.

Roberto Donna's Baked Shells with Ricotta and Eggplant

This simple main course comes together quickly and makes for a delicious Italian meal minus loads of calories.

4 servings

Ingredients

8 oz peeled and cubed eggplant, sprinkled with 1 tablespoon olive oil

8 oz low-fat ricotta cheese

2 tablespoons capers, drained (optional)

Salt and freshly ground black pepper to taste

12 fresh basil leaves

12 jumbo pasta shells, cooked, drained, and cooled

2 tablespoons olive oil (or oil spray)

1½ cups canned plum tomatoes

½ cup tomato sauce from can

¼ cup roasted, peeled, seeded red peppers

1 garlic clove, minced

4 tablespoons fat-free sour cream

4 tablespoons grated Parmesan, optional

Italian parsley leaves for garnish

Directions

Preheat oven to 450 degrees F. Place eggplant cubes on nonstick baking sheet and roast about 15 minutes until crisped and golden. Remove from oven.

Mix ricotta with capers and eggplant cubes in mixing bowl. Season with salt and pepper and 4 minced basil leaves. Set aside.

Reduce oven temperature to 400 degrees F.

Cover baking dish with foil and spray with nonstick vegetable spray.

Fill each shell with about 1 tablespoon ricotta cheese, dividing filling evenly among shells until used up. Brush tops of shells with 1 tablespoon olive oil or use oil spray. Bake 10-15 minutes or until crisped.

Meanwhile, purée tomatoes, peppers, remaining basil, olive oil and garlic in food processor. Season with salt and pepper and stir in sour cream.

Heat mixture over low heat until warmed through. Remove and set aside.

To serve, spoon one-quarter of the sauce on dish and place 3 stuffed shells on top. Drizzle a little extra sauce over each top and garnish with parsley leaf. Repeat with remaining shells and sauce. Refrigerate if not using immediately.

To reheat, place 3 shells on top of sauce on microwavable plate or shallow bowl, cover with a glass bowl or microwavable plastic, and microwave 2 minutes.

Per Serving

calories	360	total fat	17g
saturated fat	6g	dietary fiber	4g
protein	12g		

As a James Beard Award-winning chef and restaurateur in Washington, D.C., *Roberto Donna* is committed to introducing others to the real flavors of Italy. In 1984 he opened Galileo and gained a strong following, and in 1997, *Wine Spectator* called Galileo one of the "10 Best Italian Restaurants in America." The magazine has presented Mr. Donna with the "Grand Award of Excellence" every year since 1997. Galileo was also named one of the twenty finest Italian restaurants in the world by the president of Italy.

MAIN DISH SALADS

Dan Puzo's Red Wine Vinaigrette

Dan is the master of salad dressings. I can't stop eating his salads. This vinaigrette is rich, with just the right amount of tartness.

I use it on a simple tossed green salad, cucumbers and tomatoes, or as a marinade for chilled asparagus. Toss it into sliced leftover steak with some chopped vegetables.

12 servings

Ingredients

½ cup red wine vinegar
⅓ cup red wine, such as California Cabernet Sauvignon
½ cup extra virgin olive oil
1 tablespoon dried basil or ⅛ cup fresh basil
1 teaspoon dried oregano or 2 tablespoons fresh oregano
1 teaspoon sea salt
½ teaspoon garlic powder, optional
dash black pepper, optional

Directions

In deep bowl, mix red wine vinegar, red wine, olive oil, basil, oregano, and salt. Add garlic powder and/or black pepper, if desired.

Whisk until blended. Makes about 1½ cups.

Per 2-Tablespoon Serving

calories	90	total fat	9g
saturated fat	1.5g	total carbohydrate	2g
dietary fiber	0g	protein	0g

Dan Puzo is an 18-year veteran of the *Los Angeles Times,* where he won two James Beard Awards for food journalism. He is also a wine columnist with a passion for California wines.

East Coast Grill and Raw Bar's Chickpea Salad with Cumin and Mint

I love a spicy, hearty salad with a lot of different elements—crunch, tartness, sweetness, and heat. And they're all in this dish. And so are all the nutritional elements that make this a perfect one-pot meal. I bring this dish to a spring or summer pot luck and people are thrilled with the flavors. I love serving it as a main course for a simple lunch. It's a versatile recipe and can be stored in the refrigerator for a week for many meals for you and your family. Double or triple it so you'll have plenty!

4 servings

Ingredients

1 cup dried chickpeas or 1 15-ounce can chickpeas
1 tablespoon salt (if using dried chickpeas)
⅓ cup olive oil
¼ cup fresh lemon juice (about 1 lemon)
1 tablespoon minced garlic
1 red bell pepper, halved, seeded, and diced medium
½ cup roughly chopped scallions (white and green parts)
¼ cup roughly chopped fresh mint
2 tablespoon cumin seeds, toasted if you want, or 1 tablespoon
    ground cumin
1 tablespoon minced jalapeño or other fresh chili pepper of your
    choice (optional)
2 bunches fresh watercress, trimmed, washed, and dried

Directions

If you are using dried chickpeas place them in a large pot, cover with water, and let soak overnight, or for at least 5 hours. Drain and rinse 2 or 3 times.

Return the chickpeas to the pot, cover with water again, add salt, and bring to a boil over high heat. Immediately reduce the heat to medium and simmer for 1 hour to 1 hour and 15 minutes, or until the chickpeas are tender but not mushy. Drain and rinse thoroughly with cold water. If you are using canned chickpeas, simply drain and rinse them.

Place the chickpeas in a medium bowl, add all the remaining ingredients except the watercress, and toss well. Cover and refrigerate until well chilled, at least 30 minutes. When chilled, place the watercress on a platter or individual serving plates, top with the chickpea salad, and serve.

Per Serving

calories	370	total fat	21g
saturated fat	3g	total carbohydrate	36g
dietary fiber	10g	protein	11g

Chris Schlesinger is the chef and co-owner of the East Coast Grill, named one of Boston's "Top 20 Restaurants" in the *Zagat Survey 2001.* *John Wiloughby* is senior editor of *Cook's Illustrated.* Schlesinger and Wiloughby are authors of *Lettuce in Your Kitchen, Big Flavors of the Hot Sun,* and *License to Grill,* among other books.

"Chickpea Salad with Cumin and Mint" is excerpted from *License to Grill,* published by William Morrow and Company, Inc., 1997.

©Chris Schlesinger, John Wiloughby

Gerard Pangaud's Salad of Cod with Citrus

This is an elegant dish from one of the top French chefs in the country. It is a wonderful first course, but I prefer to double the recipe and the serving size for week-long main courses. The citrus fruit is a perfect accompaniment with the fish. It doesn't overpower, only complements and adds depth. You'll be transported to an island in the Mediterranean with just one bite.

4 servings

Ingredients

1 10- to 12-ounce cod filet, with skin
½ teaspoon ground dried ginger
½ teaspoon ground dried coriander
¼ teaspoon dried nutmeg
½ teaspoon anise seed
1 pinch ground clove
¼ teaspoon ground cumin
1 orange, plus zest
1 lemon, plus zest
1 lime, plus zest
¼ grapefruit
⅓ cup olive oil
¼ pound arugula

Directions

Preheat the oven to 375 degrees and mix all the spices.

Using about ⅔ of the olive oil, brush the fish and coat the baking dish. Reserve ⅓ of the oil for use later. Place the fish in the baking dish skin side down. Spread the spices on top of the fish and put in the oven for approximately 8–12 minutes, depending on the thickness of the fish.

Grate the skin of the orange, lemon, and lime, being careful to use only the colorful zest, not the white pith. Peel the orange, lemon, lime, and grapefruit and separate the fruits into sections.

Take the fish out of the oven and flake it. Deglaze the baking dish by adding the rest of the olive oil and pulling up the bits of fish left in the bottom of the pan. Put the flavored oil in a bowl and add the citrus sections, tossing well.

Arrange the cod harmoniously with the arugula on a plate and spoon the citrus relish over the fish.

Serve warm.

Per Serving

calories	260	total fat	19g
saturated fat	2.5g	total carbohydrate	10g
dietary fiber	3g	protein	14g

Gerard Pangaud opened Gerard's Place in downtown Washington, D.C., in 1993 and has been lauded by the critics ever since. Many times over he has been awarded 4 Stars in the Mobil Guide as well as by *Washingtonian* magazine. The *Zagat Survey* consistently lists Gerard's Place in the top 5 restaurants in Washington, D.C.

Najmieh Batmanglij's Persian Chicken Salad

This is a beautiful chicken salad, with a perfect harmony of flavors, colors, and textures. I love to serve it for a ladies' lunch or a summer picnic. My friends and clients who have sampled it are delighted with the unique combination of vegetables, chicken, herbs, and spices. It's a filling comfort food with the added lightness of fresh vegetables and the tang of a great dressing. I call it Nouvelle Persian!

12 servings

Ingredients

1 frying chicken, about 2 or 3 pounds, with skin removed
1 onion, peeled and finely chopped
1 teaspoon salt
4 carrots, peeled and chopped
2 cups fresh shelled or frozen green peas
2 scallions, chopped
2 celery stalks, chopped
5 large potatoes, boiled, peeled, and chopped
3 medium cucumber pickles, finely chopped (dill pickles—Polish or kosher—are best)
½ cup chopped fresh parsley
⅔ cup green olives, pitted and chopped
3 hard-boiled eggs, peeled and chopped (optional)

Dressing:

1 cup defatted chicken broth
3 cups light mayonnaise
2 tablespoons Dijon mustard
¼ cup olive oil
¼ cup vinegar
¼ cup lime juice
1½ teaspoon salt
½ teaspoon freshly ground black pepper

Directions

Place the chicken in a nonstick pot along with the onion and salt. Cover and cook for 1½ hours over low heat. (No water is added because chicken makes its own juice.) When done, allow to cool, debone the chicken, and chop finely. Set aside the chicken broth for later use.

Steam the carrots for 5 minutes and set aside.

Steam shelled peas for 5 minutes and set aside. (If using frozen peas, follow package directions.)

In a large bowl, whisk together chicken broth, mayonnaise, mustard, olive oil, vinegar, lime juice, salt and pepper. Mix thoroughly.

Combine chicken, prepared vegetables, and eggs with the rest of the ingredients. Pour the dressing over it and toss well. Adjust seasoning to taste.

Chill for at least 2 hours.

Per Serving

calories	480	total fat	29g
saturated fat	5g	total carbohydrate	29g
dietary fiber	4g	protein	26g

Persian Chicken Salad is from *Persian Cooking for a Healthy Kitchen,* by *Najmieh Batmanglij.* Persian cooking is unique in its imaginative use of spices. This book combines the best of Persian cuisine with healthy living.

©1994–2001 courtesy of Mage Publishers, Washington, D.C.

Phyllis Frucht's Black Bean and Mango Salad with Citrus Herb Dressing

This is a spicy and light salad with all the elements of a great main course—hearty beans, sweet mango, crunchy pepper and onion, tart lime juice, hot jalapeño. This dish is quick to prepare and perfect for an individual summer dinner. Double or triple the recipe so you'll have plenty for the week

6 servings.

Ingredients
2 cans black beans, drained and rinsed
2 mangos, peeled and diced
2 red bell peppers, seeded and diced
1 cup red onion, diced
½ cup lime juice
½ cup orange juice
2 tablespoons honey
2 tablespoons lime zest
2 tablespoons orange zest
2 tablespoons herbes de Provence
2 jalapeño peppers, seeded and minced
½ cup cilantro, chopped

Directions

Combine the beans, mango, red pepper, and onion in a bowl. Mix the rest of the ingredients. Toss well and serve.

Per Serving

calories	220	total fat	2g
saturated fat	0g	total carbohydrate	46g
dietary fiber	10g	protein	10g

Phyllis Frucht is a chef and teacher in Washington, D.C., specializing in international cuisine from the Orient to India, Europe, the Middle East, the Caribbean, and more.

Roberto Donna's White Bean and Shrimp Salad with Basil Dressing

I have made this recipe so many times I can't keep track. I've not met one person who can resist the flavorful combination of cold beans and shrimp lathered in basil and balsamic vinegar. I take it to picnics and use it as a main course for lunch or dinner. It's a light and flavorful summer meal.

4 servings

Ingredients

8 ounces dry cannellini beans (or 24 oz canned, rinsed)
½ peeled onion
1 celery stalk
4 sage leaves, finely diced
½ medium carrot
8 ounces shrimp
2 cups white wine
2 tablespoons balsamic vinegar
6 tablespoons extra virgin olive oil
10 basil leaves
salt and pepper to taste

Directions

Soak the cannellini beans in water for 12 hours; drain, and place in a pot of water, add salt and pepper; cover and simmer for 45 minutes.

Chop and add the onion, celery, and carrot, cooking another 10 minutes. Add the finely diced sage to the pot and drain the cooking liquid.

Wash and clean the shrimp and poach for 3 minutes, or until done, in the white wine. Add salt and pepper to taste.

Dressing: Finely chop basil and add the balsamic vinegar, salt, pepper, and olive oil. Whisk until emulsified. Place ¼ of the mixture on each plate and top with 2 ounces of the shrimp. Dress with the basil dressing.

Per Serving

| calories | 540 | total fat | 23g | dietary fiber | 15g |
| saturated fat | 3.5g | total carbohydrate | 41g | protein | 24g |

Brenda Ponichtera's Broccoli Salad

Should I admit I'm not a broccoli lover? As a nutritionist, that might make me a candidate for jail time. But since I know broccoli is so good for me—it's one of the great vegetable superstars with off-the-charts disease-fighting powers—I've been constantly on the lookout for broccoli recipes I could love. And this is one. I love it. The sweet and chewy raisins balance the salty bacon bits. The yogurt-mayonnaise dressing with just the right amount of vinegar makes it smooth, creamy, and a little tart. This recipe is so simple and quick, it's great for people who don't like to cook—and for people like me who may not even like broccoli!

3 cups (6 ½-cup servings)

Ingredients

2 ½ cups chopped broccoli
½ cup raisins
¼ cup sunflower seeds (unsalted)
2 tablespoons diced red onion
2 tablespoons bacon-flavored soy bits

Dressing:
2 tablespoons nonfat plain yogurt
2 tablespoons light mayonnaise
1½ tablespoons sugar (or the equivalent in artificial sweetener)
½ tablespoons vinegar

Directions

Combine broccoli, raisins, sunflower seeds, onion, and soy bits.
Mix remaining ingredients together and add to the broccoli mixture.
Toss well to coat. Chill 2 hours or longer for flavors to blend.

Per Serving

calories	132	fat	5g
total carbohydrate	17g	protein	4g

Broccoli Salad was taken from *Quick & Healthy Volume II*, ©Brenda J. Ponichtera, R.D., and is reprinted with permission from ScaleDown Publishing, Inc.

The *Think Yourself Thin* strategies alone will work. But if you'd like to take a more scientific approach to weight loss, these next four sections are for you.

The Metabolism Toolbox

You can use *Think Yourself Thin* in several ways. You can pick from the many simple strategies that create a slight, but consistent, caloric deficit. Or, if you're completely unsure about what and how much you should be eating, you can calculate your metabolic needs by using *Think Yourself Thin*'s formula to determine your ideal daily and meal-by-meal calorie needs.

This is important because if you eat too little, you run the risk of making weight loss even more difficult in the long run, which is just what happened to Natalie.

Natalie, like many American women, is a wounded veteran of the diet wars.

She had tried everything, especially if it promised quick results. The "cleansing fast" with 9 days of lemon juice. The cabbage soup diet. The no-carbohydrate diet. Eating only fruits and vegetables. The diets would all "work"—she'd lose weight quickly—but the pounds had a way of coming back. She would lose 9 pounds in 9 days, but gain back 15 in 4 days. After a dozen years of yo-yo dieting, she wasn't just getting nowhere, she was losing ground.

When Natalie hit 200 pounds, she finally sought help from an expert and discovered the reason for her troubles. Because of her long-term serial dieting, her metabolism—the rate at which her body burns calories—had dropped by about 20 percent. This meant that, just to stay the same weight, she had to slash her caloric intake by 20 percent. To lose weight, she'd have to cut her consumption even more—and thereby risk slowing down her metabolism again. Natalie's history of severe calorie restricting on and off for many years stripped her body of muscle. Metabolic experts believe that restrictive dieting and muscle loss are the main reasons why most people have low metabolisms. And it's especially prevalent among middle-aged women. And this is on top of the natural loss of muscle we all begin experiencing once we hit our 30s. The average person loses 30 percent of their muscle by the age of 70.

This was Natalie's harsh introduction to the complex, sometimes baffling world of the human metabolism, which holds one of the cruelest ironies in all of dietdom: Restricting calories—which is necessary to lose weight—can slow down the body's metabolism, stunting one's ability to burn calories, making weight loss virtually impossible.

It doesn't take a long history of dieting failures to affect metabolism. In fact, large increases or decreases in calorie intake for as little as several days can raise or lower your metabolism. Although for chronic dieters, because their bodies have been primed to go into survival mode, their metabolisms can lower in just 24 to 48 hours, according to studies.

It is widely accepted that, in response to starving, the body reduces levels of various hormones and chemicals that help determine metabolic rate: insulin, active thyroid hormone, norepinephrine (similar to adrenaline). This is a powerful survival mechanism, as it permits the body to slow the nervous, cardiovascular, and gastrointestinal systems to help it conserve resources of energy and calories during a period of assumed scarcity of food.

The groups most likely to have provoked their bodies into below-normal metabolism are long-term yo-yo dieters; dieters who restrict their calories too severely; and people with eating disorders such as bulimia and anorexia nervosa, who either starve or alternate starving with bingeing.

The change in metabolic rate as a result of food restriction may vary from person to person. Studies show if a 200-pound woman is limited to

800 calories a day, after 3 weeks her metabolism may decline by 15 percent—possibly prompting further, unrealistic calorie reductions that cannot be sustained. Remarkably, exercise may actually exacerbate the problem. If a person isn't consuming enough calories and is exercising, the body—which automatically does the math and reacts to an even more severe calorie deficit—will reduce its metabolism further. Most people are told to eat less and exercise more, and it may not work for every person. All people going on very low calorie diets will develop low resting metabolic rates (RMRs).

A low RMR has other consequences. The decline in metabolism makes it almost impossible to maintain weight loss. For example, if the metabolism for a sample 150-pound woman is just 6 percent below normal, that means she must eat 100 fewer calories per day to avoid weight gain. If it drops to 25 percent below normal, she must reduce daily consumption by 400 calories to stay even. This is a huge food deficit that few can maintain over a lifetime and contributes to the long-term failure rates of diets, according to the experts.

So the dilemma is this: If restricting calories lowers the metabolism, endangering health and making weight loss and weight maintenance nearly impossible, how can weight loss be accomplished without wrecking your metabolism? The answer, at the risk of appearing flip: Very carefully.

A growing body of scientific evidence confirms that the human body is an extraordinarily adaptive and delicate instrument, whose instinctive drive for survival complicates the plans of even the most dedicated dieter. Losing weight and keeping it off require a careful understanding of the body and, specifically, its metabolic needs.

The less you eat, the more your body's metabolism slows down, requiring you to eat even less. And when, out of frustration or exhaustion, you resume "normal" eating, your body grabs onto those extra calories and sends them into fat storage with a vengeance.

Your body's calorie needs are largely determined by two factors: your level of physical activity and your RMR.

About one-third of the calories you burn are the result of physical activity, which includes anything other than resting—brushing your teeth, folding clothes, working at your computer, walking around the block, or exercising in your health club.

The other two-thirds are the calories needed to sustain basic bodily functioning: maintaining body temperature, heart beat, breathing, organ repair, and basic chemical reactions. This is your resting metabolic rate. Because RMR accounts for a large majority of calories burned, keeping your RMR high is essential to losing weight and keeping it off.

All of which raises the questions: How do you find out what your RMR is? And how can you raise it?

Your RMR is influenced by a variety of factors including genetics, body size, muscle mass, age, gender, body weight, pregnancy, hormonal status and, yes, physical condition. (A fit and muscular body burns more calories while at rest than an unfit, less muscular one.) To make things more difficult, RMR naturally declines through adulthood at about 2 percent per decade, usually because of the muscle loss you experience as you age and become more sedentary. Chronic dieters exacerbate muscle loss through repeated quick weight reductions.

You can determine your estimated RMR using *Think Yourself Thin*'s formula. Then continue the calculation to account for your level of physical activity and see how many calories you need to eat just to maintain your weight. Next, subtract 250 to 500 calories to determine your best daily calorie level for producing a 1/2 to 1 pound per week weight loss. But your calorie intake should never go below your RMR and ideally, even for the lower calorie levels, should always be at least 150 calories above it.

Once you've done the math, spend at least a week—or up to a month—eating at that calorie level, to see if you are losing weight at the desired pace. If you don't lose weight, and you're sure you've calculated your calorie needs and your food intake correctly (cheating here will do you no good, folks), then that's the sign your metabolism is probably low.

A low metabolism makes it almost impossible to lose weight or even maintain a weight loss. If you think your RMR is low, you may benefit from visiting a doctor and getting tested to verify your metabolic status or check that your thyroid is functioning properly.

If everything checks out, and your doctor determines you don't need medication, eating a healthy diet, exercising, and muscle building are the only ways a low metabolism can be reversed safely and effectively.

Three factors, then, are necessary in order to lose weight:

First, raise your metabolism level with a muscle-building program. The more lean muscle you have, the more calories your body burns. The American College of Sports Medicine recommends strength training all of your major muscle groups twice a week.

Second, cardiovascular activity burns body fat and calories (and, of course, improves your heart and general health). A fit body also continues to burn more calories even after the workout has ended. Accumulate at least 30 minutes per day of cardiovascular activity for health and weight maintenance. You may need more to lose weight.

The third element is diet. If you want to lose weight without affecting your metabolism negatively, the key is keeping calories as high as possible—but still slightly lower than what is needed to maintain weight. The metabolic experts recommend a daily caloric deficit of no more than 250 to 500 calories below the calorie level necessary to maintain your weight. Using the formula that 3,500 calories equals 1 pound, a daily deficit of 250 to 500 calories would produce losses of ½ to 1 pound every week. If you're losing faster than that, you are risking muscle and water loss, and you may only be losing 50 to 60 percent fat.

Think Yourself Thin's formula* for Calculating Your Resting Metabolic Rate (RMR) and Calorie Needs

* Based on the Harris Benedict Equation for people over 17 years old.

WOMEN	
1. Begin with a base of 655 calories	655
2. Multiply your weight in pounds by 4.3	
3. Multiply your height in inches by 4.7	
4. Add together the totals from #1, #2, and #3	
5. Multiply your age by 4.7	
6. Subtract result of #5 from total of #4 (your normal RMR)	
7. Multiply #6 by your activity factor (your daily maintenance calories)	
8. Subtract 250 to 500 calories (your daily weight-loss calories)	

FOR ACTIVITY, MULTIPLY:

RMR times 1.2 for low levels of activity (sedentary)

RMR times 1.3 for light exercise (about 2-3 hours per week)

RMR times 1.4 for moderate physical activity (about 4–7 hours per week), and

RMR times 1.6 for high levels of activity (about 7+ hours per week: high levels of exercise or manual labor)

Some athletes may double or even triple their RMR to determine their daily calorie needs

MEN	
1. Begin with a base of 66 calories	66
2. Multiply your weight in pounds by 6.3	
3. Multiply your height in inches by 12.7	
4. Add together the totals from #1, #2, and #3	
5. Multiply your age by 6.8	
6. Subtract result of #5 from total of #4 (your normal RMR)	
7. Multiply #6 by your activity factor (your daily maintenance calories)	
8. Subtract 250 to 500 calories (your daily weight-loss calories)	

FOR ACTIVITY, MULTIPLY:

RMR times 1.2 for low levels of activity (sedentary)

RMR times 1.3 for light exercise (about 2–3 hours per week)

RMR times 1.4 for moderate physical activity (about 4–7 hours per week), and

RMR times 1.6 for high levels of activity (about 7+ hours per week: high levels of exercise or manual labor)

Some athletes may double or even triple their RMR to determine their daily calorie needs

EXAMPLES

1. 150-pound, 5'4" 40-year-old moderately exercising woman:	
1. Begin with a base of 655 calories	655
2. Multiply your weight in pounds by 4.3	645
3. Multiply your height in inches by 4.7	301
4. Add together the totals from #1, #2, and #3	TOTAL = 1,601
5. Multiply your age by 4.7	subtract: –188
6. Subtract result of #5 from total of #4 (your normal RMR)	RMR = 1,413
7. Calories to maintain weight (RMR x 1.4)	1,978 calories per day
8. Calories to lose weight (subtract 250–500)	1,498–1,728 calories per day

2. 200-pound, 6'1" 50-year-old highly active man:	
1. Begin with a base of 66 calories	66
2. Multiply your weight in pounds by 6.3	1,260
3. Multiply your height in inches by 12.7	+927
4. Add together the totals from #1, #2, and #3	TOTAL = 2,253
5. Multiply your age by 6.8	subtract: –340
6. Subtract result of #5 from total of #4 (your normal RMR)	RMR = 1,913
7. Calories to maintain weight (RMR x 1.6)	3,060 calories per day
8. Calories to lose weight (subtract 500)	2,560 calories per day

Think Yourself Thin
Menu Plans

For weight loss to last, it has to be enjoyable; you can't feel deprived. And this may seem surprising: *It's important to feed yourself well and often*. I've found that the biggest cause of overeating is actually undereating. For most people, it's that simple.

Most overeating is simply due to poor planning. I hear so many people say "I have no willpower" or "I hate myself because I have no discipline." These people are usually underestimating themselves and doing themselves a grave injustice. And unfortunately, when you focus on the wrong problem, you focus on the wrong solution and continually beat yourself up for "failing," instead of spending time doing constructive problem-solving.

I believe in making things easy on yourself. When you learn to plan better, willpower and discipline are a piece of cake. I've seen it time and time again...miraculous recoveries of "discipline" and "willpower." It's amazing what a well-stocked refrigerator full of prepared, delicious food does for preventing that stop at the fast-food joint. Or what a nice full tummy in the morning does for saying "no, thank you" to the cookie or doughnut trays passed around in office meetings.

Most of your craving and uncontrolled overeating will be conquered when you feed your body what it needs regularly during the day and you have the right food right at your fingertips when you need it. Even my clients with eating disorders stop most of their craving and bingeing when they plan and organize their meals and snacks.

That's why I strongly advocate what I do myself—evenly dividing your food throughout the day. For most people, this style of eating means having a larger breakfast and a lighter dinner than they're used to. But this is the style of eating that's much more likely to stoke your metabolism—that is, give your body the ability to burn calories most efficiently. You must feed yourself well and often to keep your metabolism high.

Evidence suggests a pattern of eating three large meals per day, including planned midmorning and afternoon snacks, if desired, increases metabolism slightly. After eating, food stimulates an increase in the metabolism. So increasing the number of meals eaten starting in the morning takes the best advantage of this phenomenon, called the "thermic effect of food." (And by the way, protein and carbohydrate have a higher thermic effect than fat.)

One study shows people who skip breakfast or lunch have lower metabolisms. But, most importantly, eating a breakfast, lunch, and dinner of equal size decreases food cravings and overeating in the evenings—a cardinal sin if you want to lose weight, according to metabolism experts. Other evidence suggests people who eat heavily in the evenings are heavier and have higher cholesterol than those who eat the same calories spread throughout the day.

But with today's fast-paced world, many people do just the opposite. They have a light breakfast of toast and tea or a tiny bowl of cereal, if anything. They may grab just a salad at lunch because they're "watching it." And at dinner, well, watch out! At this point, they're so ravenous, there's no telling what they'll inhale. They'll stop at the local greasy spoon and down a dinner with at least 1,600 calories. (That's what the Center for Science in the Public Interest recently found was in just one serving of General Tso's chicken!) Or they may go for a 1,550 calorie plate of fettuccine al fredo. Just a cheese quesadilla appetizer packs in 900 calories. (See the book: *Restaurant Confidential* by Michael F. Jacobson, Ph.D., and Jayne Hurley, R.D., Workman Publishing, 2002.)

Which Menus Should I Follow?

To determine which set of menus will work best for you, calculate your calorie needs, then divide by three and distribute equally among breakfast, lunch, and dinner.

If your calorie needs are 1,500, give yourself a 500-calorie breakfast, a 500-calorie lunch, and a 500-calorie dinner. If you need 2,400 calories per day, the 800-calorie meals would be best for you. For the lower-calorie levels, I recommend eating a minimum 500-calorie breakfast, with smaller meals later. So, for instance, if you want to eat 1,300 calories per day, eat a 500-calorie breakfast, a 400-calorie lunch, and a 400-calorie dinner. I've even provided examples of dinners as low as 300 calories. This will enable you to eat adequate breakfasts and lunches, a snack or two in between, and a light dinner.

I have found that people do their best, crave less, overeat less, and feel most in control when they eat adequate calories during the day. This also keeps you from attacking dinner; it enables you to eat lighter at night and wake up hungry for a big breakfast—a very successful strategy for weight loss.

I've designed these menus to be delicious, simple, quick to prepare, and perfectly balanced so you feel completely satisfied with each meal even though you're eating fewer calories than your body needs so you lose weight.

Your health and satisfaction with your meals depend on eating a wide variety of foods each day. The menu plans I've designed for you here are perfectly balanced among all of the elements: fruits and vegetables, grains, protein, and fat.

Fruits and Vegetables

Probably the most important part of your meals is the fruits and vegetables. But you already know that, don't you? That's why *Think Yourself Thin* is so full of practical tips for how you and your family can eat more of them and make them delicious additions to your meals. Think of each fruit and vegetable as a little factory of nutrients and beneficial substances (called phytochemicals) with potent powers of healing and disease prevention.

For weight loss, fruits and vegetables are critical because they add water, fiber, bulk, and volume to your meals to help you feel nice and full.

Studies show adding vegetables to meals helps you eat 100 calories fewer while still feeling quite satisfied.

Whole Grains

Most of *Think Yourself Thin*'s meals contain a whole grain, which provides fiber and satisfaction. Studies show people who eat more fiber, especially at breakfast, feel less hungry the whole day, and that means it's easier to lose weight. The nutrients in a whole grain are correlated with a decrease in many types of cancer, heart disease, and even diabetes. But 75 percent of a grain's nutritional value is removed when it is refined to make white flour. So it's worth it to make the switch to whole-grain foods, especially considering the superior flavor and texture you'll get from the whole grain.

Protein

Think Yourself Thin's menus are chock-full of protein, in the form of hearty beans, lean red meat, poultry, or seafood. I stress fish as the most ideal protein source because of the presence of important omega-3 fatty acids and the wonderful flavor. Research shows omega-3s may prevent a host of health problems such as depression, inflammatory diseases, Alzheimer's disease, high cholesterol and triglycerides, and heart disease.

Fat

Recent studies confirm that people who lose weight and keep it off successfully eat a relatively low fat diet. And since I can't argue with success, that's what I recommend. But you do have to eat healthy fat at every meal. You need it to feel full and to make your food taste good. You will find most of *Think Yourself Thin*'s menus contain about 20 to 35 percent fat calories (mainly from nuts, oils, and seafood), which is the ideal recommended by all the experts, and means that, at 1,800 calories, you'll be eating anywhere from 40 grams to 70 grams of fat daily. You might also notice that most of the fats used in these menus are monounsaturated or polyunsaturated, which are more beneficial for your health. Artery-clogging saturated fat and trans fat are definitely hard to find in these menus. I recommend minimal trans fat, found in processed foods, and minimal saturated fat, found in high levels in fatty meat and dairy products.

400-CALORIE BALANCED BREAKFASTS

Simple Breakfast
cold cereal (150)
1 cup skim milk (100)
½ oz (¼ cup) nuts (80)
4 oz fresh fruit or juice (60)

Katherine's Favorite Breakfast
½ cup old-fashioned oats (150), cooked in:
  1 cup skim milk (100) or soy milk
pinch salt
2 whole chopped walnuts (50)
Microwave 5 minutes in a large bowl (to prevent it from spilling over),
leave in microwave another minute
Stir in:
  1 tsp brown sugar (15)
On the side: ½ cup orange juice (60)

Peanut Butter "To Go" Breakfast
2 slices whole-grain bread (160)
1 tbsp peanut butter (90)
6–8 oz fat-free yogurt (90)
4 oz fresh-fruit or juice (60)

Egg and Sausage Breakfast
¼ cup egg substitute (50)
1 tbsp olive oil (120)
Or
2 eggs (150) and 1 tsp oil (40)
Scramble in:
  ½ cup chopped onion and garlic (20)
  1 oz lean sausage or ham (50)
½ whole wheat English muffin or 1 slice whole wheat toast (80)
½ cup orange juice (60)

Lox and Bagel "To Go" Breakfast
2 oz whole wheat bagel (160)
4 oz lox (140)
1 tbsp fat-free cream cheese (30)
4 oz juice (60)

400-CALORIE SIMPLE, BALANCED LUNCHES OR DINNERS

4 oz halibut or white fish (105)
1 tsp olive oil, herbs, salt (40)
sautéed or steamed vegetables (50)
1 6-oz baked potato (160)
Top with:
  2 tbsp fat-free sour cream topping or ¼ cup 1 percent cottage cheese (30)

½ cup cooked (1 oz raw) whole wheat pasta (100)
4 oz chicken breast or tuna (140)
Stirred into:
  ½ cup stir-fried diced tomatoes, capers (50)
  2 tbsp grated Parmesan cheese (50)
1 piece fruit (60)

4 oz grilled chicken breast (140)
1 slice (1 oz) whole grain roll (80)
sautéed sliced red and yellow peppers (25)
1 tbsp oil (120)
1 piece fruit (60)

3 oz grilled salmon (150)
6 oz boiled new potatoes with skin (boiled 15 minutes, check for done-ness) (160)
1 tsp olive oil with parsley drizzled over potatoes (40)
1 cup fresh greens salad (25)
low-calorie salad dressing (25)

1 small whole wheat tortilla (130)
Filled with:
  4 oz refried beans or canned, rinsed black beans (100)
  1 oz cheese (100)
  ¾ cup salsa (75)

1 cup brown rice and beans (200)
1 oz baked chips for dipping (100)
½ cup fresh salsa (50)
⅙ of an avocado (50)

Stir-Fried Shrimp (or Chicken or Tofu) and Vegetables

1 cup cooked (or 2 oz raw) brown rice (200)
4 oz shrimp or chicken breast or ¾ cup tofu (140)
1–2 cups raw vegetables (50)
Stir-fried in 1 tsp sesame oil (40)

Simple, Good Old American "To Go" Lunch

Sandwich: 2 slices bread (160), ½ tbsp mayo (50), 3 oz lean beef, turkey, seafood, or chicken breast (150)
Vegetable salad (25–50), 2 tbsp fat-free salad dressing (20)

500-CALORIE BALANCED BREAKFASTS

Simple Breakfast

cold cereal (200)
1 cup skim milk (100)
½ oz (⅛ cup) nuts (80)
8 oz fresh fruit and/or juice (120)

Katherine's Favorite Breakfast

½ cup old-fashioned oats (150), cooked in:
    1 cup skim milk (100) or soy milk
pinch salt
2 whole chopped walnuts (50) (¼ cup walnuts, about 1 oz = 200 calories)
Microwave 5 minutes in a large bowl (to prevent it from spilling over), leave in microwave another minute
Add:
    1 tsp brown sugar (15)
    1 tbsp light butter (50)
    ½ medium banana or ½ cup blueberries (50)
On the side: ½ cup orange juice (60)

Peanut Butter "To Go" Breakfast

2 slices whole grain bread (160)
2 tbsp peanut butter (180)
6–8 oz fat-free yogurt (90)
4 oz fruit/juice (60)

Egg and Sausage Breakfast

¼ cup egg substitute (50)
1 tbsp olive oil (120)

Or
2 eggs (150) and 1 tsp oil (40)
Scramble in:
  ½ cup chopped onion and garlic (20)
  1 oz lean sausage or ham (50)
whole wheat English muffin or 2 slices toast (160)
4 oz fresh fruit or juice (60)

Lox and Bagel "To Go" Breakfast

2½ oz whole wheat bagel (200)—that would be half of a large 5 oz bagel
  (bagels are 80 cal/oz)
4 oz lox (140)
1 oz cream cheese (100)
4 oz juice (60)

500-CALORIE SIMPLE, BALANCED LUNCHES OR DINNERS

4 oz halibut or white fish (140)
1 tsp olive oil, herbs, salt (40)
sautéed or steamed vegetables (50)
1 6-oz baked potato (160)
Top with: 2 tbsp sour cream or ½ cup 2 percent cottage cheese (100)

1 cup cooked (2 oz raw) whole wheat pasta (200)
4 oz chicken breast or tuna (140)
Stir in:
  ½ cup stir-fried diced tomatoes, capers (50)
  2 tbsp grated Parmesan cheese (50)
1 piece fruit (60)

4 oz grilled chicken breast (140)
2 slices (ounces) whole grain roll (160)
sautéed, sliced red and yellow peppers (25)
1 tbsp oil or 2 tbsp regular salad dressing (120)
1 piece fruit (60)

4 oz grilled salmon (200)
6 oz boiled new potatoes (boiled 15 minutes, check for doneness) (160)
1 tsp olive oil with parsley, drizzled over potatoes (40)
1 cup salad greens or grated cabbage (25)
2 tbsp reduced-calorie salad dressing (50)

1 small whole wheat tortilla (130)
Filled with:
 4 oz refried beans or canned, rinsed black beans (100)
 1 oz cheese (100)
 ½ cup salsa (50)
 ½ avocado (150)

1½ cups beans and rice (300)
Sautéed in 1 tbsp oil (120)
½ cup salsa (50)

Stir-Fried Shrimp (or Chicken or Tofu) and Vegetables
1 cup brown rice (200)
4 oz shrimp or chicken breast or ¾ cup tofu (140)
1–2 cups raw vegetables (50)
Stir-fried in 1 tbsp sesame oil (120)

Simple, Good Old American "To Go" Lunch
Sandwich: 2 slices bread (160), 1 tbsp mayo (100), 3 oz lean beef, turkey,
seafood, or chicken breast (150)
Vegetable salad (25–50), 2 tbsp low-calorie salad dressing (75)

600-CALORIE BALANCED BREAKFASTS

Easy Breakfast
cold cereal (280), 1 cup skim milk (100)
½ oz or about ⅛ cup chopped walnuts (80)
8 oz fresh fruit and/or juice (120)

Katherine's Favorite Breakfast
½ cup old-fashioned oats (150) or cold cereal, cooked in:
 1 cup skim milk (100) or soy milk
pinch salt
1 oz (¼ cup) chopped nuts (160)
Microwave 5 minutes in a large bowl (to prevent it from spilling over),
leave in microwave another minute
Mix in:
 1 tsp brown sugar (20)
 1 tbsp light butter (50)
Top with:
 ½ sliced medium banana, ½ cup blueberries or other fresh fruit (50)
½ cup juice (60)

Peanut Butter "To Go" Breakfast

2 slices whole grain bread (160)
2 tbsp peanut butter (180)
8 oz yogurt (200)
4 oz fresh fruit or juice (60)

Eggs and Sausage Breakfast

½ cup egg substitute (100)
1 tbsp olive oil (120)
Or
2 eggs (150) and 1 tsp oil (40)
Scramble in:
   1 oz lean sausages or ham
   ½ cup chopped onion and garlic (50)
whole wheat English muffin or 2 slices whole wheat toast (160)
½ cup orange juice (60)
½ large banana or other fruit (60)

Lox and Bagel "To Go" Breakfast

4 oz whole wheat bagel (300) (bagels are about 80 cal/oz)
4 oz lox (140)
1 oz cream cheese (100)
4 oz juice or fresh fruit (60)

600-CALORIE SIMPLE, BALANCED DINNERS OR LUNCHES

6 oz halibut or white fish (210)
1 tbsp olive oil, herbs, salt (120)
1–2 cups raw, sautéed, or steamed vegetables (50)
1 6-oz baked potato (160)
Top with:
   3 tbsp reduced-fat sour cream or ½ cup 1 percent cottage cheese (75)

1½ cups cooked (3 oz raw) whole wheat pasta (300)
4 oz chicken breast or tuna (140)
1 cup stir fried diced tomatoes, capers (50)
1 tbsp olive oil (120)

6 oz grilled chicken breast marinated in fat-free Italian dressing (210)
1 medium (6 oz) Yukon Gold or Idaho potato (160) shredded and
cooked in ½ tbsp olive oil (60)

1-2 cups sliced red and yellow peppers, raw or sautéed (50)
1 tbsp oil (120)

4 oz grilled salmon (200)
1 4-inch acorn squash, baked (45 minutes, check for doneness) (170)
1 tbsp olive oil and parsley, drizzled over potatoes (120)
1 cup salad greens and/or grated cabbage (25)
2 tbsp reduced-calorie salad dressing or 1 tbsp regular (75)

1½ cups beans/rice (300)
1 oz cheese (100)
1 cup salad greens and/or grated cabbage (25)
⅓ of an avocado (100)
2 tbsp reduced-calorie salad dressing or 1 tbsp regular (75)

Stir-Fried Shrimp (or Chicken or Tofu) and Vegetables
1½ cups brown rice (300)
4 oz shrimp or chicken breast or ¾ cup tofu (140)
1–2 cups raw vegetables (50)
Stir-fried in 1 tbsp sesame oil (120)

Simple, Good Old American "To Go" Lunch
Sandwich: 2 slices whole grain bread (160), 1 tbsp mayo (100), 3 oz lean beef or turkey or chicken breast (150)
Vegetable salad (25–50), 2 tbsp regular salad dressing (130)

FOR PEOPLE WHO EAT DINNER TOO LATE (AND DON'T WANT TO ATTACK IT)

600-calorie dinner divided into:
300-calorie afternoon or early evening snack plus 300-calorie dinner

300-CALORIE SIMPLE, QUICK, AND EASY SNACK IDEAS

Snack 1: Fruit, crackers, or bread (100) with 2 tbsp peanut butter (180)
Snack 2: Fruit (60) and yogurt (240)
Snack 3: Fruit (140) and 1 oz (1/4 cup) nuts (160)
Snack 4: Frozen dinner (300)

300-CALORIE SIMPLE, BALANCED LUNCHES AND DINNERS

3 oz halibut or white fish (105)
2 tsp olive oil, herbs, salt (80)
1 cup raw, sautéed, or steamed vegetables (25)
1 3-oz potato (80)

½ cup cooked (1 oz dry) whole wheat pasta (100)
3 oz chicken breast or tuna (105)
Stirred into:
   ½ cup diced tomatoes, capers, or 50 calories' worth of tomato sauce (50)
   2 tbsp grated Parmesan cheese (50)

3 oz grilled chicken breast (105)
1 slice (1 oz) whole grain roll (80)
1–2 cups sautéed, sliced red and yellow peppers or other vegetables (50)
1 tsp oil (40)

3 oz grilled salmon (150)
1 cup green salad or grated cabbage (25)
2 tbsp regular salad dressing (130)

1 small whole wheat tortilla (130)
4 oz refried beans or canned, rinsed black beans (100)
½ cup salsa (50)

½ cup brown rice and beans (100)
½ cup fresh salsa (50)
1 oz baked chips (100) for dipping
2 tbsp reduced-fat sour cream (50)

Stir-Fried Shrimp (or Chicken or Tofu) and Vegetables
½ cups cooked (1 oz raw) brown rice (100)
3 oz shrimp or chicken breast or ½ cup tofu (105)
1–2 cups raw vegetables (50),
Sautéed in 1 tsp sesame oil (40)

700-CALORIE BALANCED BREAKFASTS

Easy Breakfast
Cereal (230)

1½ cups skim milk (150)
1 oz (¼ cup) nuts (180)
8 oz fresh fruit and/or juice (120)

Katherine's Favorite Breakfast

½ cup old-fashioned oats (150), cooked in:
  1 cup skim milk or soy milk (100)
pinch salt
1 oz (¼ cup) chopped walnuts (160)
Microwave 5 minutes in a large bowl (to prevent it from spilling over),
leave in microwave another minute
Add:
  2 tsp brown sugar (30)
  2 tbsp light butter (100)
  ½ large banana or 1 cup blueberries or other fruit (60)
½ cup orange juice (60)

Egg and Sausage Breakfast

½ cup egg substitute (100)
1 tbsp olive oil (120)
Or
3 eggs (225) and 1 tsp olive oil (40)
Scramble in:
  ½ cup chopped onion and garlic (25)
  3 oz lean sausage or ham (130)
whole wheat English muffin or 2 slices toast (160)
½ cup orange juice (60)
½ large banana or 4 oz other fresh fruit (60)

Peanut Butter "To Go" Breakfast

8 oz low-fat yogurt (210)
2 slices whole wheat toast (160)
2 tbsp peanut butter (200)
8 oz fresh fruit or juice (120)

Lox and Bagel "To Go" Breakfast

4 oz bagel (320)
4 oz lox (140)
1 oz cream cheese (100)
8 oz fruit and/or juice (120)

700-CALORIE DINNERS OR LUNCHES

6 oz halibut or white fish (210)
1 tbsp olive oil, herbs, salt (120)
1–2 cups raw, sautéed, or steamed vegetables (50)
1 9-oz baked potato (240)
2 tbsp reduced-fat sour cream (40)
3 oz wine or 4 oz fruit or juice (60)

1½ cups cooked (3 ounces dry) whole wheat pasta (300)
5 oz chicken breast or tuna (175)
1 cup stir-fried diced tomatoes, capers (100)
1 tbsp olive oil (120)

6 oz grilled salmon (300)
6 oz boiled new potatoes (boiled 15 minutes, check for doneness) (160)
1 tbsp olive oil and parsley, drizzled over potatoes (120)
1 cup salad greens and/or grated cabbage (25)
2 tbsp reduced-calorie salad dressing (75)

4 oz sliced chicken breast (140)
2 cups red beans mixed with rice (400)
sautéed vegetables in (25) ½ tbsp oil or 2 tbsp salad dressing (120)

Stir-Fried Shrimp (or Chicken or Tofu) and Vegetables

1½ cups (or 3 oz dry) brown rice (300)
6 oz shrimp or chicken breast or 1 cup tofu (210)
1–2 cups raw chopped vegetables (50)
Stir-fried in 1 tbsp sesame oil (120)

Simple, Good Old American "To Go" Lunch

Sandwich: 2 slices bread (160), 1 tbsp mayo (100), 6 oz lean beef or
turkey or chicken breast (210)
Vegetable salad (25), 3 tbsp regular salad dressing (225)

800-CALORIE BALANCED BREAKFASTS

Simple Breakfast

cereal (400)
1 cup skim milk (100)
1 oz (¼ cup) nuts (160)
8 oz fresh fruit and/or juice (120)

Katherine's Favorite Breakfast
¾ cup old-fashioned oats (225) or cold cereal, cooked in:
1½ cup skim milk (150)
pinch salt
1 oz (¼ cup) chopped walnuts (160)
Microwave 5 minutes in large bowl (to prevent it from spilling over),
leave in microwave another minute
Mix in:
1 tbsp brown sugar (45)
2 tbsp light butter (100)
Top with:
½ large banana or 3/4 cup blueberries or other fruit (60)
½ cup orange juice (60)

Peanut Butter "To Go" Breakfast
3 slices whole wheat toast (240)
3 tbsp peanut butter (270)
8 oz fresh fruit and/or juice (120)
yogurt (170)

Egg and Sausage Breakfast
¾ cup egg substitute (75)
1½ tbsp olive oil (180)
Or
3 eggs (225) and 1 tsp olive oil (40)
Scramble in:
½ cup chopped onion and garlic(25)
4–6 oz extra lean sausage or ham (230)
whole wheat English muffin or 2 slices whole wheat toast (160)
½ cup orange juice (60)
½ large banana or fruit (60)

Lox and Bagel "To Go" Breakfast
4 oz bagel (320)
6 oz lox (210)
1 oz cream cheese (100)
8 oz fresh fruit and/or juice (120)

800-CALORIE DINNERS OR LUNCHES

whole wheat tortilla (250)
Stuffed with:
  4 oz canned, rinsed refried beans or black beans (100)
  1 oz cheese (100)
  2 oz chicken breast (70)
  2 tbsp reduced-fat sour cream (50)
1 cup greens salad (25), with:
  ½ avocado (150)
  2 tbsp reduced-calorie salad dressing (75)

8 oz halibut or white fish (280)
1 tbsp olive oil, herbs, salt (120)
1–2 cups raw, sautéed, or steamed vegetables (50)
1 9-oz baked potato (240), topped with:
2 tbsp reduced-fat sour cream or ¼ cup cottage cheese (50)
3 oz wine or 4 oz fruit juice (60)

2 cups whole wheat pasta (¼ pound dry) (400)
4 oz chicken breast or tuna (140)
1 cup stir-fried diced tomatoes, capers (100)
1 tbsp olive oil (120)
½ oz or 2 tbsp grated Parmesan cheese (50)

7 oz grilled salmon (350)
6 oz boiled new potatoes (boil 15 minutes, check for doneness) (160)
1 tbsp olive oil and parsley, drizzled over potatoes (120)
1–2 cup greens salad or shredded cabbage (25)
2 tbsp regular salad dressing (150)

Stir-Fried Shrimp (or Chicken or Tofu) and Vegetables

1½ cups brown rice (300)
8 oz shrimp or chicken breast or 1½ cups tofu (280)
2–3 cups raw vegetables (75)
Stir-fried in 1 tbsp sesame oil (120)

Simple, Good Old American "To Go" Lunch

Sandwich: 2 slices bread (160), 2 tbsp mayo (200), 6 oz lean beef or
turkey or chicken breast (210)
Vegetable salad (25), 3 tbsp regular dressing (225)

Think Yourself Thin
Food Diary

Keeping a food diary is the most important tool for self-examination of your eating habits. Socrates told us the road to wisdom is to know ourselves. This is never more true than in your eating habits.

It is important that you begin observing objectively what you eat and the way you eat, for this is the cornerstone of your program: your own observations. Don't make any judgments at this point. There is no good or bad behavior, only objective self-observation, which leads to learning. To learn more about the effectiveness of a food diary, check out Tip #46, Write It and Lose It.

The success of your nutrition program depends on how accurately you describe *all* the food you eat and *all* the drinks you consume. Please keep the record every day until you reach your goals and/or periodically to check yourself. During the first week, *do not* change your normal eating habits. Just list everything you eat and drink. Once you start making changes, using a variety of the *Think Yourself Thin* tips or cooking some of the batch recipes, for example, then start to record some of the other things you want to keep track of, for instance, calories, water, fiber grams, saturated fat grams, feelings, hunger levels.

The "location," "mood" and "hunger" columns will help you keep track of behavioral issues that may influence what and how much you eat. Under "location," some examples might be: dining room table, kitchen table, parking lot of fast-food restaurant, office desk, living room couch while watching TV, in bed while reading, in car while driving, etc. Under "mood," some examples might be: happy, sad, lonely, angry, mad at spouse, feeling disrespected by boss, enjoying friends, rushed, relaxed, etc. Under "hunger," refer to Tip #87, Fight the Beast, and record how physically hungry you feel before and after you eat to help you analyze whether you're feeding yourself appropriately.

Print carefully, one food item per line. For instance, added butter, sugar, mayonnaise, salad dressing, ketchup, oil in cooking, and other condiments should be recorded on separate lines.

Accurate portion size is very important in making a valid assessment. Use common measurements to describe the amount of food you are eating. The following examples may help:

Measures	Examples
ounces (oz)	meats, fish, cheeses, liquids
teaspoons (tsp)	butter, oil
tablespoons (tbsp)	salad dressings, mayonnaise
cups (c)	cereals, pasta, rice, vegetables, soups

Recording Hints

Read weights and measures on sides of packages and/or cans to determine the weight or amount you are eating or use a kitchen scale. To determine the amount of the food, weigh it or put the food in a measuring cup or spoon before cooking with it or eating it to determine the amount.

Date: _____

Time	Food	Quantity	Physical Activity	Calories	Location	Mood	Hunger Level
Total							

Optional Entries

(Goal Reached vs Low or High)

Body Mass Index (BMI) Chart

Body Mass Index (BMI) Chart

Height	Weight in Pounds											
4'11"	94	99	104	109	114	119	124	128	133	138	143	148
5'0"	97	102	107	112	117	122	128	133	138	143	148	153
5'1"	100	106	111	116	121	127	132	137	143	148	153	158
5'2"	103	108	114	119	124	130	136	142	147	153	158	164
5'3"	107	113	118	124	130	135	141	146	152	158	163	169
5'4"	110	115	121	127	133	138	145	151	157	163	169	174
5'5"	114	120	126	132	138	144	150	156	162	168	174	180
5'6"	118	124	130	136	143	149	155	161	167	173	179	185
5'7"	121	127	134	140	147	153	159	166	172	178	185	191
5'8"	124	130	137	143	150	156	164	171	177	184	190	197
5'9"	128	135	141	148	155	162	169	176	182	189	196	203
5'10"	133	139	146	153	160	167	174	181	188	195	202	209
5'11"	135	143	150	157	164	171	179	186	193	200	207	215
BMI	19	20	21	22	23	24	25	26	27	28	29	30

Alphabetical Tips Index

Numerical Tips Index

Index